Health Services Privatization in Industrial Societies

HEALTH SERVICES PRIVATIZATION IN INDUSTRIAL SOCIETIES

EDITED BY

Joseph L. Scarpaci

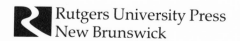
Rutgers University Press
New Brunswick

Library of Congress Cataloging-in-Publication Data

Health services privatization in industrial societies / edited by
   Joseph L. Scarpaci.
      p.   cm.
   Includes bibliographies and index.
   ISBN 0-8135-1437-1 (cloth) ISBN 0-8135-1438-X (pbk.)
   1. Medical policy.   2. Privatization.   I. Scarpaci, Joseph L.
   [DNLM: 1. Health Policy—economics.   2. Health Services—
economics.   3. Health Services—organization & administration.
4. Ownership—trends.   W84.1 H4379]
RA394.H44   1988
362.1'042—dc19
DNLM/DLC
for Library of Congress   88-36764
                                                              CIP

TP

To Cristina Alessandra

Contents

List of Figures

List of Tables

Contributors

JOSEPH L. SCARPACI is Assistant Professor of Urban Affairs and Planning at Virginia Polytechnic Institute and State University.

J. ROSS BARNETT is Senior Lecturer in Geography at the University of Canterbury, Christchurch, New Zealand.

PAULINE BARNETT is Scientist in Charge at the Health Planning and Research Unit, Christchurch, New Zealand.

JAMES R. BOHLAND is Professor of Urban Affairs and Planning at Virginia Polytechnic Institute and State University.

JOHN EYLES is Professor of Geography at McMaster University, Hamilton, Ontario.

WILBERT GESLER is Associate Professor of Geography at the University of North Carolina, Chapel Hill.

MICHAEL R. GREENBERG is Distinguished Professor and Co-director of the Public Health Program at Rutgers University.

PAUL L. KNOX is Professor of Urban Affairs and Planning at Virginia Polytechnic Institute and State University.

GLENDA LAWS is Assistant Professor of Geography at Pennsylvania State University, University Park.

SARA L. McLAFFERTY is Associate Professor in the Department of Geology and Geography at Hunter College, CUNY.

JOHN MOHAN is Lecturer in Geography at Queen Mary College, University of London.

CHRISTOPHER J. SMITH is Associate Professor of Geography and Planning at the State University of New York, Albany.

Chapter 1

Introduction

*The Theory and Practice of Health
Services Privatization*

JOSEPH L. SCARPACI

This is a particularly appropriate time for those in the field of human geography and social sciences to publish a collection of original essays that treat health services privatization in comparative perspective. Industrial societies in the 1980s have pursued the sale of public goods and services more single-mindedly than any other social public policy in the postwar era. This process, commonly called privatization, has stirred the imaginations of policymakers and the electorate around the world. It has become a household word—as did the term *welfare state* in postwar Europe. The dialectical process of creating the welfare state, on the one hand, and implementing privatization, on the other, underscores the dynamic political economy of today. The sale or administrative transfer of public goods and services to the private sector portends savings, equity, or efficiency for governments perennially caught in fiscal straits.

Examples of privatization are varied yet nearly universal, including the sale of public utilities and National Weather Service satellites in the United States; of British Telecom and British Gas; of Japanese telephone, tobacco, and railway monopolies; of a Spanish automobile manufacturer; of French television channels; and even of the bridge over the Bosporus in Turkey. Governments in North America, Western Europe, South America, and Australasia spearhead efforts to roll back the welfare state and its attendant social programs; and even the USSR, under Mikhail Gorbachev's policy of *perestroika* (restructuring), and Fidel Castro's Cuba have begun promoting small-scale free enterprise and the profit principle.

Only a few years ago the power and size of governments were growing steadily, independent of the kind of political regime in power. On the eve of the 1990s, however, privatization stands high on the agendas of national, state, and local governments. It is one response to the global economic downturn of the late 1970s and 1980s. What started in the 1970s among municipal governments in the United States as the contracting-out of, for instance, waste-removal services and fire protection to the lowest private bidders, has grown to include such controversial endeavors as corrections-facility management, schooling, and health services (Abramowitz 1986). Since the mid-1970s in Great Britain the promotion of private health insurance has expanded to include certain electrical and railroad workers. Under Margaret Thatcher's Conservative tenure, the proportion of National Health Service users has declined from 97 percent in 1979 to 93 percent in 1984 (Mohan and Woods 1985). The privatization movement in Great Britain stems from public discontent over the expanding role of government since the Second World War and from a growing consensus that the unfettered marketplace can effectively regulate health services. Such sentiment about privatization represents a backlash against liberal welfare policies. Its great popular appeal is that it proposes to curtail public spending, increase cash reserves, and reduce taxes.

The privatization of health care is, to say the least, a controversial issue that elicits strong emotions about the proper role of government. Yet our knowledge about the ways in which governments seek to privatize health care is meager. For this reason, in this book we examine recent experiences in the privatization of health services of selected industrial societies and their organizational and ideological extensions from around the world. An understanding of the process of health care privatization can be useful when examining the potential privatization of other social programs, the delivery of health services, and theories of the state. This collection of essays addresses a newly emerging political economy that rearranges the ways in which the state, capital, and the private sector confront the high costs of health care in the advanced capitalist and developing countries. These essays are a critical response to the growing consensus worldwide that the unfettered marketplace effectively regulates the availability and accessibility of health services. However, the authors do not suggest that health services privatization is merely a response to the fiscal crisis of the state nor that it stems from a global conspiracy to roll back the welfare state. We instead argue that health services privatization depends on the specific nature of conflict among the state, the private sector, health care consumers, and capital. Through the use of detailed case studies of a wide array of health services that are set in clearly defined historical and geographical contexts, these chapters show the inherent limits to the dismantling of state-sponsored health services. Indeed, health services privatization may have reached its peak in the late 1980s in light of the mounting opposition to the trend, the empirical evidence indicating its deleterious outcomes, and the inherent weaknesses of a full transfer of health programs to the private sector. We argue that while the line between public and private health services is in the process of being redrawn in many advanced capitalist nations, fiscal retrenchment will be checked by certain structural constraints identified in the chapters ahead.

In selecting health services as an industry that is undergoing a certain degree of privatization, several caveats about the nature of providers, consumers, and markets in the industry should be noted. Unlike other markets, unless referrals are made to other specialists, entrance into the health care market rarely goes beyond general encounters with physicians or nurses (primary-care providers). Health care consumers (patients) face special problems not encountered by consumers of transportation, housing, or education in that they often lack the clinical competence to judge the adequacy of the service rendered. Nor is health care a uniform product or service. Curative and preventive services produce very different responses from government, providers, and consumers. Historically, mixed economies developed programs of curative-care regulation, subsidy, or provision mostly for the infirm, infants and children, and indigents. These vulnerable populations have traditionally constituted the core of welfare state consumers. More controversial, however, is the provision of health services to able-bodied men and women who are capable of incurring considerable out-of-pocket charges for health services. Less controversial is preventive care such as infectious disease or epidemic prevention, which can be thought of as a pure public good; that is, it cannot be easily subdivided for the benefit of a few individuals. Public health education and publicly provided immunization and vaccination are examples of preventive health services that benefit the entire population and are less polemical than curative health care (Roth 1987, 130). To be sure, the state serves as mediator in both constraining and encouraging the provision of private health services.

Scope and Nature of This Book

Theoretical debates on the merits of public versus private provision of health services are not resolved in the chapters ahead, but these chapters do identify the merits and weaknesses of health care privatization among certain preventive and curative services. They represent both the first international review of the privatization of health services and the first placement of spatial concerns on equal footing with other structural elements such as access to capital, the political economy of a particular country, multinational-corporate capital, class, and gender. In doing so, the case studies illustrate how international, national, and local economies have altered the geography of health services delivery. The extent to which health services are spatially and socially distributed deserves greater attention in both human geography and social science research because they are key outcome measures in the privatization debate.

The chapters that follow are perhaps best characterized in what Marmor, Hoffman, and Heagy (1975) describe as a "most similar systems" approach to comparative health studies. This approach draws on the similarities of either sector-specific aspects of health care (i.e., ambulatory care, hospital care, health education, mental health care) or organizational traits such as health care financing, service organization and delivery, models of use and satisfaction, and other topical areas. In this work privatization serves as a vehicle for examining the common structures of health services. In choosing this approach, we are cognizant of the pitfalls that lie ahead, for a major criticism of health services research and medical geography is that such analyses are inherently descriptive. The descriptive emphasis derives in part from the relatively new perspectives that social science has brought to the health care field and the increasing difficulty that lies in introducing comparative or complementary paradigms to the predominant biomedical model.

The dilemma of linking descriptive health care studies with more theoretical concerns has been well documented in international health studies (Wilensky et al. 1985) and medical geography (Knox 1986). There is agreement that comparative studies of health care delivery often adopt a case-study approach, which is predominantly descriptive and not analytic, because it is often directed toward policy planners, who value pragmatic goals rather than theory construction (see, for example, Roemer 1985). This focus explains why many researchers "have limited themselves to detailed examinations of a small number of countries" (Wilensky et al. 1985, 53) and why applied and basic researchers of health and social behavior often direct their findings to restricted audiences (Levine 1987). Unfortunately, failure to place case studies in geographical and historical contexts deprives others of potentially rich insights into the behavior of health care users, the relationship between local and national governments, the politics of health care, and changes in the built environment. The task, therefore, is to provide a much-needed bridge between theory and practice.

We argue that the process of health services privatization is a diverse phenomenon that defies a simple interpretation. We reject the notion that health services privatization is part of a global conspiracy, that it is launched solely as a fiscal response to mounting debt and deficit spending, and that it is intended to float the state through financial crisis. While these aspects of the economic restructuring of social programs are crucial in understanding privatization, they fail to specify exactly how restructuring manifests itself over space and time. Our premise is that there are limits to rolling back the welfare state. In the current crisis, industrial societies may seize on privatization as a tactic for ameliorating some problems, but this is bound to be a short-term strategy. To date, there is no wholesale retreat of the state from essential social services (see Vernon 1988). The historical evidence brought forth in this book shows that privatization is not new, but tends to be cyclical in nature. Our goal is not to predict its occurrence, but to better understand its origins and consequences.

Four brief definitions should help the reader of these essays. First, *privatization* of health services refers to reduced levels of public provision, subsidy, or regulation of either preventive or curative health services (cf. Dunleavy 1986, n. 1). This tripartite emphasis on provision, subsidy, or regulation is noteworthy because privatization is generally associated only with the private provision of public services (Roth 1987), as evidenced, say, by the sale of British Telecom (*Economist*, 6 October 1984, 88–89). A county commissioner from the state of Iowa echoed this popular misconception before voting on the transfer of a county home for the aged to private management: "I was like most people when I heard about this privatization business—I was dead set against it. . . . But when I heard all about what privatization really entailed and the savings that would accrue to the county because of private-sector eligibility for federal dollars, I realized it was the best thing for the county" (author's notes, Johnson County Commission, public hearing, July 1987). Rarely, as we shall see, does health care privatization entail the sale of an entire health program to a private fee-for-service provider. Rather, it is much more subtle and frequently includes reductions in government regulation (allowing more providers into the health care market), subsidy (increasing monthly coinsurance payments, out-of-pocket charges, or the cost of medical vouchers), or provision (substituting private providers for public ones).

Second, *health services* includes a broad gamut of curative and preventive services. The case studies that follow examine hospital and ambulatory-care financing and regulation (chapters 2–6 and 10), mental health services (chapters 7 and 8), long-term care for the elderly (chapter 6), pharmaceutical industries (chapter 11), environmental health services (chapters 9 and 10), and cancer prevention programs (chapter 9).

Third, the term *industrial societies* encompasses those advanced capitalist countries whose gross national product is generated mainly from industrial and manufacturing production. While some level of privatization is evident in the Soviet bloc nations, this book focuses on the advanced capitalist or mixed economies that lie outside the Soviet bloc. These countries tend to have long histories of industrialization. We exclude the post-World War II phenomenon, the newly industrialized countries (NICs), except for Chile (chapter 10). Great Britain, Canada, the United States, the countries of Western Europe, and New Zealand are all nations that achieved economic growth through some combination of the production of associated consumer durables, a deepening commitment to Keynesian macroeconomic policy, capital goods exports to other countries, and an emerging military-industrial complex (Storper and Scott 1986, 4). These industrial nations also have similar medical models of health care and similar age and mortality profiles. They all operate modern, Western, biomedical systems of health care, and their mortality profiles exemplify the culmination of the epidemiological transition: in their aging populations death results mainly from chronic, degenerative diseases such as heart disease and neoplasms. Such diseases are costly to treat and can place economic hardship on the hospital and environmental health services that treat them.

Finally, the *state* refers to aspects of social control in a particular society that are embodied in public institutions and laws and are reflected in ideology. In health services the state manifests itself most clearly in the complex interactions among the various participants: physicians, health service workers, patients, labor unions, the drug industry, social classes, and the legislative and executive branches of government.

Although exhaustive documentation about all health services undergoing some form of privatization among industrial societies is not feasible in a book of this nature, we do attempt a certain representativeness based both on well-known cases (the United States, Canada, Great Britain, and Western Europe) and on those less well known (New Zealand). Furthermore, we present two case studies where the transfer of free-market ideology and multinational corporate activity from the industrial societies to less industrial ones is apparent (part 4, Developing Countries: Privatization in the Periphery). These case studies examine how each country attempts to open up opportunities for private accumulation or, as Miller (1978) describes, to allow for the "recapitalisation of capital." However, the manner in which privatization is carried out varies. As Le Grand and Robinson note, "Privatization is not simply a matter of the full transfer of ownership from the state to private enterprise." Indeed, such views simply "pander to the needs of political rhetoric" (1984, 25). Theoretical views on the roles of privatization and the welfare state, to which we turn in the following section, provide background against which the case studies are examined.

Privatization and the Welfare State

Historical Overview

Privatization takes many forms, so a simple interpretation is rarely sufficient. Nonetheless, there is a strong consensus that privatization is effectively a *political* process (Barnes 1986; Mohan 1986b; Hirschoff 1986; Dunleavy 1986; Pirie 1985; Heald 1985). Because it includes both collective provision and more privatized systems, it can appear in several forms in the health care sector. Most health care privatization, however, tends to reduce state participation and increase private-sector activity. The state attempts to keep itself at arm's length while fewer public monies and personnel provide health services. Not-for-profit organizations have long existed in the health care field. Consumer cooperatives, community associations, and charities are examples of these private services. Only in extreme cases does the market replace the state in a completely unregulated environment and without a floor of protection.

Private health services can flourish without major policy and legislative restructuring. For instance, free-standing ambulatory centers that provide urgent care (sometimes referred to as "doc-in-the-boxes") are appearing in suburban areas of the United States as alternatives to emergency rooms and physician offices. Referrals are not necessary, and urgent care at these facilities is quicker and, usually, less expensive than care at other facilities. These centers can be established like any other retail activity, as long as they satisfy licensure requirements.

The need for medical and health services has increasingly been met and satisfied in the marketplace. In many places these services are changing from an inalienable right of the citizenry to being treated as a commodity. This process, which we will refer to as the commodification of health services, is tied to technology that greatly enhanced the exchange value of such services. Until the advent of germ theory in the nineteenth century, private services were the predominant mode of medical care delivery around the world. Historically, only selected populations received state-funded curative care, and these populations tended to be strategic civil servants such as soldiers, politicians, and government administrators. Parts of Africa, Asia, and Latin America are still untouched by the influence of modern medical care; these populations interact with traditional healers (shamans, witch doctors, *curanderos*) on a totally fee-for-service basis or as part of traditional community structure (Good 1987; Chávez 1977).

The demise of the feudal system and city-state structures of medieval Europe and the subsequent development of a world capitalist system cast governments into greater spheres of service delivery. As artisan guilds gave way to labor unions during the Industrial Revolution of Western Europe, workers pressed employers and the state for pensions, social security, worker's compensation, and health care benefits. During the Industrial Revolution, working conditions for those who toiled in factories and sweatshops were unhealthy and unsafe. Many of these workers became radicalized through union activities and placed demands upon their employers that eventually cast European governments into health services provision (Kaser 1976).

German chancellor Otto von Bismarck was among the first European leaders to attempt to stifle labor unions and the perceived threat of socialism by mandating employer- and employee-funded health and social security programs. Bismarck reasoned that if employers could meet certain health care and social security (retirement) needs, union demands would be weakened and union quest for worker control, inspired by the writings of Marx and Engels, would be quelled. By the end of the nineteenth century, most of the industrialized European nations had installed some form of health care and social security programs financed by general tax revenues or employer funds (Sigerist 1947). A century later, what had begun as small-scale welfare state services during the era of Bismarck had evolved into a labyrinth of social programs.

The role of the state in health care provision in the United States evolved quite differently than in Europe. Although scattered accounts of public-sponsored health care in the United States exist, health services generally remained in the hands of private providers. Paul Starr (1982) has demonstrated that private insurance firms emphasized five-cent and ten-cent weekly withholdings for life insurance policies, which, from the industry's vantage point, were more lucrative than health insurance policies. Low-skilled workers in the manufacturing and service sectors of the United States economy at the turn of the century, many of them European-born, were persuaded to leave something behind in the form of life insurance instead of worrying about health insurance. Thus, a high social value was placed upon individual initiative and responsibility, as personified by Horatio Alger's fictional character, and life insurance was favored over health insurance in the United States.

Patterns of Convergence: An International Perspective

Colonization and imperialist expansion transferred new systems of health care financing to Asia, Africa, and Latin America. The development of vaccines and antibiotics against tropical diseases was funded by private philanthropic institutions for the health of the colonizers and, later, the indigenous population—especially as wealth from the colony accrued to the parent state. Such care was most often provided by the private sector—large trading companies and merchants—and by colonial governments (Brown 1982; Eyer 1984). Private charities, many of them church groups, spread modern medical care based on the principles of germ theory and the identification of transmission routes of infectious diseases. Missionaries in Third World countries still use modern healing practices as a means of converting locals to their religious organizations. What little modern public health care existed in the Third World before the middle of this century was, for the most part, confined to special occupational groups, unions, or public workers (Gesler 1984). Health ministries and departments in these developing nations were created to integrate fragmented health care services and to coordinate the financing of health services among employees, employers, dependents, and the state. Through centralization of these small, private health care programs, governments sought to maximize the efficiency and equity of these services, if only in a normative bureaucratic manner (Romero 1977; Roemer 1985).

The trajectories followed by the poor and rich nations are converging because of the strained world economy. Independent of modes of production or per capita wealth, many nations are trying to ensure minimum levels of health care while maintaining fiscal solvency. The current fiscal dilemma derives in good measure from the loosening of credit during the post-1973 OPEC (Organization of Petroleum Exporting Countries) price escalation in the form of finance capital (see chapter 2). A glutted Eurocurrency market made lending at lower rates of interest more attractive. Third World nations borrowed huge sums of capital in hopes of fostering economic development, and many of these nations are now burdened with foreign debt. Furthermore, lending nations cannot afford default on these debts. Both lender and borrower nations strive to agree on the structure of domestic expenditures in the borrower nations. The International Monetary Fund, the World Bank, and other lending agencies have issued strict domestic expenditure guidelines, and it is not surprising that "the general thrust of these programs is to promote market-oriented, open economies geared to export production" (Loxley 1984, 29). The borrower nations, for their part, must deal with mounting domestic demands for social services while confining domestic expenditures to guidelines set by foreign lending agencies.

It is at this critical junction—the dependency between borrower and lender—that controls on public domestic expenditures affect the beneficiaries of health, education, and housing programs in the Third World. Witness, for example, Brazil's near-total default on its $143 billion debt in early 1987. The ensuing speculation on the major stock and exchange markets wreaked havoc on commodities and capital flows to and from Brazil; small lending institutions in scores of cities in the United States and Western Europe were on the brink of closure; and the value of the Brazilian cruzeiro plummeted in major foreign currency markets. While the size of Brazil's foreign debt is spectacular, this precarious scenario is commonplace in nearly eighty countries around the world (de Janvry 1985).

The wage and monetary devaluations, inflation, and shortages of basic vital goods and services generated by Third World debt have been devastating to the masses in these nations, who often take their protest to the street. John Walton has documented the impact of this new political economy of debt and underdevelopment in twenty-two developing nations. He observes somewhat graphically that "intentional IMF 'shock treatments' produced unprescribed fits as electrified patients turned on their tormentors" (Walton 1987, 302). In a critical way, therefore, these are the social and fiscal climates that bind national economies in unprecedented ways. The privatization of social programs provides yet another remedy for coping with the etiology of this crisis.

Privatization's challenge to welfare state functions cannot, however, be construed as part of a global conspiracy. Likewise, privatization is not a monolithic process that responds solely to the fiscal crisis of the state. Instead, the role of the state changes in response to numerous pressures, challenges, and ideologies. The pressure for the state to become more economically efficient in social program delivery has been ever present, most centrally in the conceptual issues that are central to public-choice theory. Challenges for lower-cost private-sector service delivery have perhaps been most dramatically apparent in electoral politics among the advanced capitalist nations. There is strong electoral appeal in the state's abdication of services and production that are either perceived to be inapplicable to certain classes (jobs programs, relief, Medicaid for "middle classes") or can be provided at lower cost by the private sector. Lastly, ideology plays a key role in how privatization is perceived by scholars and the public. For example, the Left has long criticized the client dependency on the state that results from welfare state functions (Doyal and Pennell 1979). At the same time, there is much debate about the rolling back of the welfare state and the deleterious effects such a process imposes on the poor. A more accurate appraisal is that privatization is neither a new process, nor a process that develops uniformly across space and time.

Trends in Central Government Expenditures on Health Services

The comparison of international data on public and private health expenditures reveals several problems. Suffice it to say here that the major ones include different definitions of what constitutes health services, the great diversity of employer insurance programs, and data unavailability. These caveats notwithstanding, several general trends are evident. First, in all groups of countries except industrial market economies, the proportion of central government expenditures on health services declined between 1972 and 1985 (table 1.1). Greater out-of-pocket expenditures due to rising incomes, more over-

Table 1.1. Central Government Expenditures on Health Services

Groups of Countries	1972 (%)	1985 (%)
Developing economies	6.6	4.2
Oil exporters	4.9	4.3
Exporters of manufactures	9.7	4.2
Highly indebted countries	8.5	4.6
Industrial market economies	10.0	11.4

Industrial Market Economies	1972 (%)	1985 (%)
Spain	0.9	0.6
Italy	13.5	12.1
New Zealand	14.8	12.8
Belgium	1.5	1.7
United Kingdom	--	12.2
Austria	10.1	12.7
Australia	7.0	9.5
Finland	10.6	10.4
West Germany	17.5	18.7
Sweden	3.6	1.2
Norway	12.3	10.8
Switzerland	10.0	13.1
United States	8.6	11.3

Source: World Bank 1987. Reprinted by courtesy of The World Bank.

Notes: "Health [services] cover[s] public expenditure on hospitals, medical and dental centers, and clinics with a major medical component;. on national health and medical insurance schemes, and on family planning and preventive care. Also included is expenditure on the general administration and regulation of relevant

the-counter medications, and increased employer-sponsored care are likely to contribute to this decline in central government expenditures. A second and perhaps more curious trend is the rise in central government expenditures in the industrial economies, the great majority of the case studies identified in this book. What accounts for this increase in central government expenditures on health services in the more developed countries?

The World Bank (1987, 278) lists several qualifiers in comparing these data. First, central government data alone do not always represent the contributions of state, provincial, county, local, or other intranational data. Thus, for example, state contributions to the United States Medicaid program (which usually entails a fifty-fifty state/federal partnership) are not included here. Second, like data from table 1.1., slightly different measures of health services enter into these cross-national comparisons. Third, differences in how coverage is defined will determine the nature and amount of expenditures. Fourth, since 1972 the health care industry in these nations has been much more capital intensive. New technology such as CAT scanners and MRI (magnetic resonance imagery) did not exist in 1972. Finally, environmental legislation passed in this period of time (before the 1980s) is an outcome of the ecological movement of the 1960s and 1970s. The costs of environmental health services mask the more commonly associated health services categories of hospitalization and ambulatory care.

---

government departments, hospitals and clinics, health and sanitation, and national health and medical insurance schemes; and on research and development" (World Bank 1987, 278).

The World Bank categorizes the groups of countries as follows: "*Developing economies* refer to countries with 1985 per person incomes of $400 or less. *Oil exporters* are middle-income developing countries with exports of gas and petroleum accounting for at least 30 percent of merchandise exports. These countries include Algeria, Egypt, Cameroon, Ecuador, Gabon, Indonesia, Iraq, Iran, Mexico, Nigeria, Oman, People's Republic of the Congo, Syria, Trinidad and Tobago, and Venezuela. *Exporters of manufactures* are developing countries with exports of manufactures (based on most of the SITC codes 5, 6, and 7) with at least 30 percent of exports of services and goods. They include Brazil, China, Hong Kong, Hungary, India, Israel, Poland, Portugal, South Korea, Rumania, Singapore, and Yugoslavia. *Highly indebted countries* include the following seventeen countries: Argentina, Bolivia, Brazil, Chile, Colombia, Costa Rica, Côte d'Ivoire, Ecuador, Jamaica, Mexico, Morocco, Nigeria, Peru, Philippines, Uruguay, Venezuela, and Yugoslavia. *Market economies*, commonly referred to as the 'industrial economies' or 'more developed countries' and members of the Organisation for Economic Co-operation and Development, except Greece, Portugal, and Turkey" (xi).

Summing up these global trends, in the vast majority of countries the proportion of central government expenditures has fallen. Curiously, the proportion of expenditures among the industrial economies has increased for the reasons alluded to above. The essays that follow focus mainly on this last group of countries and further clarify the nature of health services expenditures and delivery by addressing specific types of health services. The point to remember is not that some countries listed in table 1.1 have increased health services expenditures slightly (Belgium, Austria, Australia, West Germany) while others have not. Rather, we should note that the broad process of privatization (changes in subsidy, regulation, and provision) can best be understood by examining economic restructuring in greater detail.

In the section that follows, we turn to some of the central arguments in the privatization debate. My aim is to provide a backdrop to the chapters ahead so that those case studies might inform us about the theory and practice of health services privatization.

The Privatization Debate

The Merits of Privatization

The public-choice school, represented by James Buchanan, Anthony Downs, Gordon Tullock, and writers associated with the Institute of Economic Affairs and the London-based Adam Smith Institute, argues against the welfare state and for privatization (Tullock 1970; Pirie 1985). Friedrich von Hayek and Milton Friedman of the Department of Economics at the University of Chicago share similar views (Friedman and Friedman 1980; Will 1983). They contend that the invisible hand of the market is more efficient and responsive to consumer needs and that public administrative budgets consume large portions of tax monies that could otherwise be used for service delivery. Although the arguments that follow are not unique to the above writers and institutions, many of the arguments in favor of privatization can be traced to them, and their influence in shaping policies in Western Europe, North America, and parts of the Third World has been formidable.

The state is inefficient, they argue, because it fails to provide services at minimal cost. Managers confront different challenges in state settings. They are not easily fired or hired and they do not share in dividends or other monetary incentives as do private managers. This absence of accountability results from the lack of shareholders, who would be free to remove incompetent administrators. Many mid-level managers and bureaucrats are politically appointed or pro-moted by civil service exams. Salaried providers are insensitive to costs, which may be high if care for the indigent is widely adminis-tered. By resurrecting competition, many of these pitfalls can be avoided. A growing hospital-management literature is addressing how incentive compensation can be implemented among salaried medical staff while holding down costs (Broadbent 1987).

Madsen Pirie, England's so-called privatization tsar, identifies some twenty-two types of privatization. He claims that successful privatization schemes employ a good share of the managers and workers from the former public agency. Efficiency and greater com-pliance under new management is enhanced by offering employees stock options and discounted goods and services (Pirie 1985). Gov-ernment can gradually release stock to the open market so as not to overvalue it (Gwynne 1987), but should still retain about half of all stock (sometimes called the "golden share option"). This option serves two purposes: it grants the state considerable discretion in the operations of the company, and it dampens antiprivatization protest. Efficiency, however, may be reduced in companies that remain quasi-independent government-owned enterprises, or quangos (Barnes 1986), thus further compounding the public/private debate.

Centralized health care services under state control are not an unqualified blessing. The World Health Organization's pursuit of complete physical, mental, and emotional well-being for everyone is a nebulous goal that can consume enormous public resources (Coo-per 1975). Escalating consumer demands may drain public treasuries or lock health services in a stranglehold of political influence if benefi-ciaries gain political strength. These problems have been identified in governments ranging from the democratic United States (Califano 1981) to the authoritarian regimes of Turkey, Greece, South Korea, and some South American nations. These latter governments have dealt with the problem of using public monies for health services by severely curtailing social spending (Remmer and Merkx 1982; O'Donnell, Schmitter, and Whitehead 1987; Scarpaci, Infante, and Gaete 1988). Such a draconian tactic, however, is rarely an option in electoral politics.

Many of the arguments against the public provision of goods and services are subsumed under the public burden thesis, which

contends that the public sector is wasteful, inefficient, and unproductive. The thesis relies on the conceptual distinction between
"unproductive" social relations and "productive" economic ones.
Accordingly, domestic policy is cast into social and economic camps.
It follows, then, that most human capital investment in the area of
health and education (long-term ventures) is less profitable than investment in mining, industry, manufacturing, and transportation
(short-term ventures). However, this dichotomy of "unproductive"
social programs and "productive" economic programs tends to
oversimplify the public/private debate.

Large and competitive health care markets should allow prices to
reflect the tastes and incomes of their patients. Private health insurance can offer alternatives to patients who both prefer and can pay
for the amenities of private hospitals and doctors' offices versus the
crowded, less alluring ones of public systems. Besides the attractiveness of these "hotel" aspects of private health care, private providers
often evoke confidence in both the providers and the system (Battistella 1987). To date, however, there is no strong evidence that economies of scale in the private health sector have reduced costs for
significant numbers of patients in the United States (Spann 1977),
Great Britain (Le Grand and Robinson 1984; West 1984). Chile (Scarpaci 1985b), New Zealand (Barnett, Ward, and Tatchell 1980), and
several developing nations (Lee and Mills 1983). Supporters of private health care argue that such failures are partially attributable to
government intervention and that skyrocketing medical costs "can
be corrected only by restoring the natural incentives of the market
and letting immutable economic laws work their way" (Freeman
1981, 268).

Several empirical and theoretical studies indicate that free public
medical care tends to pump up demand for medical services (Stockman and Gramm 1980). Patients are insensitive to price when they
make little or no copayment at the time of service delivery. As a result, superfluous use ensues, driving up costs (Boland and Young
1983). Moreover, state medical care can be illiberal or coercive because the preferences of patients for certain providers, facilities, and
even treatments may be overruled in nationalized health systems.
Also, free medical services, whether they are supplied by public providers in Tanzania, by missionaries in Kenya, or by the National
Health Service in Great Britain, can produce psychological dependence (cf. Turshen 1984; Good 1987; Doyal and Pennell 1979), thus
reducing patients' abilities to make their own choices. Seen in this

perspective, any accretion of power to the state results in a corresponding reduction in the liberty of individuals.

While nationalized health services may ostensibly provide universal coverage, the quality and outcomes of health care vary. Equality in health care persists as an illusive policy objective, but there is no guarantee that nationalized health systems can attain that goal. The removal of financial barriers does not necessarily lead to equal health status. Witness, for example, studies in Great Britain that show that while national indicators of health status are improving, differences in mortality and morbidity by social class persist (U.K. DHSS 1980; Doyal and Pennell 1979). Nor has the Soviet Union resolved problems of equity; infant mortality actually increased in the 1970s despite greater state expenditures (Davis and Fesbach 1980), and fee-for-service medical care still exists (Maxwell 1974; Ryan 1978).

The geographic maldistribution of health personnel is not always remedied by state intervention either. Government attempts in the United States to remedy maldistribution through Title XIX of the Social Security Act (to lure physicians to inner cities) and the Hill-Burton Act (to enhance hospital care in rural areas) have had mixed results. Nor has public intervention in Great Britain been entirely successful in eradicating maldistribution problems. More powerful and culturally advantaged areas continue to attract more personnel (Maxwell 1974; Battistella 1987).

A seminal international review of curative-care financing by Kohn and White (1976) showed that partial payment for primary and secondary care increases both patient use and satisfaction. Two factors seem to be at work here. First, partial payment may enhance the credibility of the delivery system, since fees help to legitimize medical services in market economies, and patients feel they have something at stake when they invest travel and waiting time. A second alleged benefit of charging for medical services is that patients are more likely to carry out subsequent curative and preventive care when they incur some out-of-pocket expenses.

A recent study of the empirical aspects of demand for primary care in the Third World drew similar conclusions. John Aken and colleagues found that free public medical care may draw off charity clients from private providers and allow patients simply to experiment with alternative forms of care. Based on their own research in the Bicol region of the Philippines, they concluded that "not charging for care did not necessarily increase the probability of capturing the target group, and it turned out that many of the services reached people who could reasonably have paid." The policy relevance of this find-ing in the study of health care privatization is that "partial or self-financing of local PHC [primary health care] projects . . . reduces dependence on national government and donor agency funds for survival" (Aken et al. 1985, 175–176).

In synthesis, arguments for privatization and private health ser-vices rest on several key points. Privatization promotes, or at least preserves, individual liberty. Managers are more accountable and sensitive to consumer needs when they are subject to removal by stockholders and paid according to the success of their enterprise. Program innovation and implementation are more likely to occur in small private firms than in large public bureaucracies (which may be attributable more to the scale of production than to public versus pri-vate management per se). The removal of health services from the public sector alleviates the state's financial burden, which in turn can foster capital formation and promote economic development. Incur-ring cost at the time of delivery often enhances the patients' use of and compliance with a specified regime.

The Detriments of Privatization

Despite the growing literature on the role of the state in providing goods and services, ideology once again surfaces as a prevailing force in assaying the merits of privatization. While there are no neatly de-lineated schools of thought that argue against privatization per se, in-sights into the issue can be gained from the writings on theories of the state and its role in providing health services.

Doyal and Pennell (1979) have analyzed the creation of national health systems and programs with regard to the political economy of advanced capitalism. They have found that state intervention in the provision of curative and preventive health services is a necessary ally of industrial capitalism. The restructuring of Western European economies after the Second World War depended upon public in-vestment in sectors of the economy where private capital would not, or could not, be placed. Thus, state-sponsored health care facilitates the process of capital accumulation by guaranteeing employers mini-mum levels of health services and productivity for their workers. State health care expenditures also augment labor's real wages. Seen in this light, the state legitimizes intervention in health care as media-tor and keeper of the social contract. However, Doyal and Pennell ar-gue that the National Health Service in England has been careful not to support a labor force that is too healthy, one that might demand a more active role in the production process. They find strengths and weaknesses in England's National Health Service, stating that it is "commonplace of left wing rhetoric that 'capitalism causes disease,' but a generalised statement of this kind, uniformly applied to all ill health in all places and at all times has very little theoretical or political content" (Doyal and Pennell 1979, 24).

To be sure, many public services are provided under the guise that the state might otherwise have to apply direct repression. For example, welfare services can be conceptualized either as the struggles of the working class to wrestle programs from an unwilling state or as the actions of a benevolent state. On the one hand, fiscal pressures from the state to try to arrest public expenditures that maintain social investment and social consumption. Thus, providing health care augments private-sector profits, but it necessarily taps tax revenues in the process (O'Connor 1973). Public health programs provide a level of social stability that is difficult to measure, especially when they temper social movements against the state (Castells 1978). On the other hand, state health care programs ensure the reproduction of labor power, which is essential for capitalist development. Arguments over the merits of privatization become moot if one assumes that the state must necessarily be involved in social program provision. Ian Gough comments on this immutable obligation:

> The social contract permits the private wage, the 'social wage', and 'collective consumption', plus the level of and direction of taxation, to be simultaneously negotiated on a tripartite basis between business, union leaders and the state. This could dampen down some of the conflicts over financing welfare expenditures that have proved harmful to the stability of capitalist economies in recent years. At the same time, by combining this with policies to restructure industry, aid the private sector and channel funds to stimulate investment, this could lay the basis for a renewal of capital accumulation and growth, without encountering some of the risks and adverse consequences of the alternative, right-wing strategy. (1979, 149)

In this way, privatization remains part of the ongoing give-and-take between the state, capital, and labor in promoting economic development.

Although criticisms of national health systems abound, privatization is not a panacea. Health services are not always the proper means for tackling the ill effects of industrial capitalism. The spheres of occupational and environmental health, for instance, are often blurred with curative-care services. Curative care may be provided as compensation to the proletariat when occupational and environmental services are appropriate. Emphasis on curative care leads to what Illich (1975) calls the "medicalization" of the current era, with its diversionary emphasis on the physician and medical technology as the primary determinants of people's health status. Promises by national health services often go unfulfilled because of two kinds of unforeseen constraints. External constraints stem from the pressures exerted by hospital supply and pharmaceutical industries that promote inappropriate drugs (Bodenheimer 1984). Internal constraints derive from the demands brought on by political groups who wish to dismantle health services after their inauguration (Carpenter 1980, 76).

The inextricable bond between the state and capitalist production has changed the way in which the state barters with labor. Recent European labor relations are illustrative. The governments of Belgium, West Germany, Norway, and Italy bargained arduously with organized labor in the late 1970s. Wage concessions were made in return for health and social security compensation (Barkin 1977; Offe 1984). Increasingly, the relationship between real and social wages becomes the central issue in labor-contract negotiation. Once again, issues of privatization are germane to this struggle because changes in state provision, subsidy, and regulation determine levels of public service. As John Eyles, Glenda Laws, and others in this book argue, the welfare state cannot be rolled back without a total collapse of social relations. Accordingly, the golden age of the welfare state has not ended, it has merely taken a new course, one that leads to the scaling back of social programs. This suggests that in the long run, advanced capitalism can neither live harmoniously with nor live without the welfare state. The welfare state functions as an arbiter of crisis management in capitalist development while performing two contradictory tasks: on the one hand, it is limited in gaining access to capital and labor because they lie mainly in the private sector; on the other hand, it seeks to compensate labor for the inefficiencies of the market by subsidizing employment, housing, education, and health care. Although the state attempts to encourage private-sector investment in particular areas, it ultimately gives private capital preferential treatment to ensure the social reproduction of classes (Offe 1984; Piven and Cloward 1971).

Those who take less theoretical positions on the weaknesses of privatization point to the administrative advantages of public-sponsored health services. They highlight the benefits of the central coordination of health services. In developing countries where smaller, private markets exist, national administration of health services can coordinate overall investments more efficiently than market-oriented criteria to which private health care organizations respond. Support for this arrangement has been found in World Health Organization studies of developing nations (Mach 1978). More developed countries also benefit from national-level planning and coordination. In their study of the social geography of health services in Greater London, Mohan and Woods (1985) identified unprecedented health services investment in high-income sections of the city under the Conservative government. They contended that the circumvention of traditional planning procedures squandered millions of pounds on new hospital construction and diagnostic equipment. A similar problem may emerge in the United States if the certificate-of-need review process by Health Systems Agencies, despite their questionable efficacy (Bice 1984), is not assumed by state or local governments in the 1990s.

It is also a contentious issue whether state-provided services are coercive or illiberal. In the United States this thinking may stem from the association of nationalized health systems with the communist nations of Eastern Europe (Battistella 1987). While the neoclassical economic assumption that consumers should purchase goods and services according to their incomes is unquestioned in most retail markets, such logic is challenged in the health care arena. The notion that individual behavior determines financial success in the labor market is also difficult to apply to the health care consumer. There is little doubt that accidents and life-style behaviors such as smoking, diet, exercise, and stimulant consumption are responsible for the lion's share of deaths in developed industrial societies (Dever 1980). But it would be unwise to adopt the functionalist view that all ill health is the direct outcome of individual life-style. Such victim blaming is laden with class bias because it fails to recognize that the poor and disenfranchised cannot easily overcome disease that is derived from squalor and poverty (Eyer 1984).

The criticism that state provision of goods and services is coercive is ahistorical because the state has not been the only agent to make decisions on behalf of others. Parents, social classes, and private firms constantly influence the fate of others. Indeed, the entire history of social work is founded on the premise that individuals have the right to be protected from the tyranny of their families and communities (Bremmer 1968). The accusation that state intervention is an infringement must therefore be tempered.

Collective provision of goods and services promotes noneconomic benefits that might otherwise fail to develop under private systems. Free-market approaches to social programs may be undemocratic or unfair because they promote differentiation of individuals as opposed to social integration. Market forces fail to create altruistic behavior that generates social cohesion. Rather, the market allocates goods and services in terms of status, power, and resources. Public activities can generate a sense of social cohesion and altruism; many people feel good about providing certain services for the general welfare of the country, especially for the needy (Berkowitz 1980).

To illustrate, we turn to one of the most (symbolically) altruistic behaviors: donating blood. Richard Titmus (1970) studied national blood-donation programs in terms of economic efficiency, administrative efficiency, cost per unit to the patient, and quality per unit. Using 1960s data he examined publicly and privately financed systems in England, the United States, the USSR, Japan, South Africa, and twenty-seven other countries. He found that England, Ireland, and other countries with no payment to donors performed the best among the outcome measures employed. At the polar extreme were Sweden, Japan, and the United Arab Republic, where nearly all donors were paid. Most countries that had about 50 percent paid donors, including the United States and the USSR, performed less well than voluntary systems (Titmus 1970, 174–176).

The level of payment required to enhance proper use and follow-up care remains a difficult empirical question. The determination of reasonable levels of payment varies among and within nations. Recommendations that partial payment is advisable in all places would impact hardest on the poor because their disposable income for health care is meager after food, clothing, and housing needs are met. One study of 140 users of a National Health Service System (SNSS) clinic in Santiago, Chile, showed that household expenditures on food consumed on average 80 percent of household income, leaving the remainder for clothing, shelter, transportation, education, and other goods and services (Scarpaci 1985a). In Latin America, Africa, and Asia, the size of the informal sector precludes the application of nominal fees for medical attention because employment and income levels are so low and erratic. Chris Birkbeck (1979) has shown that although the garbage pickers of Cali, Colombia, are the main suppliers to one of the city's largest industries, paper recycling, they are denied benefits of health care, disability, and workers' compensation because of their informal status. Their scavengerlike occupation generates considerable revenues for both the national government and the private sector even though they remain disenfranchised from formal benefits.

The foregoing arguments on the privatization debate have necessarily involved issues of method and ideology, and have cast the debate into two (perhaps artificially-defined) perspectives. There are strengths and weaknesses on each side of the debate, but the polemics surrounding the debate hamper our understanding of health care privatization. As Pommerhene and Frey have stated, "Theoretical reasoning alone cannot settle the dispute of whether public or private production is more efficient" (1977, 227), nor can it point to broad policy or structural changes while ignoring local contexts. The chapters that follow aim to inform us about the processes of health services privatization so that we may better understand the chasm between its theory and practice.

PART ONE

Hospital Services

Chapter 2

Growth of Proprietary Hospitals in the United States
A Historical Geographic Perspective

JAMES BOHLAND AND PAUL L. KNOX

Growth in the number and influence of for-profit (proprietary) hospitals has been one of the more important structural changes in the United States medical care system in the last two decades (Ginzberg 1985). Between 1975 and 1983 the number of proprietary hospitals increased by 103 percent, from 378 to 767, while the number of proprietary beds increased by 95 percent. As a result, by 1983 over 13 percent of the hospitals were owned by private investors. The rates of increase are impressive, yet they do not fully convey the magnitude or scope of the restructuring. With privatization has come greater horizontal and vertical integration in the health care sector of the economy. Multihospital chains, both for-profit and non-profit, have expanded under the stimulus of privatization. Expansion by hospital corporations into new ventures—hospital-management firms, insurance, long-term care facilities, among others—has characterized the for-profit movement in medicine. Numbers aside, the controversy sparked by the growth in investor-owned hospitals has prompted serious debate over the role of profit taking in medicine. This debate has raised questions about the ethical dimension as well as the quality and cost dimensions of privatization (see Eisenberg 1984; Rafferty 1984; Relman and Reinhardt 1986; and Veatch 1983 for differing ideas about the ethical aspects of for-profit ventures in medicine). Our purpose is not to add to the ethical debate over privatization but rather to examine the historical pattern of growth and spatial distribution of proprietary hospitals in the United States to better understand the relationships between privatization and social transformation.

What does the future hold for the privatization movement in the hospital industry? Was the growth in the 1970s and early 1980s a harbinger of a future where for-profit enterprises will dominate the hospital system, or was it simply a short-term manifestation of a unique convergence of economic, medical, and policy conditions? Relman (1980), when he coined the term "medical-industrial complex," was describing a future (as he described it, a dangerous future) in which our health care system would become increasingly dominated by a few large medical corporations. The eventuality of continued growth in investor ownership seems to be a view held by both those who see the trend as a positive, in fact, necessary, move for cost containment and those who have a less sanguine interpretation of such a future (see Gray 1986 for a discussion of these opposing views).

Recent financial problems of many of the larger for-profit firms suggest, however, that expansion is less assured than was previously thought, and that large corporate hospital firms may have reached a size and degree of diversity that cannot be sustained by the economic and policy conditions in the later half of the 1980s or in the 1990s. In 1987, for example, HCA (Hospital Corporation of America) reported a loss of $58.4 million compared to a profit of $174.6 million in 1986 (Mayer 1988a), despite disinvesting 104 of its less profitable hospitals. Financial distress has not been limited to HCA. Humana's financial problems, created by overexpansion in health insurance, lower dividends for shareholders in hospital corporations such as American Medical International, and an overall decline in the value of corporate hospital stocks suggest that the future of for-profits is less optimistic than was predicted in the early 1980s (see Horowitz 1988; Mayer 1988b).

Speculation about the future of for-profit hospitals requires an understanding of the conditions that led to their recent growth. Interpretations of this recent growth of proprietary institutions must be viewed, in turn, against a history of medicine in which for-profit hospitals have at various times been as important or more important in the structure of the American hospital system than they are today. In the early 1900s, for example, proprietary hospitals constituted nearly 60 percent of all hospitals. Although this represented the zenith in proprietary ownership, twenty years later investor-owned hospitals still constituted over 30 percent of the nation's hospitals (Bays 1983).

The growth of proprietary hospitals that occurred in the late nineteenth and early twentieth centuries provides an excellent opportunity to further our understanding of the contemporary surge in for-profit hospitals. Principal differences were that at the turn of the century proprietaries were smaller, independent enterprises rather than part of a large multihospital system, and ownership was typically by one or two individuals, usually physicians, rather than by many investors. Proprietary hospitals in that earlier period differed in important ways from their contemporaries, but similarities can also be found. Similarities exist in their distributional characteristics and in the social class of patients they serve. Also, in both periods the appropriateness of for-profit institutions in medicine was heatedly debated. A 1922 editorial in the *California State Journal of Medicine* on the issue of profit taking in medicine could easily summarize the views of those who currently question the expanded roles of investor-owned hospitals: "The real problem is whether the practice of medicine, including the prevention and treatment of disease and control of its essential agencies shall be constituted a 'business' run by 'business men' for business results, or whether medicine shall continue to be a profession—a great humanitarian profession, conducted by men who are specially educated for their work; who are endowed with altruism, love of service" (26:103).

The purpose of this chapter is to examine the importance of access to investment capital in influencing the growth and distribution of proprietary hospitals in two periods: 1890 to 1930 and 1970 to 1985. Our premise is that the distributional patterns of proprietary hospitals in the two periods will share certain common characteristics because for-profits responded to a basic concern in both periods: the need to adjust to new sources of investment capital. Our view is not that history repeats itself in predictable cycles of events, but rather that there are important parallels in the two periods that can be used to better understand the dynamics underlying the growth of for-profits and the consequence of those dynamics for their distribution.

Our conceptual framework stresses the reciprocal, interdependent linkages between the hospitals as institutions and the larger social context in which they function. The increased importance of for-profits was a result, we argue, of a transformation in the set of relationships between four structural elements—providers, clients, managers, and capital—that have always linked the hospital to the larger social context. The chain of events forging the new conditions that eventually created a context favorable to for-profits began in both periods with restructuring of conditions in the larger social context. These transformations provided for-profit hospitals with the opportunity to expand their market share and influence relative to non-profit enterprises. Furthermore, we argue that the expansion process had a distinctive geography that reflected the imperatives responsible for the growth.

Hospitals as Service Institutions

Histories of specific hospitals (Rosenberg 1982; Rosner 1982; Vogel 1980) and of the American hospital system (Rosenberg 1987) have documented the radical changes in the design, function, and organization of hospitals since the end of the American Civil War. The early nineteenth-century almshouse, one of the earliest forms of hospitals in the United States, bears at first glance little resemblance to the modern research and teaching hospital. Yet, despite obvious differences, the two share a core function that has been the basis for hospitals throughout their existence. Hospitals have always functioned to deliver a particular bundle of medical and health services in an inpatient setting to a client population. What constitutes the bundle of services to be provided, how the institution is managed (including type of ownership), where services are to be located, and to whom they are provided have changed significantly through time, but the core function has remained in place.

Historic changes in the who, how, and where of hospitals can be explained in terms of four structural elements that are necessary to the performance of the core function of any hospital. The relationships among these four establish the character and conduct of hospitals at any point in time. Redefinition of the relationships among the four caused by structural changes in the larger social context creates change in a hospital's character (ownership and location, for example) and conduct. These four elements are: client population, providers, managers, and capital.

1. *Client population*—A hospital needs a client population whose demand for services is sufficiently predictable that the institution can make a long-term commitment to the provision of services.
2. *Providers*—A group of individuals with the skills and knowledge necessary to provide services at a level of quality and cost that clients find satisfactory. Over time, if the services are deemed valuable to society, this group takes on the stature of a professional class.
3. *Managers*—This group administers the operation of the hospital and sets institutional plans. One important duty is to define

what bundle of services will be made available by the institution.

4. *Capital*—Money to be invested in technology, facilities, or programs that is necessary to ensure the continued existence of the institution.

The four structural elements are bound by a complex but volatile set of relationships. The nature of those relationships defines the structure, conduct, and performance of the hospital (fig. 2.1). How the relationships among the four are structured is influenced by the social context in which the hospital operates. Conditions in the local economy will determine, for example, the availability of capital. Society's technological level will influence the type of medical services provided and the management skills to be used in organizing and running the hospital. The size of the local population and its class and family structure will define who uses the hospital and how frequently.

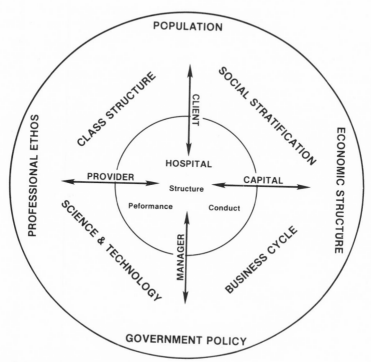

Fig. 2.1. Model of Hospital Transformation

In this model of hospital transformation, the hospital is an institution whose form and function are shaped by the relationships among the four basic components and the larger social context in which hospitals are located. As the contextual contours of the hospital's external environment change, new relationships between the external environment and the hospital are forged. These, in turn, lead to internal restructuring. For much of history, the restructuring of relationships among a hospital's four components have been minor and only small organizational adjustments have occurred. Growth in the elderly population of the local region, for example, may require a change in the provider component such as procuring a geriatric specialist. At other times, social transformations have caused a more radical realignment of the hospital's elements and a very different institution has emerged.

The major shifts in ownership patterns around the turn of the century and in the 1970s and 1980s were in response to a new set of relationships among capital, managers, providers, and clients that was engendered by a transformation of the social context within which hospitals functioned. All four of these components had a role in the growth of for-profits, but our thesis is that the ownership changes occurred principally in response to forces affecting the availability of investment capital for hospitals. Changing conditions within society meant that old relationships between hospitals and sources of investment capital had to be redefined. Different financial conditions gave investor-owned hospitals a comparative advantage in accessing investment capital. To capitalize on this advantage, however, it was necessary to pursue a particular locational strategy. As a consequence, a distinctive distributional pattern of for-profits became evident in both periods. Furthermore, there were important similarities in the geography of for-profits in both periods because the locational imperatives for securing investment capital were similar in both. To understand the link between capital acquisition and location requires an understanding of the manner in which hospitals have historically acquired capital.

Role of Capital

Like all institutions, hospitals require large investments in new technology, programs, or facilities to meet demands for new services and to remain competitive for patients or staff physicians. All forms of hospitals—non-profit, public, and proprietary—need capital for new services, facilities, and technology. Who makes or has the greater influence in investment decisions is an important consideration in the for-profit and non-profit distinction of hospitals and has been a subject of different theoretical interpretations. The differences revolve around the relative power of the provider in provider-manager relationships. One theory holds that hospitals' capital investments are in response to the demands of patients (Ginsburg 1976) and that managers make investment decisions to maximize the availability of services for patients. An opposing view is that physician demands, rather than those of patients, are principally responsible for investment decisions and that, consequently, investment decisions are influenced by physicians rather than managers (Pauley and Redisch 1973).

Taking the latter view, Bays (1983) has argued that, historically, non-profit, as opposed to for-profit, hospitals have prevailed in the United States because they are favored by physicians. Physicians, through their professional organizations, have acted as a cartel to reduce competition and increase their profit-making ability, according to Bays. Moreover, non-profit hospitals provide the best opportunity for achieving these ends because in non-profit settings physicians have more influence on decisions regarding services, technology, and capital investment by virtue of their professional stature. They use their power to "lower the total cost of the complementary hospital inputs and therefore increase the prices that physicians can charge" (Bays 1983, 377). According to this interpretation, for-profits are transitory forms of hospitals that arise to take advantage of expanding markets but which cannot be sustained for long periods of time because physicians will eventually exert their power and limit the growth of for-profits.

The emphasis on the relationship between providers and managers in hospitals is implicit in Bays's interpretation. In non-profits the provider class dominates the relationship. In for-profits, however, the managerial class seems to have a greater voice and greater control of investment decisions that influence services. Alexander, Morrisey, and Shortell (1986) support this view and note that physicians in investor-owned hospitals are less integrated into the managerial process than is true in non-profits.

The investment decision is also important in the cyclical model of for-profit growth presented by Schlesinger, Marmor, and Smithey (1987). Like Bays, they assume that non-profits provide doctors with greater control over hospital investment decisions because non-profits are more compatible with the nonpecuniary interests of professional providers. In their life-cycle model, new services prompted by technological or social innovations in medicine will initially be supported by non-profit agencies because innovators generally require subsidization. Subsidies must come from either government or philanthropic sources because nonpecuniary goals are more easily met in non-profits. As the demand for the innovative services expands, however, a niche in the market is created for for-profits. When growth in the market for the new services slows, non-profits and for-profits converge in their behavior and a relatively stable market is established (Schlesinger, Marmor, and Smithey 1987).

The Bays and the Schlesinger interpretations of non-profit and for-profit growth patterns share three common assumptions: (1) physicians prefer non-profits because of the greater power they have in influencing investment decisions; (2) for-profits are transitory because their market niche depends on securing acceptable profits, and profitable market conditions are highly volatile in the medical industry; and (3) there is a relationship between hospital ownership and the structure of the provider-manager-capital association.

While the Bays and Schlesinger models stress the role of capital investments in influencing ownership, their approaches, particularly Bays's, emphasize the investment stage of capital decisions (i.e., how to spend capital). Equally important is the finance decision (i.e., where and how capital is obtained). The two stages are, of course, interdependent. Ease in raising capital can encourage a higher rate of capital investment by hospitals, while how capital is to be invested will influence which sources will be more readily available to the hospital. Historically, capital financing of hospitals has come from philanthropy, debt financing, government grants or tax benefits, equity financing (sale of stock certificates), or surplus from operations. Several factors determine hospitals' access to these sources of capital, including type of ownership. Equity financing, for example, is an option only for proprietary hospitals, and for-profits are thought to have an advantage in debt financing (Cohodes and Kinkead 1984). Capital from philanthropic and governmental sources, however, is principally accessible to non-profits and public hospitals. The comparative advantage of one form of ownership over another in obtaining lower cost capital financing has varied throughout history as the amount of capital and ease of access to these five sources have changed. Conditions in several periods have favored access to capital by non-profits; at other times, the advantage has been with for-profit institutions. These shifts in capital accessibility have been the consequence of restructuring of national or local economic conditions. A reorganization of capital sources occurred, for example, in the latter half of the nineteenth century because of the urban/industrial transformation of the United States. Since the 1960s, the national economy has been undergoing a structural change of considerable magnitude. That transformation, along with the expanded role of government in the social agenda of the nation, has restructured the medical system to one based more on a competitive market model. With this redefinition, conditions favoring the appropriation of capital by investor-owned rather than non-profit hospitals were created.

Our conceptual framework emphasizes the role of capital-financing markets in influencing the growth of for-profits. The importance of capital-finance sources has important spatial consequences because reliance on specific capital sources creates locational imperatives for hospitals. The locational consequences of these strategies became clearly manifested in the distributional pattern of for-profit hospitals in the different historic periods. If, for example, operational surpluses are to be a principal source of capital, it is imperative that hospitals locate where they can maximize that surplus. In the remaining portion of the chapter we describe the associations among societal transformation, access to capital by hospitals, and the national and intrametropolitan distribution of proprietary hospitals for the periods 1890 to 1930 and 1970 to 1985.

Proprietary Hospitals:
The Urban/Industrial Transformation

For most of the nineteenth century, the hospital, or its precursor, the almshouse, was marginal to the United States medical system. Most medical care, including surgery, was practiced in either the patient's or the provider's residence. Hospitals were established primarily to serve the poor and were not acceptable for persons of higher social status (Rosenberg 1982). Because of the prevailing views on the etiology of poverty, most of the early hospitals served the moral as well as the medical needs of patients. Moral redemption was as important as curing the patient's health affliction. Because patients were principally from the lower socioeconomic strata, most hospitals were either public institutions or were operated by charitable trusts, many with religious ties (Starr 1982). From its narrow and peripheral role, however, the hospital moved to the center of the medical care system by 1910. In so doing, it moved from a social welfare institution to one whose foundation was a scientific medical paradigm. Accompanying this transition was a shift in the pattern of ownership from the nine-teenth-century standard—public and charitable trusts—to one in which proprietary hospitals were a significant component of the system. The shift, remarkable in scope and speed of occurrence, was en-twined with the general transformation of medicine that occurred between the end of the Civil War and the 1920s.

Much has been written on the history of the evolution of modern medicine and the role of the hospital in that transformation. Most observers have emphasized the importance of technological and sci-entific innovations, but the importance of the broader social and eco-nomic restructuring of society in the period has been given greater accord recently (see, for example, Knox, Bohland, and Shumsky 1983, 1984; Reverby and Rosner 1979; Rosner 1982; Starr 1982; and Vogel 1980). These researchers have attempted to link the evolution of the medical system, including the role of hospitals, to the social and economic dynamics of the urban/industrial revolution. While not denying that new technological developments were important to the development of modern medicine, researchers emphasize how the social transformation of the period created conditions supportive of a change to a science-based medical model and of the professional-ization of physicians.

Growth of Proprietary Hospitals

The forces shaping a new social and economic order in the United States altered the structure of the medical system, the role of the hos-pital in that system, and the standard of ownership in hospitals. The causal connections in this process involved a complex set of recipro-cal, interdependent processes. It is not our purpose to offer a com-plete definition and explanation of these processes; our concern is with those processes principally responsible for the growth of for-profit hospitals. That growth can be traced to four important di-mensions of the medical transformation that were outcomes of the broader social restructuring: increased demand for medical services, commodification of medical care, increased role of science and tech-nology in medicine, and the vulnerability of philanthropic capital. These dimensional transformations were necessary for the growth of for-profit hospitals. Taken individually they were not sufficient for the shift in ownership; collectively, however, they created a context that supported the growth of proprietary hospitals. Their combined effect was to expand the opportunities for securing capital from the operational surpluses of hospitals, an expansion that provided proprietary hospitals with a new source of capital that heretofore had not been important.

In response to the labor requirements of industrialization, the nation's urban population grew rapidly between 1870 and 1920, reaching 50 percent of the total population in 1920. Although urban growth was important in increasing the demand for medical services, more significant were transfigurations in the traditional family structure, which were a consequence of the new urban/industrial order. The rationalization of everyday urban life that accompanied the industrialization process meant that many of the traditional roles of the family were no longer possible (Pred 1981). Moreover, many immigrants to the city came without any family support. Young males seeking employment and greater social mobility than was possible in rural areas or small towns became part of the "bachelor" movement, which fueled the demand for services in the industrial city (Risse, Numbers, and Leavitte 1977; Warner 1972). Tasks previously performed by family members now had to be purchased, thus creating a demand for new service occupations. Providing care for sick family members could no longer be done easily in the new conjugal family. Not only were there cost and time constraints, but the emotional drain was greater than was true in an extended family structure (Parsons and Fox 1952). The hospital of the mid-nineteenth century could not meet these needs. What was required was a new institution that could respond to the demands of the city's working and middle classes.

Initially, the increased demand for medical services fostered an increase in the supply of physicians as the laissez-faire regulatory environment of the period enabled "medical" schools to respond quickly to the demand for physicians. However, as providers mobilized, the professionalization of physicians led eventually to strong regulatory constraints on medical education and licensure. By the early twentieth century, there were relatively fewer physicians in urban areas (Burrow 1977). In response to the increased demand for and the reduced supply of physicians, the cost of medical care inside and outside the hospital rose, but the new techno-interventionist view of medicine (Eyles and Woods 1987) found willing consumers in the middle classes of the new industrial city.

The mutually supporting union of a new medical ethos and the demands of the urban middle class led to further legitimization of the view that medical services were commodities to be bought and sold in the market like other goods. It is true that physicians had always received compensation for their services, although prior to 1890 the poor were routinely provided medical care at no cost in dispensaries or almshouses. By 1920, however, the tone of the medical profession toward fees and reimbursement solidified into a more rational approach to the issue. Concern was routinely expressed by the medical profession about the demoralizing effects of free medicine (the target was the moral behavior of patients, although lower payments were undoubtedly demoralizing for physicians) and how it encouraged laziness and deceit (Gay 1905). An editorial in 1919 in the *California State Journal of Medicine* is indicative of how far the profession had moved toward viewing medical services as commodities: "It is no more incumbent on the physician to disburse his service free than it is on any other *seller* [emphasis added] to disburse his wares or services free" (17:104). Not all physicians shared this view, of course, but efficiency rather than stewardship had come to medicine and the hospital as it had to education, business, and industry (Rosenberg 1987).

The continued legitimization of medical services as commodities enabled hospitals to shift costs to patients. The middle class, who were becoming patients in significant numbers, were willing to purchase hospital services provided they were carefully packaged in settings (private rooms, attractive surroundings, and good food, among others) that were comfortable and supportive. Hospitals became increasingly reliant on patient charges for operating expenses and as a source of capital investment. In Brooklyn Hospital, for example, the share of total income from patient fees increased from approximately 16 percent in 1892 to over 50 percent in 1917 (Rosner 1982).

The increased importance of payment from patients as a source of hospital revenue came at a time when hospital costs were rising. While total costs rose partially in response to the increased numbers of patients, average costs per patient were also rising. In Brooklyn the average cost per day for a patient was only $.78 in 1885 but rose to $2.78 in 1915 despite a decline in the average length of stay from 31.7 to 15.6 days over the same period (Rosner 1982). The rise in average costs was in response to the higher cost of providing medicine in a scientific/technological medical paradigm. It was no longer feasible to practice medicine in the lower-cost settings that had been common prior to 1890. New equipment (X-ray machines, for example), new procedures (sterilization), maintaining a qualified nursing staff, and accommodating the middle class's demands for better facilities were all expensive. By the early twentieth century, hospitals had become capital intensive, and although the intensification increased productivity and improved the quality of care (a subject of some debate at the time), it placed a greater burden on management to obtain investment capital. Without continued investment in more suitable facilities, new technology, and the scientific trappings now essential to medicine, physicians would be less likely to join staff and the paying patients would seek care elsewhere.

The principal sources of capital for hospitals prior to the twentieth century were philanthropic capitalists, local governments, and charitable donations. The importance of philanthropic capital during the Progressive Era in supporting institutions with a strong social agenda, such as hospitals, has always seemed to be a contradiction between the strident advocacy of free enterprise by capitalists and their strong belief in social protectionism. According to Polyani (1957), however, the support by paternalistic philanthropists for social welfare institutions was a means of protecting capitalism from its internal contradictions, such as rising wealth in the midst of life-threatening environments and negative externalities rising from greater productivity. Reforms in government, the public health movement, and medical care, among others, were underwritten by many of the eminent capitalists of the day in order to legitimize their role in the industrial society. Andrew Carnegie, for example, funded the Flexner Report of 1910, which set out the reform agenda for medical education. Hospitals were particularly important beneficiaries of philanthropists. The relationship between hospitals and philanthropists was not, however, asymmetrical. Philanthropy "gave legitimacy to the wealth and position of the donors, just as the associations with prominent citizens gave legitimacy to the hospital and its physicians. Hospital philanthropy, like other kinds of charity, was a way to convert wealth into status and influence" (Starr 1982, 153).

Paternal philanthropy was the most important source of capital for hospitals until the late nineteenth century. However, with the growth of the industrial economy it became increasingly more vulnerable as a source of funds. Fluctuations in the economy caused philanthropic donations to hospitals to rise and fall with business cycles. The depression of the 1890s in particular caused severe economic distress in hospitals that had come to base their finances on philanthropy. Philanthropic capital was also susceptible to shifts in the interests of the donor. Projects that could accord the donor with greater status—universities or libraries, for example—were in competition with hospitals for capital. Also, to maintain access to capital, hospitals gave philanthropists important policy roles, such as board membership. Their influence on management decisions increasingly became a source of conflict with physicians, who had in their minds achieved sufficient status to be granted greater authority in the operation of the hospital. In other words, the mid-nineteenth-century provider-manager relationships were being redefined.

The increased vulnerability of hospitals to fluctuations in philanthropic money reduced its importance as a source of investment capital. An alternate source was necessary to meet the investment demands of the new medical paradigm. The sale of medical services in hospitals had become legitimized, and the increased demand for service provided hospitals with a new source of capital: operational surpluses. Proprietary hospitals had been at a disadvantage in securing capital from previous sources (philanthropists and government), and the new source was consistent with for-profit enterprises. Moreover, the increased stature of the medical profession allowed physicians to mobilize their strength effectively and to obtain greater control over medical practices and policies in the hospital. This authority could be attained in hospitals owned by physicians—singly, in partnerships, or as a group of investors—without forfeiting access to what was becoming the principal source of capital in all hospitals, the paying patient.

Spatial Distribution

We analyzed the spatial distribution of proprietary hospitals in this period at the national and intrametropolitan scales. At the national scale, we used states as the unit of analysis; while for the intrametropolitan analysis, we analyzed the location of proprietary hospitals in San Francisco. San Francisco was used because, like most West Coast cities in this period, it had a large number of proprietary hospitals and because the historical geography of the city's health care delivery service has been documented (Bohland, Knox, and Shumsky 1987; Knox; Bohland, and Shumsky 1983, 1984).

Proprietary hospitals in the late nineteenth and early twentieth centuries were owned primarily by individual physicians, were small in size, and entered and exited the health care system relatively quickly (Rosner 1982; Starr 1982; Steinwald and Neuhauser 1970).

Their size meant that their investment-capital demands were less than those of the larger non-profit or public hospitals of the period; however, their inability to access philanthropic capital meant that a location with improved access to paying patients was important to their success.

Because of the importance of philanthropic capital in this period, its distribution had a significant influence on the distribution of non-profit and for-profit hospitals. If philanthropic capital was unevenly distributed across the nation during the period, well-defined distribution patterns of proprietary and non-profit hospitals should be evident. Where philanthropic capital was available, one would expect to find a higher proportion of non-profit and public hospitals; and where it was scarce, one would expect to find more proprietary hospitals. Since the transformation to an industrial economy had led to the accumulation of capital in the industrial and commercial centers of the nation, states that were more fully integrated into the new industrial order should have a higher percentage of non-profit hospitals. In the absence of sufficient surplus capital to foster philanthropic giving, hospitals had to rely more heavily on patient fees. Reliance on patient fees as a major source of revenue came to characterize hospitals throughout the country as philanthropy declined and the investment demands of hospitals increased. However, patient fees, of necessity, were the principal source of revenue in states marginal to the urban/industrial transformation because they had neither the philanthropic capital nor a sufficient history of urban, public involvement to support non-profit or public hospitals. In such states, proprietary hospitals should be more prevalent in the hospital system.

At the intrametropolitan scale, proprietary hospitals would be influenced by the income distribution of urban neighborhoods. Middle- to upper-income neighborhoods would be favored locations for proprietary hospitals, while public and non-profit facilities would be situated in the older sections of the city, reflecting their earlier histories as sources of care for disadvantaged members of urban society.

National Scale. Historical geographic analyses of proprietary hospitals are hampered by the absence of reliable data prior to 1920. Surveys conducted by the American Medical Association are the principal source of information on hospitals prior to 1910; but the data do not differentiate ownership, nor are they at a scale suitable for detailed geographic analysis. In 1905, the U.S. Bureau of the Census published a special report on benevolent institutions that enumerated by state and city hospitals providing charitable care. Proprietary hospitals, however, were excluded from the tabulation because of their "non benevolent" character. Steinwald and Neuhauser (1970) used the tabulation of benevolent hospitals to estimate the total number of proprietary hospitals in 1910 (estimated at 2,441, or 56 percent of the total), but they did not break down the total by states.

The most comprehensive and reliable data on proprietary hospitals for the period appeared in 1925 in a U.S. Bureau of the Census report, *Hospitals and Dispensaries, 1923*. According to that report, of the 4,863 hospitals in the country in 1923, 36 percent were proprietary, 17 percent were financed and administered by a government, and 47 percent were non-profit. Of the proprietary hospitals, 65 percent

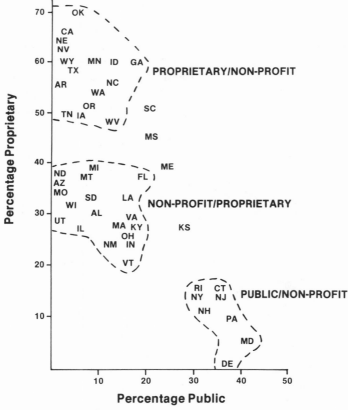

Fig. 2.2. Classification of States by Hospital Mix, 1923

were owned by individuals rather than corporations or partnerships. Although by all accounts (Bays 1983; Starr 1982; Schlesinger, Marmor, and Smithey 1987) the number of proprietary hospitals had begun to decline after 1910, the absence of reliable data prior to 1923 necessitated the use of the 1923 data in our analysis. We have assumed that the distribution in 1923 reflects the geographic pattern, if not the intensity, of proprietary hospitals throughout the period 1890-1930.

To analyze the spatial distribution of hospitals according to type of ownership, we calculated the proportions of proprietary, public, and non-profit hospitals in each state. States were classified, according to the percentage of hospitals in each of the three ownership categories, into three distinctive groups (figs. 2.2 and 2.3). One group consisted of states where public and non-profits constituted the majority of hospitals, and proprietary hospitals represented a very small proportion of the total facilities. Geographically, all members of the group were either New England states or were part of the industrial core of the Mid-Atlantic region.

In the second group, non-profit and proprietary hospitals formed

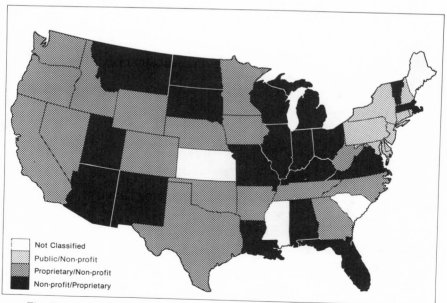

Fig. 2.3. Distribution of Dominant Hospital Combinations, 1923

the majority combination, although proprietary facilities generally constituted a smaller percentage (20 to 40 percent) than non-profits. Public hospitals were less than 20 percent of all hospitals in any state in the group. Geographically, members of this group were more widely distributed than were those in group one, but the majority of states in the non-profit/proprietary group were located in the Midwest or in adjoining Plains or Border states. The third combination was characterized by a predominance of proprietary hospitals (45 to 70 percent) mixed with non-profits. Again, public facilities were a small share of the total in any state (less than 20 percent). The majority of members of the group were western or southern states, although two states were in the Midwest (Iowa and Minnesota).

The spatial distribution of the three groups conforms closely with our hypothesis regarding the influence of capital on the location of proprietary hospitals. In eastern states, where industrialization began earlier and where public involvement in social welfare processes had a longer history, public hospitals were more prevalent and proprietary hospitals were a smaller proportion of the hospital system. In the Midwest, non-profit hospitals were more prevalent, reflecting in some measure the importance of ethnic and religious groups in many of the industrial centers in this region; but proprietary hospitals had also emerged as a major component of the system by 1920. The larger number of proprietary hospitals here in comparison to eastern states reflects the rurality and low population density in many states and the more recent history here of the industrial and medical transformations. Proprietary hospitals were most prevalent in states on the margins of the urban industrial transformation and where the settlement pattern was primarily smaller cities and towns. In such states, the availability of philanthropic capital was limited and the recency of the urban development had not contributed to a strong public responsibility in the provision of health care. As a consequence, patient fees had become, of necessity, the principal source of capital funds for hospitals.

Intrametropolitan Scale: San Francisco Hospitals. Although a geographic outlier to the industrial core of the nineteenth-century United States, San Francisco offers an excellent opportunity for describing the intrametropolitan distribution of proprietary hospitals in a large urban center. From 1860 to 1920 the city's growth was spectacular. From a relatively small city of 56,000 in 1860, it grew to nearly 234,000 by 1880 (an increase of over 310 percent), and to 417,000 by 1910. The extraordinary growth came in conjunction with the city's rapid economic development during the industrializing period. By the early 1900s it had become the leading industrial city in the western United States and had most of the social and spatial characteristics of the industrial city.

By the late nineteenth century, San Francisco had all the conditions necessary for the development of segregated housing areas. A generalized housing market had existed in the city as early as 1849, and residents had accepted residential mobility as a means of social mobility by the 1860s (Shumsky, Bohland, and Knox 1986). Industrial areas adjacent to the wharves created the work-home linkages to encourage the development of working-class neighborhoods around the city's core, while externalities there encouraged the relocation of the city's middle classes to newly developing neighborhoods to the west of the central core of the city. Bowden (1967) has chronicled the rapid growth of the central business district in the latter half of the nineteenth century and its effect on the geographic structure of the core area. The development of the city's trolley system during this period was the final element that enabled city residents, primarily the middle class, to move to more remote neighborhoods while maintaining their places of business in the central core of the city. By the 1870s, immigrants (national and foreign) to the city and the indigenous population had sorted themselves into a residential mosaic whose spatial structure persisted until the 1920s (Issel and Cherny 1986).

By 1900 the social geography of the city had a general north to south trend, with Market Street as a pivotal boundary (fig. 2.4). To its south, neighborhoods were generally of lower social status and had higher levels of deprivation. The South of Market District had some of the most densely populated neighborhoods; almost 20 percent of the city's population lived in the area (Issel and Cherny 1986). Neighborhoods with high density, poor housing stock, a low proportion of families, and a high level of deprivation contributed to the poor quality of health of their residents (Klee 1983). The Mission District south of Market Street was composed primarily of working-class neighborhoods, which had high proportions of Irish and German families. Some residents of the Mission District were middle class, but the largest number of middle-class neighborhoods was in the Western Addition. Here is where the growing urban middle and upper-middle classes concentrated initially before spreading further west into the areas north of Golden Gate Park. Adjacent to the Western

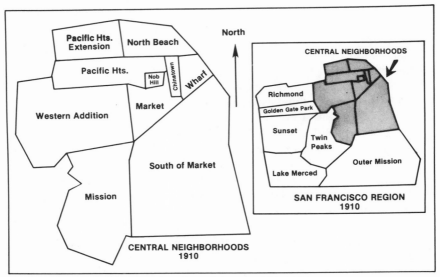

Fig. 2.4. San Francisco Residential Areas, 1890–1920

Addition to the north and east were the upper-class neighborhoods found in Pacific Heights and Nob Hill, respectively. Exceptions to these higher-status neighborhoods north of Market Street were the Chinese quarter and the North Beach District. The Chinese quarter was unique in both its physical and social organization and had the highest density of population at this time. It stood in sharp contrast to the low-density, ostentatious Nob Hill neighborhood immediately to its west. North Beach, like Mission, was a working-class neighborhood, but Italians instead of Irish or Germans were the major ethnic group.

It was within the context of the city's social geography that the spatial distribution of the city's health care delivery system emerged. The geography of that system changed significantly during the industrialization of the city. In the early stages of the transformation (1870s), medical care providers were widely distributed in the city's neighborhoods with less regard to the social status of neighborhoods than was to be true in later years (Bohland, Knox, and Shumsky 1987). By the late nineteenth and early twentieth centuries, however, a large concentration of providers had developed in the city's central business district, occupying offices in new multistory medical centers, and secondary clusters of physicians were distributed throughout most of the working-class and middle-class neighborhoods to the west of the central business district. This redistribution of physicians was in response to a number of factors, including the commodification of medicine, the increased demand for medical care by the middle classes, and the new spatial structure of the city's commercial and residential areas. (Bohland, Knox, and Shumsky 1987; Knox, Bohland, and Shumsky 1984; Shumsky, Bohland, and Knox 1986).

Although existing studies provide an understanding of the locational shifts in physicians' offices, hospitals were not included in the analyses. Information on the location of hospitals in the city is available from city directories beginning in 1870; yet, as at the national scale, analysis of proprietary hospitals is difficult because there was no standard reporting of hospitals by type of ownership within the city. A survey of hospitals in 1923 did report on the distribution of beds by ownership type. According to that report, proprietary hospitals constituted 24 percent of the total beds in the city; public hospitals, 30 percent, and non-profit, 46 percent (Emerson and Phillips 1925). The percentage for proprietary hospitals is low compared to the percentage of proprietary hospitals reported for California (66 percent) in the national figures for the period (U.S. Bureau of Census 1925). The discrepancy appears to be a function of two factors. For one, the survey appears to have ignored the smaller (fewer than twenty-five beds) facilities, which comprise a large number of the proprietary hospitals. Second, their small size means that their proportion of the total hospital system will be significantly smaller when bed size rather than number of facilities is used as the measure of system size.

Because the earthquake of 1906 in San Francisco had a major impact on the physical arrangement of the city for years afterward, we felt that any distributional analysis of hospitals should be for a year prior to the earthquake. Unfortunately, no systematic tabulation of hospitals by ownership type is available for earlier years. However, it was possible to estimate the number and distribution of proprietary hospitals in 1910 by use of the urban directory and the list of benevolent hospitals in the city (U.S. Bureau of Census 1905).

From the list of hospitals and clinics in the 1910 directory, we excluded all specialized (asylums, animal hospitals, homes for aged, as examples) hospitals and all facilities for specific groups (veterans, unwed mothers, as examples). The abbreviated list was further shortened by eliminating all facilities that received either public funding or charitable donations, a determination made from the list of benevolent hospitals in San Francisco (U.S. Bureau of Census 1905). The final list represented the estimated number of proprietary hospitals for the city in 1910. Because some for-profits were probably too small to be listed in the urban directory, the list is a conservative estimate of the total number of proprietary hospitals. We believe, however, the list included the largest share of proprietary hospitals and thus provided a representative sample of proprietary facilities in the city.

We located proprietary and public or non-profit hospitals for 1910 by their address in the city directory. By our estimate there were twenty-seven for-profit hospitals in 1910, representing 53 percent of all hospitals in the city. The majority of the for-profits, 78 percent, were located in the middle- and upper-class neighborhoods that had been developing west of the city core (fig. 2.5). The largest number were situated in the Western Addition, which was the rapidly expanding middle-class district of the city. In contrast, only one for-profit was located in the central commercial district of the city, and

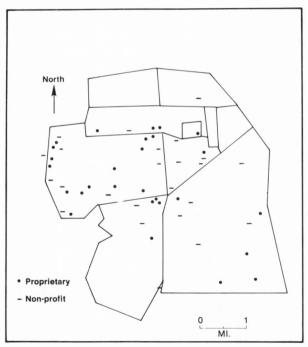

Fig. 2.5. Distribution of Hospitals in San Francisco, 1910

none were situated in densely populated Chinatown or the North Beach working-class district. Only five were located in South of Market, despite the large number and poor health status of residents of the area.

Public and non-profit hospitals were also located primarily in the middle-class districts of the city, although not to the same extent as the for-profits (53 versus 70 percent). The principal difference in the geography of the public/non-profits and the for-profits was the larger number of the former in the central commercial district. The hospitals here represented older non-profit facilities that had developed earlier in the city's history, several prior to the western migration of the city's central business district (Bowden 1967).

Given the reliance of proprietary hospitals on patient fees, it is not surprising to find them concentrated in areas of the city more accessible to paying consumers. In this sense their distribution paralleled the decentralization of physicians to outlying areas during this period. The concomitant trend for physicians to concentrate in the central district was not clearly evident with proprietary hospitals, however. The accessibility and status afforded physicians by a central location would have been an advantage for proprietary hospitals, but the high cost of space made the area unsuitable for proprietary hospitals, which required more space than a physician's office. The need for physicians in the central district to have relatively easy access to hospitals was accommodated by the existence of the public and non-profit facilities in the area. Non-profit and public hospitals, because of their earlier development in the region and philanthropic support, could maintain their location within the core of the city.

Proprietary Hospitals: Contemporary Growth Patterns

Between 1920 and 1970 the number of proprietary hospitals declined significantly. The reduction can be traced to several factors. Increased authority of physicians in the industry, the economic depression of the 1930s, major government intervention in hospital capital financing (the Hill-Burton Act in 1946), and the increasing importance of third-party vendors in hospital reimbursement were some of the more important factors contributing to the decline. The role and dominance of non-profit hospitals in the nation's medical system seemed assured by 1960.

The growth in investor-owned hospitals since 1970 has demonstrated the volatility of the medical system and its structure. The post-1970 period has become a time of major restructuring of a system that earlier had seemed resistant to change. The magnitude of the changes cannot be overestimated. As Starr noted, "Medical care in America now appears to be in the early stages of a major transformation in its institutional structure, comparable to the rise of professional sovereignty at the opening of the twentieth century," (Starr 1982, 420).

The contemporary restructuring of the medical system, as was the case at the beginning of the century, has its roots in a broader socioeconomic transformation. That transformation has several dimensions that have influenced the restructuring of the medical system. Changes in family structure (size and composition), for example, have been comparable in scope to the shift from extended to conjugal family associated with the urban industrial transfiguration (Bogue 1985; Sternlieb, Hughes, and Hughes 1982), and their impacts on demand for medical care have been far-reaching (Pegels 1980; Rice and Estes 1984). The more important aspects of the transformation, however, are related to the emergence of a "disorganized" capitalism that is characterized, among other things, by the increasing scale and interconnectedness of industrial, banking, and commercial enterprises; shifts in the international division of labor; changes in the nature of economic, social, political, and cultural relations in the world's core economies; and in the midst of all these changes a much greater fluidity and flexibility in both corporate and governmental activities (Lash and Urry 1987). Two aspects of this disorganization have been particularly important in redefining the ownership and organizational structure of hospitals. First has been the sectoral shift in the structure of the United States economy, and second has been the expanded role of the government in the nation's social welfare.

Since the end of World War II, the United States economy has been moving away from an industrial/agricultural economy to one in which the tertiary and quaternary sectors have become more central to the nation's economic growth (Gershuny and Miles 1983; Bluestone and Harrison 1982). That shift has accelerated in the last two decades. In this new economic stage (sometimes referred to as advanced, late, or corporate capitalism), professional services, such as health care, have increased their share of the nation's gross national product (GNP). Health expenditures as a share of GNP, for example, rose from 5.3 percent in 1960 to 11.0 percent in 1986.

Accompanying the sector shift has been a concentration of economic activity in fewer corporate hands. Horizontal, vertical, and diagonal expansion through friendly and unfriendly takeovers has created corporate oligarchies that require increasing amounts of capital to sustain their growth and diversification. The demand for capital has been readily accommodated as capital has become international in scope, as the federal and state governments have adopted policies to increase its availability (tax-exempt bonds, broadening tax expenditures, reducing regulations on financing monopolistic practices, as examples), and as finance capital has accumulated precipitously in the aftermath of the 1973 OPEC oil embargo (Thrift 1986). Meanwhile, investment in traditional industries, such as durable-goods manufacturing, has become less attractive because of their poor growth performance, and investment in key service industries such as health care has made them targets of opportunity for investors. For example, for much of the 1970s and early 1980s, health-related stocks, particularly hospital-management stocks, outperformed the market in general (Wallace 1988) and even many of the more visible high-tech industries. By the early 1970s, equity financing was becoming a viable option for health care organizations that wished to shift to investor ownership.

The government's role in increasing the availability of capital was but one of the important roles it has played in the transformation. In the postwar era, the federal government has become a major force in setting and implementing the nation's social agenda. That expanded role has taken many forms—regulatory, monetary, judicial activism—but a clear indicator of the new role is the growth in government resources expended on social programs in the postwar period. Total outlays (measured in constant 1972 dollars) by the federal government grew from $143 billion in 1960 to $364 billion in 1984 (a 154 percent increase); while nondefense spending grew at an even greater rate, from $64 billion to $270 billion (321 percent). Nowhere has the expanded governmental role been more evident than in health care. Direct federal expenditures for health care rose from $13 billion in 1970 to $143 billion in 1987, and an additional $24 billion in tax expenditures from the federal government have been allocated annually to health care in recent years (Scarpaci 1988a; U.S. Health Care Finance Administration 1987; U.S. Bureau of the Census 1985).

The expanded role of government caused a shift in the locus of power within the health care industry from professional provider organizations to the federal government (Havighurst 1987). Programs such as Medicare and Medicaid increased the demand for health services and set in motion a long-term trend of rising health care costs and substantial government oversight of the financial affairs of hospitals. Across all components of the system (hospitals, physicians, and ancillary services) annual increases in health care spending were, on the average, 12.4 percent between 1964 and 1985—increases that were generally above those of the consumer price index throughout the period. The increased demand stretched the capacity of the existing providers, a condition that led to federal policies of providing large subsidies to medical schools and students to increase the number of physicians.

Ironically, greater involvement by the government eventually increased privatization in the health care industry. The government's inability to control the health care cost spiral stimulated by Medicare and Medicaid and the oversupply of physicians that resulted from the federal funding of medical education helped create a social-economic context in which the allocation of health care resources was influenced more by market conditions than by government or provider directives. In this new context, many of the traditional ideas and values that were the foundation of the earlier system (pre-1970) underwent redefinition, including the belief that the government could efficiently manage health resources. The eventual outcome of the redefinition has moved the health care industry to a more competitive market model rather than one influenced primarily by the authority of the professional provider or the federal government. (L. Brown 1987; Havighurst 1987; Feldstein 1986; Starr 1982).

Growth Factors in Proprietary Hospitals

The consequences for hospitals of the broader structural changes and the transformation of the health care system have been profound. Reductions in length of stay, declining revenues, changes in reimbursement systems, hospital closings, increased cost of technology, and new organizational structures are some of the more important consequences of hospitals' new role in the health care system (Hanft 1985; Goldsmith 1985). In trying to establish their position within this more competitive health care environment, hospitals are faced with a difficult dilemma: how to be cost competitive in a market where demand for inpatient services has been declining and where large amounts of capital need to be invested in very costly technology in order to retain their status and remain competitive.

Estimates, for example, of the capital needed by hospitals in the eighties range between $100 and $200 billion (Cohodes 1983). Management technology alone (primarily computer hardware and software) cost hospitals $2.4 billion in 1984 and was projected to double within four years (Goldsmith 1985). With those capital needs and an increasingly competitive industry, the ability of hospitals to secure affordable capital has become paramount to their survival.

Although the Hill-Burton Act provided direct financial support for the construction and expansion of hospitals, direct federal government support was being phased out by the 1960s. At the same time, capital from philanthropic sources was declining. With money from these two sources limited, hospitals shifted to the remaining sources: equity capital, surplus from operating funds, and debt financing. The ownership and organizational structures that could best access these sources would gain a comparative advantage in the increasingly competitive environment in which hospitals had to operate.

Equity capital is, of course, available only to proprietary enterprises. With a national economy shifting to the service sector, profitable service industries such as health care were becoming attractive options for investors. The sale of stocks has not been the "money pump" that some have suggested, but it does provide investor-owned hospital corporations with greater flexibility in selecting sources of capital (Gray 1986). Having a choice between equity or debt capital enables for-profit institutions to take advantage of differential market conditions for bonds and stocks, shifting their investment strategy depending on the cost of capital in either market. While equity financing of long-term capital improvements has become important, the increasing reliance of hospitals on debt financing is one of the most important and dramatic changes in hospital investment in the postwar period. Prior to 1950, less than 25 percent of hospital construction was financed by long-term borrowing. By 1983, that percentage had increased to 70 percent (Cohodes and Kinkead 1984). The growing dependency on debt capital was partially influenced by growth in third-party reimbursement to hospitals. Their cost-based reimbursement policies increased hospitals' operating surpluses and made them a better risk in the financial markets. However, it was two government initiatives that had the greatest effect in spurring debt financing: the Medicare and Medicaid programs and the introduction of tax-exempt bonds for hospitals by state governments.

Medicare and Medicaid helped hospitals underwrite their debt capital in several ways. The cost-based reimbursement systems of both further assured hospitals of a stable operating surplus and reduced their risk as long-term borrowers of money. Both programs also encouraged debt financing by allowing hospitals to include depreciation and interest expenses in calculating reimbursable costs. Even with the change to prospective reimbursement in 1983, Medicare continued to reimburse hospitals for capital expenditures, albeit at a reduced rate. Medicaid and Medicare increased demand and ensured a stable operating surplus, and state policies that made hospitals eligible for tax-exempt bonds opened a large new source of debt financing: public money markets. Now, rather than relying on banks, mortgage companies, or large corporations for loans, individual investors could be accessed since tax-exempt bonds could be issued in amounts small enough to attract them (Cohodes and Kinkead 1984). Their tax-exempt status make the bonds competitive in the money market because they provided investors with a good return even though interest rates were below those of taxable securities.

In these new capital markets, investor-owned hospital corporations have had a significant advantage over public and non-profit facilities. However, at issue is whether that advantage is a function of proprietary ownership or of the multihospital organizational structure associated with today's for-profits. It seems clear that investor-owned, multihospital systems have less difficulty in securing debt capital, but Hernández (1981) argues that the organizational structure is the principal reason. Multihospital chains, for-profit or non-profit, have greater assets, can distribute risk more widely, and have demonstrated greater cost efficiency than independent hospitals, all of which improves their credit rating with lenders (Hernández and Henkel 1982).

Although membership in a chain or hospital association enhances a hospital's ability to secure debt capital, most observers of the contemporary hospital industry believe for-profit hospital-management corporations have had easier and less-costly access to debt capital than have non-profits (Cohodes and Kinkead 1984). Although non-profit and public facilities can take advantage of tax-exempt bonds more readily than for-profits (for-profits can apply for tax-exempt bonds, but there is a ceiling on the total dollar amount allowed, which effectively limits their use) and do not pay taxes, these advantages are offset by several conditions favoring proprietary hospitals.

While both non-profits and for-profits are allowed to compute depreciation and interest costs in determining reimbursable costs, for-profits can also take into account the return on their equity capital. And, although for-profits are not exempt from federal, state, and local taxes, they are permitted to compute depreciation on an accelerated basis for tax purposes. The recent tax reform has limited this advantage, but the reduction of the tax rate by the Gramm-Rudman-Hollings Act from approximately 45 percent to 35 percent offsets the depreciation loss. Finally, the financial community has the view that for-profits can better use their acquisition and management strategies to control many of the factors that influence an institution's credit rating, the more important being quality of management control, size of bad debt, size of operating surplus, and location (Alexander, Lewis, and Morrisey 1985).

The higher profit margin of for-profits is particularly important because it not only reduces risk in the debt market, but also provides them greater flexibility in using operating surplus to finance capital expansion if they choose. The size of the profit margins and the strategies used to achieve them by investor-owned corporations are points of considerable controversy. National studies of profitability between non-profits and for-profits give conflicting results, while regional studies indicate important variations in the profitability of for-profits and non-profits (see Becker and Sloan 1985; Coelen 1986; Hollingsworth and Hollingsworth 1987; Watt et al. 1986). Taken in their totality, the studies indicate slightly higher profit margins for investor-owned systems, but the size of the profit margin is influenced by a number of factors equally important as ownership.

One explanation for the higher profitability of investor-owned hospitals has been patient selection. In contrast to public hospitals and many non-profits, for-profits need not accept unprofitable patients. The extent to which they skim the cream of the patient population has been the subject of considerable research, which clearly indicates that public hospitals provide significantly higher amounts of charitable care than either for-profits or non-profits. Differences between for-profits and non-profits, however, are less clear—in part because of difficulties in differentiating between bad debt and charitable care in the data. If reported uncompensated care is used as the measure of free care, studies in five different states show that for-profits provide significantly lower uncompensated care in four of them (Gray 1986). Comparisons must be made with caution, however, because several other factors—teaching/nonteaching status, number of competing hospitals, location, and service mix—influence the amount of uncompensated care. In Virginia, for example, smaller for-profits (fewer than 100 beds) situated in areas without competing facilities had 15.6 percent of their revenue as uncompensated, while larger (251–500 beds) hospitals in locales with competing facilities had only 3.3 percent. In the former, for-profit percentages were higher than those for non-profits, while in the latter the reverse was true (VHA 1985).

The practice of dumping patients on public or non-profit hospitals is a more visible means of patient selection, but hospitals can also reduce their charitable care through the mix of services they provide and the reimbursement systems they accept or by locating facilities in middle- to upper-income areas. The extent to which these strategies are used is, like most aspects of for-profits, heatedly debated. Studies of reimbursement systems indicate little difference in the mix of Medicare, Medicaid, Blue Cross, and private insurance programs between for-profits and non-profits (Gray 1986; Hollingsworth and Hollingsworth 1987). Other studies indicate, however, that for-profits are less likely to provide services that are more frequently used by the medically indigent (Shortell et al. 1986).

Beginning in the 1970s, hospitals began to reorganize themselves to access different sources of capital as government funding for facilities and philanthropic sources of capital shrunk. Securing money from these alternative sources—equity, debt financing, and operating surplus—required different strategies than had been true previously. Hospitals that could develop and effectively employ new strategies would gain greater access to capital from these sources. Investor-owned hospital corporations, in part because of their ownership structure, gained comparative advantage in using these sources, which they then used to increase their share of the market. In fact, what emerged was an escalating, reinforcing system of capital acquisition and expansion. To expand, for-profits required more hospitals, which in turn required large amounts of capital. With expansion, capital became easier to acquire, which enabled firms to expand horizontally, vertically, or diagonally even further.

Spatially, the capital/acquisition/capital cycle did not proceed randomly. Care in the selection of hospitals to be acquired was necessary to ensure that a corporation's ability to access further capital was not jeopardized. Thus, location became an important element in capital access strategies used by hospital-management corporations. As a consequence, a definable geographic pattern of proprietary hospitals emerged in the postwar period as it had in the early 1900s.

Contemporary Spatial Distribution

The corporate structure in which contemporary proprietary hospitals exist has important consequences for their distribution. In a corporate organization, location decisions are highly structured and detailed analyses of market and management factors carefully assessed before acquisition decisions are confirmed. This contrasts with the local reactive decision-making that appeared to characterize the creation of proprietary hospitals in the early period. In the early period, many proprietary facilities were created in response to the absence of certain sources of investment capital, while in the contemporary era, location decisions are an integral part of the strategy for ensuring access to future capital. Contemporary location decisions for proprietary hospitals are national rather than local in scope. With a corporate structure, local capital is not required for acquisitions. Also, with a national focus, state regulatory policies (certification of need, rate setting, licensing, among others) and the business climate promoted by the state (tax policies and right-to-work laws, as examples) become important considerations.

Finally, with the current corporate structure, the collective good of the organization takes precedence over the viability of an individual hospital. As a consequence, corporations base some acquisition decisions on the absence rather than the presence of profitability. Alexander, Lewis, and Morrisey (1985), for example, identified four types of hospitals that fit the long-term acquisition strategies of for-profit firms. One type is the community hospital in a growing, middle-income area: the ideal acquisition. A second is the teaching and research hospital, which may not be profitable itself but which provides the entire system with a prestigious flagship facility that can be used for referrals and tertiary care. The remaining two—declining urban hospitals and competing unprofitable facilities—are useful because they can be closed or consolidated with existing hospitals owned by the firm in the area. Closings not only reduce competition, but they can be used to rationalize the need for expansion of hospital beds in more profitable locations in an area (McLafferty 1982). In states where certificate-of-need reviews pose a barrier to expansion, selectively reducing beds in one area to justify expansion in another is a useful corporate strategy.

National Scale. Despite the difference in the organizational structure of proprietary hospitals today and at the turn of the century, the distributions of proprietary hospitals in the two periods are similar. In fact, the national distribution of proprietary hospitals has remained remarkably consistent since 1900. Southern and western states have been the principal regions where proprietary hospitals are concentrated. After World War II, concentrations of proprietary hospitals were developing in Florida, California, and Texas (Hollingsworth and Hollingsworth 1987). By 1980, 60 percent of all proprietary hospitals were located in California, Florida, Texas, and Tennessee (Erman and Gabel 1984). Using a different measure, the percentage of all hospital beds in proprietary ownership, proprietary hospitals represented over 30 percent of the market share in ten states in 1985 (fig. 2.6). The only state outside the South or West of the ten was Minnesota.

The recent concentration of proprietary hospitals in southern and western states is a combination of a number of conditions that vari-

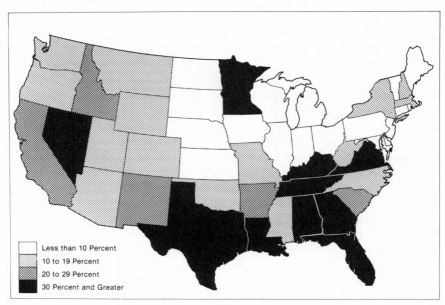

Fig. 2.6.   Percentage of Beds in Proprietary Ownership, 1985

ous studies indicate are important to investor-owned hospital companies wishing to expand their holdings (Alexander, Lewis, and Morrisey 1985); Cohodes and Kinkead 1984; Ermann and Gabel 1984; Haberlein 1988). These include communities with growing populations, low labor costs, high household incomes, low elderly proportions, a small percentage of population below the poverty level, a small Medicaid population, few restrictive regulations, and a lack of competing facilities. With the restructuring of the nation's economy and consequent redistribution of population, many rural and suburban communities in the South and West have the demographic and economic characteristics that are attractive to investor-owned hospital firms. In addition, the regulatory and business climates in these states are conducive to expanded activity by proprietary entreprises. Finally, as we have shown, these regions have a long history of involvement with proprietary hospitals, and, as a consequence, there is greater acceptance of the concept of profit making in medicine, which appears to be less acceptable in states where proprietary hospitals have not been a major part of the history and tradition of the medical care delivery system.

Intrametropolitan Scale: Richmond, Virginia. Like many southern SMSAs (Standard Metropolitan Statistical Areas), Richmond has experienced significant growth in the last twenty years. Between 1970 and 1980 the metropolitan population increased by 16 percent, and a similar growth rate has been forecast for the 1980–1990 period (VDPB 1986). As with most moderate-sized metropolitan areas in the South (1980 pop., 590,000), growth in Richmond has been clearly differentiated between central city and suburbs. The city of Richmond experienced a loss in population of 2.2 percent between 1970 and 1980, and a loss is expected in the 1980s. In contrast, the suburban counties (politically, Virginia is organized by counties and independent cities) adjacent to the city, Henrico and Chesterfield, increased their population by 40 percent over the last census period and are expected to do so again in the 1980s.

Contrasts between the city and the suburban counties extend beyond population growth rates. Flight from the city to suburbs and differential growth rates for whites and blacks have created a duality in the social structure of the metropolitan area. Blacks represent 51 percent of the population within the city, but only 13 percent in the adjacent suburbs. In part because of the racial composition of the two areas but also because of class differences, the income gap between the city and suburbs has widened. In 1986, for example, median household incomes in the city and suburbs differed by more than ten thousand dollars (TMI 1986).

Richmond is typical of many southern metropolitan areas. The metropolitan area's population grew at higher rates than the national average for metropolitan areas of similar size. Growth has increasingly become concentrated in the urban fringe. And, because of intrametropolitan mobility and the locational selectivity of recent immigrants, socioeconomic contrasts between city and suburbs have sharpened over the last twenty years. While such contrasts fostered economic and social problems between city and suburbs, they also created an excellent environment for investor-owned hospitals. With the appropriate locational strategy they could ensure a patient mix and financial balance sheet that would improve their ability to secure capital for long-term investments.

In Richmond, the central feature of the medical care and hospital system is the Medical College of Virginia (MCV) and its 1,058-bed teaching and research hospital. One of three publicly funded medical schools in the commonwealth, MCV receives the largest amount of funds from the state and serves the most patients of the three. As a teaching and research institution, the college and its hospital have a very large indigent-care patient population. Situated in the old central core of the city, the hospital provides charitable care to most of the metropolitan area's medically indigent. In 1986, for example, uncompensated care was in excess of 40 percent of total hospital revenues, and the college, physician, and hospital costs provided an estimated $63 million in health care to the medically indigent (GTIC 1987). The large uncompensated-care patient load carried by the college enables other hospitals in the area to provide less charitable care than would be the case without the teaching hospital.

Including the MCV hospital, there were eleven general hospitals in the study area (the city of Richmond and the adjacent counties of Henrico and Chesterfield constituted the study area) in 1985. Of the eleven, six were proprietary hospitals, which between them had 42 percent of all general hospital beds in the area. If beds from the teaching hospital are excluded, the percentage is 59. One hospital-management company, Hospital Corporation of America (HCA), owned the largest percentage of the proprietary beds, 68 percent. In addition to HCA, the other two largest hospital-management corporations, Humana and Charter Medical Corporation, also owned hospitals in the study area.

The distribution of the proprietary hospitals supports the premise that investor-owned hospital-management companies have used a locational strategy to enhance their investment potential (fig. 2.7). Eighty percent of the proprietary beds were located in middle- to upper-income suburban neighborhoods, and all beds owned by the two major companies, HCA and Humana, were there. The two proprietary hospitals located within the inner city were older than the for-profits situated in the suburbs. Both were located in the same

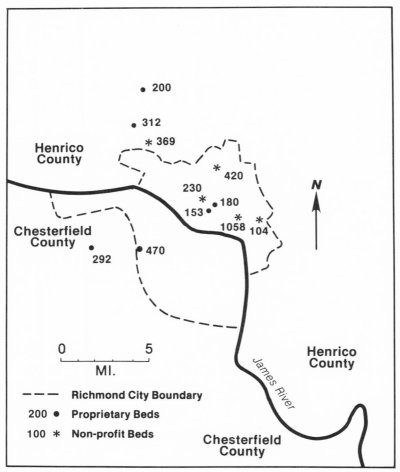

Fig. 2.7. Distribution of Hospital Beds, City of Richmond, 1985

neighborhood, an area known as the Fan. Located west of the central business district, the Fan was one of the most prestigious neighborhoods in old Richmond. With the postwar expansion of the city and the movement of the middle class and upper class to the suburbs, many of the old brownstone houses in the district deteriorated. Much of the old housing stock was converted to rental units for lower-income residents and students. The historic nature of the area and its proximity to the expanding Virginia Commonwealth University campus stimulated a revitalization of the district in the 1970s. Gentrification became so widespread that by 1985 the district had become one of the city's most popular neighborhoods for younger middle-class residents. Professionals such as physicians began to relocate in the district. With the influx of middle-class professionals, the Fan had become a risky but potentially advantageous location for proprietary hospitals. The risk stemmed from the sizable lower-income neighborhoods still numerous in the district. However, a large non-profit hospital in the Fan has been able to shoulder much of the charitable care for the residents of the surrounding lower-income neighborhoods, releasing the for-profits from a potential drain on their financial status.

The number and market share of proprietary hospitals in Richmond attest to the attractiveness of the metropolitan area for investor-owned hospitals. A spatially differentiated patient population and the presence of a large public teaching and research hospital that provided large volumes of charitable care enabled investor-owned hospital companies to successfully pursue a locational strategy that would ensure a desirable patient mix, thus making each hospital, and collectively each corporation, a more attractive investment risk.

Conclusions

Proprietary hospitals have long been a feature of the American health care system. Their numbers and market share have fluctuated in response to financial and professional factors that have either nurtured or retarded their growth. A significant factor in their growth historically has been their ability to secure financing for further capital investment, and sources of investment capital have changed both temporally and spatially. As sources of capital more easily accessed by proprietary medical enterprises became more important, for-profits hospitals increased in number.

The principal sources of capital used by proprietary hospitals varied in the two periods. In the late nineteenth and early twentieth centuries, transformations in society and the medical profession increased the use of patient fees by hospitals. Unable to access capital from either public or philanthropic sources, proprietary hospitals were able to use patient fees as a source of capital, and their numbers grew significantly. As the competition for patient fees increased among proprietary, non-profit and public hospitals, the numbers of for-profits began to decline by the 1920s. The recent increase in proprietary hospitals was facilitated by the increased availability of debt financing for investment capital. Investor-owned hospital companies had a comparative advantage not only because of their ability to sell stocks for capital, but also because investors were more willing to loan money at lower interest rates to the large investor-owned companies than to either non-profits or independent for-profits. The need to secure capital as inexpensively as possible has been a powerful force in influencing the distribution as well as the growth of proprietary hospitals. In both periods analyzed in this study, distinctive spatial patterns of proprietary hospitals were evident at both the national and intrametropolitan scales. In fact, the distributions for the two periods shared similar characteristics. Nationally, western and southern states had the preponderance of for-profits in both periods. Within metropolitan areas, proprietaries have historically shown the same locational tendencies: a preference for middle-class residential areas.

The similarities in the national distribution of proprietary hospitals, while the result of the distributional aspects of investment capital, differed in the degree to which national locational strategies were formulated and implemented. In the period from 1890 to 1920, proprietary hospitals were local in organization and scope. Investor-owned, multifacility companies were a feature only of the contemporary period. In the early period, the distribution of for-profits was a consequence of a large number of uncoordinated, individual community responses to the need to secure capital for hospitals. In many communities the absence of public or philanthropic funds forced hospitals to rely on the only other source available, patient fees, for capital. In such communities, proprietary hospitals were an alternative that came to be widely accepted. Thus, in the early period the national distribution of for-profits reflected the mirror image of the national distribution of accumulated capital. Where the accumulation was greatest, and thus where public and charitable funds were greater, non-profits and public hospitals prevailed. Where accumulations were limited, in large measure because the area had not been fully integrated into the industrial economy, proprietary hospitals were common if not predominant.

The contemporary national distribution, in contrast, reflects a coordinated, strategic implementation of policies used by investor-owned management corporations. Again, a key factor in explaining the spatial pattern is capital financing. The importance of location to management corporations is well documented. To ensure that debt capital is available at suitable costs, for-profit systems must demonstrate efficiency and profitability. Careful selection of hospital locations can help ensure the patient and service mix, the level of uncompensated care, the market competition, and the labor costs necessary for efficient management and profitability. In the contemporary period, those locational conditions most suitable to for-profits again have been in western and southern states.

At the metropolitan scale, there appear to be greater similarities in the two periods in both geographic outcome and the process underlying the distribution. In both periods, the locational objective appeared to be maximization of patient fees. Whether it was associated with the corporate decision making of the modern for-profits or that of the independent hospital at the turn of the century, proprietary hospitals clearly showed a preference for middle-class residential areas in the two cities examined in this study. In both periods, access to paying patients and avoidance of neighborhoods with large charitable-care responsibilities were locational imperatives.

Our analysis of proprietary hospitals and their growth has stressed the role of capital and its availability. While other factors have been important, we believe that changes in the availability of capital from different sources has been the principal reason for historical trends in the growth and distribution of proprietary hospitals. It follows that the future of investor-owned hospitals in the United States will continue to be a function of their ability to obtain financing of new capital investments at lower costs than non-profits or public facilities, and that this will be reflected in the changing geography of medical care.

Chapter 3

Privatizing the Health and Welfare State

The Western European Experience

JOHN EYLES

Marmor (1986, 617) begins his discussion of American medical policy and the crisis of the welfare state by saying that "most policy debates in most countries are parochial affairs," addressing national issues, citing historical and contemporary national developments, and assessing the different policy forms and visions that a particular country should adopt. This parochialism seems as much a potential issue in the debate on privatization as it does in pensions, inner-city problems, and health policy in general. It is, therefore, an initial contention of this chapter that we, especially in the Anglo-American world, which suffers particularly from empirical (if not theoretical) myopia, should look at privatization and its context, namely, the nature of social expenditures and the delivery of health and welfare services, comparatively. Indeed, the case for comparative research has been well made in social science and social policy. In the context of sociology, Durkheim (1938, 139) argued that "comparative sociology is not a particular branch of sociology; it is sociology itself, insofar as it ceases to be purely descriptive and aspires to account for facts." In other words, it is the approach that enables generalizations to be made. These generalizations result when the approach entails the study, side by side, of different groups, collectivities, institutions, communities, and environments (see Eyles and Woods, 1983). In the field of social policy, Heclo (1972, 95) comments: "To speak of comparative analysis suggests not only that one will be looking at variables which actually vary, but also that one will be doing so in contexts which themselves vary. . . . It is only through such comparative analysis that one can appreciate what are truly unique and what are the more generic phenomena." In health policy, this allows for a recognition of alternative courses of action and an identification of fashions in social policy. As we shall see, privatization is but one option in the near universal concern for cost containment. Thus, is privatization as a response culturally or systemically conditioned? What are the different economic and political conditions that shape policy responses to perceived expenditure problems? Comparative analysis may help provide an answer to such questions.

As Klein (1983) has commented, we may obtain policy learning and policy understanding for comparing social policies across nations. By policy learning we mean that social policies of other countries are examined so as to derive lessons or models for application. We should add that the lesson may be to not apply a particular policy. Policy understanding emphasizes explanation. To understand a contemporary state of affairs, it is unlikely that the key factors in one society will tell all the story. For example, the case for the importance of New Right ideology in privatization can be made for England, but the presence of that ideology in France and West Germany had led to somewhat different outcomes. As Klein (1983, 13) comments, "Comparative studies may be essential if misleading conclusions are not to be drawn from what are single case studies in the making, or evolution, of social policy." It is with this in mind that we turn to an examination of the nature and evolution of welfare states in Western Europe to discover why they are as they are so that we may further understand the policy options realistically available to them and the significance of privatization among those options.

The Evaluation of Welfare States

In their discussion of the development of welfare, Carrier and Kendall (1977) point to four potential problems: the "fetish of the single cause"; seeing history as a combination of hagiography and biography, of institutions and individuals; a search for "turning points" or key dates; and a tendency to "grand" or "a priori" theorizing on the basis of limited evidence. It may be possible to avoid these dangers by examining broad processes in specific historical contexts. Thus, for example, Flora and Alber (1982) use the ideas of Rokkan (1974) on political development as a starting point, particularly his views on the restructuring of the state through the extension and redefinition of citizenship. Political rights become equalized through participation, and this forms the basis of redistribution or the development of welfare states and the establishment of social rights through the redistribution of resources, goods, and benefits. But Flora and Alber (1982) suggest that there are institutional variations —namely, the level of enfranchisement, the significance of monarchical as opposed to democratic government, and the relative importance of liberal and mass democratic systems—that can affect the nature of welfare state development. Thus, they suggest that liberal democracies tend to restrict government intervention and public assistance, while mass democracies are more likely to develop extended and centralized welfare systems based on social rights and compulsory contributions.

Similar welfare systems are likely to develop in constitutional monarchies with extended suffrage. While it is not our intention to rehearse the actual historical development of welfare states, the importance of political, institutional, and constitutional features can be laid down. Variations in these features (for example, between contribution and entitlement, localization and centralization of provision) will result in variations in the contemporary configuration of welfare states, and hence in their propensity to be amenable to privatization.

Other dimensions must, however, be highlighted. We should not take as a given that the welfare state is a product of a particular level of economic development and primarily of industrial capitalism. Although good arguments for the relationship between capitalism and the welfare state have been made (Habermas 1976; Gough 1979; Offe 1984), it is important to recall tensions in this relationship. First, there is tension between security and equality (Flora and Heidenheimer 1982). The relative importance of these two objectives, pursued through regulation and minimum standards and redistribution and equality of opportunity, respectively, has varied over time and between nations. In some instances, the objectives may supplement each other; in others they contradict one another. In fact, the relationship between the objectives may depend in part on the other: tension between legitimacy (a basis of political authority) and efficiency (a basis for judging economic performance). In pursuing mass legitimacy, the state may employ measures to enhance both security and equality; but if greater efficiency is a primary goal, then the development of measures to improve opportunity may militate against security. In general terms it is possible to conclude that privatization is more likely to occur in states that pursue equality of opportunity to enhance efficiency. As Offe (1984, 137–138) comments: "The capitalist state is efficient . . . to the extent that it succeeds in the universalization of the commodity form. The ideal state of affairs is a situation in which every citizen can take care of all of his or her needs through participation in market processes, and the inherent test of rationality of policy-making in the capitalist state is the extent to which it approximates this situation." To this must be added, all things being equal. But are all things equal? As an examination of the evolution of welfare states reveals, they most certainly are not.

We have already noted variations in political, institutional, constitutional, and economic criteria that affect welfare state development and policy possibilities. Along with these we must consider the nature of professional and bureaucratic organizations (how, for example, does the evolution of medical practice and employer organizations affect the shape and delivery of health policy?) and the political mobilization of the working class (particularly vis-à-vis other classes and significant social groupings such as those based on religion). For Esping-Anderson (1985, 223) the degree of power mobilization is in fact the key variable shaping distributional outcomes, although she correctly notes that "similar levels of power mobilization may yield widely different outcomes given the structure of power." In fact, the welfare state is itself central in the structure of power. Not only do welfare states grant entitlement outside market regulations, institutionalize collective political responsibilities for individuals' living standards, redistribute income and resources, and provide goods and services outside the cash nexus, but they also can alter the balance of class power in favor of the disadvantaged. This is their strength and weakness. This ability to alter the power balance means that their development will be resisted and, if possible, retarded and retrenched by privileged groups. But it also means that, once established, welfare states become very hard to shift as long as political and ideological support remains, whatever the temporary economic circumstances.

In a persuasive analysis, Esping-Anderson (1985) argues that this establishment depends on a high and durable level of power mobilization and on the formation of cross-class alliances, the latter capacity varying greatly from nation to nation. From this perspective too, "social and health policies emerge as important ways of raising working-class power resources" (Esping-Anderson 1985, 228). This "social democratization" of capitalism involves the decommodification of wage earners and consumption, a restratification of society along solidaristic principles, redistributive corrections of market-induced inequalities, and institutionalizing sustained full employment. Particularly important for our discussion of privatization of health care delivery are decommodification and redistributive corrections.

Decommodification means extending citizen rights so that medical care and the social wage become independent of the market. It means that these services are received as of right and are not dependent on poor relief (welfare or means-tested benefits). There has been convergence on the social wage for most of the postwar period in Europe among conservative Catholic societies and social democratic societies. Anglo-Saxon nations have been the laggards, and it is with the laggards that means testing and the removal of services from the public domain first started and have been most intensely applied. As we shall see, the welfare state has been least challenged and weakened in those nations (Norway, Sweden, and Finland) where its accomplishments have gone furthest.

With redistributive corrections, great reliance is placed on progressive and heavy taxation to provide the state with resources to transfer from one group, program, or region to another. The greatest commitment to transfers and universal services, and hence to fiscal redistribution, may be found in the Scandinavian nations, and the lowest in France, the United Kingdom, and Austria. There are, however, other ways of paying for universal, if unequal, benefits and services, mainly through occupational programs. Such schemes were promoted by conservative forces to preserve established status privileges and differences and to direct working-class loyalties away from socialism, as evidenced by Austria, West Germany, and Italy. These programs themselves then help to generate vested interests in a particular mode of provision and policy, such that Esping-Andersen (1985) found a negative correlation between levels of corporativism and levels of privatization. In other words, corporatist interests—employers, providers, and financiers as well as consumers—have resisted moves towards privatization, which suggests that privatization may be easier to achieve in some types of welfare states than in others.

This finding calls attention to the diversity among welfare states. It is important to avoid the notion that welfare states are convergent or that one has more welfare services or more working-class power mobilization than others. Much depends, as we have seen, on the nature of the economic, ideological, and political context (Rimlinger 1971). It should be noted that other authorities have also identified different types of welfare and welfare states (e.g., Wilensky and Lebeaux 1965; Titmuss 1976), but we require a scheme that emphasizes modes of distribution and delivery so as to see better where privatization fits in. Esping-Andersen (1985) has suggested three distributional regimes: the social democratic, which is integrative, comprehensive, and societal in scope and universal and public in provision; the conservative, which is based on statist, paternalistic reform, promoting individual subordination and loyalty to state and employer with most welfare being occupation based; and the liberal, which stresses private market provision, voluntary membership in insurance, individualistic actuarialism, and means-tested, targeted social policy.

These regimes are ideal types, although in general terms the conservative model is preeminent in nations where the church was important in welfare and where bourgeois developments were weak or absent (Austria, France, West Germany, Belgium, and Italy). Conservative regimes are similar to social democratic ones in their willingness to grant benefits and care, but these attach to occupation and status rather than to citizenship. The liberal model most closely approximates the situation in societies that underwent a bourgeois revolution: the United Kingdom, the United States, and the remaining Anglo-Saxon New World. The boundaries have shifted for all distributional regimes, as have decisions on what should or should not be in the public domain. The types of boundary shifts possible are dependent upon the existing nature of welfare states and the state of tension between security and equality and legitimacy and efficiency. These dimensions and the relative status of power blocs will shape the effects of boundary pressures. Thus, for example, the neoliberal Right's thrust for privatization and financial self-reliance will have a different impact on societies dominated by conservative church institutions (e.g., West Germany) than on those with strong bourgeois and co-opted labor-based organizations (e.g., the United Kingdom and Denmark). But all of the West European welfare states have had to confront the boundary question, the impetus for which has been increasing health and welfare expenditures.

Cost Containment, Policy Options, and Health Services Privatization

The growth in the proportion of national incomes in industrialized countries given over to health and welfare is now well documented (OECD 1977; Maxwell 1981), although the relative positions of different nations can only be roughly assessed because of the lack of standardized data. To be sure, there is variation in health spending and the public proportion. In 1983, nearly 11 percent of GDP (gross domestic product) in the United States was expended on health care (OECD 1985a), of which some 40 percent was in the form of public expenditures. Health expenditure in France was 9.3 percent of GDP, of which 71 percent was public spending. The respective figures for Sweden were 9.6 percent and 90 percent, for Belgium 6.5 and 91, for Italy 7.4 and 85, and for the United Kingdom 6.2 and 88. Thus, despite the roughly doubling of health expenditures since the early 1960s and the view that emphasis be placed not on the cause of rising costs but on the development of cost-containment policies, we are able to ask several questions. First, in what sense is increased expenditure on health care a problem? Are we consuming more health care than we need? Is health care provision ineffective? Is the health care sector inefficient? Or is it a problem because governments find it difficult to control overall budget deficits and are primarily concerned with the cost of public health care? In the main, it has been the last two questions that have been central and have inspired the notion that the state must be rolled back. This option makes sense in a society like England in which the rhetoric has addressed reducing the size of the public sector, increasing incentives to work by increasing the gap between market-derived and social wages; reducing consumption expenditure; and increasing individual freedom and choice by providing more scope for nonstate provision of services (O'Higgins, 1983). This rhetoric is particularly powerful in a liberal as opposed to conservative or social democratic climate. Second, with Gray (1984) we may ask at what point does increasing health care expenditure become and then cease to be a problem? The United Kingdom feels it has a problem with health expenditure of 6.2 percent of GDP. If that is the case, how much must France or Sweden reduce their health expenditures to cease to have problems? The question seems fatuous, but it points up the need for comparative analysis, the problems of evaluating cost-containment strategies, and the specificity of national contexts and therefore of policy options and practices.

But a problem was perceived to exist. Bearing in mind the arguments about the welfare state in crisis in chapter 1 and elsewhere (Mishra 1984; OECD 1985b), we note that slower economic growth and the fact that mature welfare programs cannot continue to grow as rapidly as developing ones without imposing significant costs mean that all OECD (Organization for Economic Cooperation and Development) countries have reduced their rates of increase in social spending (Marmor 1986). None, however, have actually reduced real total social expenditures, although reductions in the rate of increase were higher in some countries than in others. For example, the Netherlands decreased the rate of expansion far more than did France, reflecting both the relative maturity of the welfare system and the relative intensity of economic problems in the late 1970s and early 1980s. As should perhaps be expected, different political systems responded differently in social expenditure terms to the need for cost containment, although in general terms most restrained expenditure growth in health and education rather than on pensions. And if we turn to the health sector specifically, we can outline the various options that were available. In this examination, it must be noted that American (and British) political discourse sets itself apart from the rest of the OECD world (Marmor 1986). It is in these societies that the liberal rhetoric of increasing competition and reestablishing the private sector to help roll back the state was first heard and has been most felt. However, even then privatization is but one market option; Abel-Smith (1985) suggests that there are three ways in which the market can be introduced into the health care industry: deinsurance, mainly through copayments and cost sharing; the removal of insurance concessions from beneficiaries so that they pay the market cost; and privatization, putting services out to contract or removing public provision.

The first two of these market strategies affect the demand for health care services. The evidence on the effects of increased charges is variable; they appear to have acted as disincentives in ophthalmic services in Denmark, dental care in England, and hospital services in Belgium, but have not reduced demand in France or the United States (Gray 1984). Most countries have increased user fees for pharmaceuticals. With respect to supply, privatization has the effect of altering the point of delivery, removing it from the public sector and placing it in the private sector. But there are more commonly used and more direct ways of affecting the supply of health care other than through the introduction of the market. For example, hospitals may be closed (e.g., in the United Kingdom and Italy) and other services rationalized. More common still are limits placed on current and capital expenditures. Global spending controls are in place in, for example, England, Ireland, and Italy. In Denmark, central government grants to local authority–run hospitals have been reduced, as has expenditure on primary health care (Abel-Smith 1985). West Germany, France, and the Netherlands have imposed strict financial limits on capital spending: Germany and the Netherlands with respect to government grant-aided capital schemes, and France on the introduction of new technology (Gray 1984). More long-term, many countries have begun to affect the supply and remuneration of physicians. For example, of the twelve EC (European Common Market) countries, only Belgium and Italy do not have quotas operating in medical schools, and income ceilings have been put into place in the fee-for-service systems of the Netherlands, Belgium, and West Germany. These strategies are aimed at reducing the rate of increase in the supply of medical care; other planning strategies include examining the effectiveness of existing supply through programs that may lead to the redistribution of resources among regions, among health programs, and between health policy and other sectors of the economy. Italy and the United Kingdom have developed regional resource-allocation techniques; while, among others, the Netherlands and Luxembourg have searched for alternatives to hospital care for a variety of illnesses and disabilities. Regional and program redistributions can be and have been used to contain costs, but sectoral shifts perhaps require a degree of ideological commitment to publicly funded health and welfare services found primarily in Scandinavia.

From this overview of cost-containment and policy options we can see that privatization in the form of the direct sale of a public agency to a private firm is only one possible strategy. Far more important is budget planning and regulating demand, supply, fees, and remuneration. As Abel-Smith (1985) comments, West European states have used regulation (budgetary and other) very innovatively to contain costs. To be sure, those innovative actions have been at the expense of consumer provision and expectations. We can see this clearly if we adopt Therborn and Roebroek's (1986) list of measures to ensure redistribution from labor to capital and from the poor to the affluent; namely, changes in the indexing of benefits; stricter entitlement to benefits; certain tendencies toward privatization; a tendency toward deindividualization of rights on social insurance through family principles and means testing; rationalization and closure of services and facilities; and shifting costs to fees and direct payments. But there has only been, they suggest, a fundamental reappraisal of the nature of the welfare state in three countries: Belgium, the Netherlands, and the United Kingdom. The welfare state remains fully entrenched in Sweden and Austria. Reappraisal of the nature of welfare policy need not lead to privatization of provision. The results of any reappraisal (or attempt to contain costs) will depend upon the configuration of political, economic, constitutional, ideological, and social forces. Our discussion will be better advanced by examining some examples of policy practice from Western Europe from the age of cost containment.

Selected Examples of Policy Practice

We have seen that all Western European nations have been concerned with health costs and have adopted a range of strategies to combat this perceived evil. We have, however, been loathe to see much of this state endeavor as changes in provision, subsidy, and regulation. Le Grand and Robinson (1984) have noted that private provision and contracting-out are somewhat limited in extent. There has certainly been a reduction in subsidies through increased fees and cost sharing. Whether subsidy reduction or removal is privatization is a moot point necessitating an extension of *privatization* to include family, community, and voluntary care in which the state may or may not have been involved in the past. Further, there has been an extension of state activity in regulation, especially over the establishment of budgets, fees, and, increasingly, the supply of medical personnel and infrastructure. In perhaps where it matters, in personnel and finance, the state appears to have extended its hegemony. In doing so, it may use the private sector as a partner, as with joint-care ventures in England or the increased use of private insurance in the Netherlands, but through regulation it maintains control. This is not, however, to say that the state acts universally in every Western European society in this way or that it is an independent actor. The coalescence of forces around the state apparatus will in large measure shape the nature of the state and its policy practice. With respect to health policy, this practice is further constrained by the established methods of organizing and financing health care.

Health care in Western Europe is funded either through central or local taxation or through some form of compulsory insurance (Maxwell 1981; Gray 1984). This distinction appears to be increasingly unimportant, largely because of increased state intervention and regulation. An important difference, however, is the method of hospital financing and physician remuneration. Where the former is budget limited and the latter on a salaried or per capita basis, it seems easier to contain costs; but where hospitals are recompensed by per diem financing and doctors by fee per item, then cost containment becomes more difficult. This is especially the case when the physicians are private practitioners. Then, the fee per item of service is a power-ful incentive to maximize work volumes (Pauly 1970; Rodwin 1981). If many of the providers of care are already in private practice, there is little point in suggesting that services might be privatized. Where there are strong private and local interests in the funding of health care, the extension of private-sector involvement is likely to be un-welcome. To illustrate these cases, West Germany and France will be used as examples.

West Germany

In West Germany, a national consensus has developed over statu-tory health insurance (National Health Insurance, or NHI), which over the last one-hundred years has been changed into an all-inclusive health insurance and income-maintenance program (Alten-stetter 1987). In fact, NHI insures over 90 percent of the population and provides a range of benefits, including comprehensive coverage for chronic or temporary illness and for physical, mental, or emo-tional instability. Patients may choose their primary-care doctor and also their hospital, although much depends on their physician's referral practice. While NHI is subject to state supervision and regula-tion, it is self-administrated. Insurance funds are organized by local-ity, occupation, or enterprise, and NHI obtains its monies through payroll taxes levied equally on employers and workers. But despite its pluralism, comprehensive coverage, and almost universal enti-tlement, costs in terms of percentage of GNP spent on health insur-ance have remained fairly stable since the mid-1970s (OECD 1985b, 1986).

Cost stability was in part achieved through cost-containment legis-lation passed in 1977, demonstrating that it was possible for a federal government to legislate against providers and the pharmaceutical in-dustry. The legislation was itself helped by the national consensus on health care, which further led to the establishment of a national coun-cil to advise on cost containment. This does not mean that the West German government has not reduced and withdrawn health subsi-dies nor that cost sharing has been introduced for hospitalization ex-penses. Worst affected, however, have been the elderly (Altenstetter 1987). The federal government has also tried to limit hospital costs and investments (Vollmer and Hoffman 1985, 1986); but, while it can lay down legislative and regulatory details, the decentralized admin-istration of the hospital system means that the German provinces can assert their own interests. The spirit of compromise lurks beneath these assertions. Although conflicts exist, virtually all interests are vested in that compromise; as Abel-Smith (1985, 8) comments, "The system works as well as it does because the key provider groups are well aware that if the system does not work reasonably well over the years, more drastic compulsory action would be likely to follow." This leads Altenstetter (1987) to conclude that political rather than economic judgments have determined important features of NHI and that political constraints leave little leeway to depart substantially from past patterns.

Altenstetter's conclusions apply to suggestions made in the mid-1980s to privatize elements of the financing, organization, and production of health services and to strengthen competitive forces. While health economists (Pfaff 1986; Thiemeyer 1986) suggest that the removal of professional and financial monopolies and additional cost sharing and competition would reduce cost increases (at the expense of abolishing insurance coverage for children and nonworking spouses); political structures (especially the provinces), sickness funds, and doctors are against change. Disagreements among them must hide the continued existence of a national consensus, which makes privatization an unlikely broad-based project. As Altenstetter (1987, 527) perceptively notes, "For the present coalition to endorse and applaud competition and incentive on principle is one thing, but to undermine the economic interests of their own political supporters by acting according to the ideological script is something else."

France

France presents a different story, one in which privatization is almost meaningless (Baker 1986). In France, though the state regulates and has in recent years reduced the burden on other agencies by helping patients with costs incurred with independent doctors and hospitals, little tax revenue goes into health. In fact, universal health provision is a post-1945 phenomenon. Despite attempts to harmonize services and unify funds, there still exists a mosaic of insurance funds (Dumont 1982), although over three-quarters of the population is covered by the General Fund. This fund is financed by compulsory employer and worker contributions and is administered by 129 autonomous local boards (De Pouvoirville and Renaud 1985). There is no clear chain of command between the national government and the local boards or between the government and the hospitals, which greatly increased in number during the 1960s and 1970s. The picture is further complicated by a mix of salaried and private practitioners. Seventy-one percent of doctors are in private practice (Baker 1986). Such a complicated and pluralistic system has meant that health expenditures in France have risen at one of the fastest rates in Europe (Levy et al. 1983), while planning has been greatly hindered.

Health expenditures rise despite cost sharing at all levels of the health system. In other words, consumers obtain only a partial subsidy or refund. As in most Western European societies, pressures for cost containment began in the 1970s, which saw a weakened economic base and therefore a weakened financial basis for health insurance. This structural change was associated with other problems; namely, the tendency of the funds to go into deficit, the alarm at the effects of growing insurance contributions, no apparent mechanism for self-regulation in health care costs, and doubts about the effectiveness of increased expenditure (Baker 1986). But the nature of the system (and its containing society) make cost-containment strategies difficult to implement. There has been a small, reluctant movement to use taxation contributions (Abel-Smith 1984); but there has been fierce opposition to and political defeat for those trying to raise insurance contributions and increase cost sharing. The private, liberal-based physician system means that passing on costs to the patient is the only way to control consumption because all practitioners have a vested interest in maximizing consumption of care up to the permitted ceilings.

But as with the West Germans so with the French: they seem to be too strongly attached to the existing system for revolutionary change. Reluctance to restructure the system has meant that the search for economy has been wide-ranging, including "increasing charges, reducing refunds on drugs, reducing the income of practitioners, introducing tighter controls in hospitals and limiting increases to their staff, trimming profit margins on drugs, compelling chemists to hand over a part of their turnover, restricting medical training and limiting career opportunities of doctors, increasing competition between sectors and promoting prevention" (Baker 1986, 229). Block budgets have been introduced for hospitals, and some hospitals have been closed (De Pouvoirville and Renaud 1985). The government's attempts to modernize hospital management are also meant to rationalize the use of resources (De Pouvoirville 1986). While some of these measures appear to increase broadly defined privatization through reducing subsidies, increasing community care, and raising

charges, the most significant change has been increased state intervention through the regulation of finance and personnel. Indeed,
much of the cost inflation of the French system appears to have been
caused by its liberal and private nature. Charging consumers has not
limited cost or improved the efficiency of health care delivery. The interest of providers in increased use has overpowered the resistance of
patients to pay. While the French system certainly gives consumers
more power and choice, that choice has not been extended beyond
the affluent (see Morel et al. 1985). For the proponents of privatization, therefore, France provides a cautionary tale: private care has developed inflationary mechanisms, and it is state control that has been
used to limit rising health care expenditures.

The Netherlands

To continue the cautionary tale that context is all, we may turn
briefly to the Dutch system. In the Netherlands, a generous if diffuse
health and welfare system (Brenton 1982; Idenburg 1985) has been
run with minimal state involvement, financed by health insurance,
and run by private organizations. But throughout the late 1970s and
early 1980s, it was increasingly recognized that the Dutch economy
could no longer support such a system. The election of a neoliberal
government has led not to direct controls but to a questioning of the
efficacy of welfare itself and to suggestions of deregulation, decentralization, and privatization. The ideological commitment to welfare, perhaps not assisted by the reluctance of earlier governments to
support health and welfare services, has been weakened, and retrenchment is now the key economic and social policy initiative in the
Netherlands.

Sweden

As a final example, we will briefly examine a society in which ideological commitment seems ever present: Sweden. From the 1930s,
Sweden has aimed at achieving egalitarian social and economic security within a framework of solidarity among the different social
classes and financed through progressive taxation (Nasenius and
Veit-Wilson 1985). The view that social welfare expenditure is not a
burden has not been seriously challenged in Sweden. The bourgeois
parties that held power from 1976 to 1982 criticized the health care
system for its heavy bureaucratization and its removal of the price

mechanism (Diderichsen 1982). They suggested competition and privatization as ways of improving the service, but they did not receive wide public support. Indeed, the main attempts to limit the rise in health and welfare expenditures have been in trying to fit resources more closely to need through better planning, meaning a greater emphasis on prevention, community care, and primary care. Such a strategy is necessary given the expensive nature of the Swedish health system, the costs of which are financed mainly through local and national taxes on income and consumption and on employer contributions. Employee contributions were in fact abolished in the 1970s, and the nature of financing in general is intended to make services free or low-cost at the point of delivery. In fact, the real level of most benefits and services was maintained during the recession of the early 1980s, meaning that people have a very positive perception of public welfare. Wealthier Swedes support, use, and value the comprehensive, universal services; and Sweden has not experienced a taxpayer's revolt that would be resonant with neoliberal ideology. But while the planning strategy has been successful, reducing health's share of GNP to 9.5 percent in 1987, there has been some discontent with the system (Rosenthal 1986).

Rosenthal (1986) notes four elements of disquiet in the Swedish health care system: increasing economic constraints on the public sector, a growing pool of physicians, a new emphasis on individual freedom and choice, and some criticisms of public-sector health care. These concerns are in part responsible for the emergence of a small private sector in the Swedish health system. There exist two private clinics and hospitals in Stockholm and Göteborg, and Rosenthal estimates that about a quarter of Swedish doctors offer private medical care through insurance plans. She also estimates that about 6 percent may offer care strictly in the private market. These figures seem high compared with Swedish government estimates, which suggest that about 10 percent offer private care on the side and about one-half of one percent are exclusively in private practice. In fact, the Swedish government controls the numbers of doctors who can practice privately and is sensitive to charges of profit making from illness. It is also not likely to allow private, foreign, for-profit hospital chains into Sweden or to grant tax breaks for subscribers to private insurance. While there is increased freedom for the individual within the public system, the public commitment to the existing health system and the ideological commitment of the state to control and regulate delivery (forged by Left power and aided by a fragmented Right) mean that adaptation will occur, but with private care a minor option for wealthy Swedes.

Indeed, privatization is unlikely to be an important policy alternative in states with strong welfare and employment commitments (e.g., Norway and Austria). In Finland, for example, the nationally planned and subsidized but municipally funded and run health system is concerned with the efficient use of its limited resources, but its strategy is to reward those areas and functions that act efficiently with some of the scarce new posts (Saltman 1988). Privatization is not considered in a system that is based on municipal socialism; that is, the concentration of Left power at the local level. As Therborn and Roebroek (1986, 334) argue, the rollback of the welfare state (and the increased likelihood of privatization measures) is more likely where there is "a division, demoralization, decomposition, and an at least partial political marginalization of the broad coalition of socio-political forces that supported and sustained the welfare state expansion in the 1960s and 1970s." Political marginalization is assisted by high unemployment, a dualistic economy and society, and an elitist political system. Such conditions are found in England and the United States in particular, although we must be wary of such apparent convergence and of underplaying specific historical and societal circumstances.

Conclusions

This chapter began with the suggestion that comparative analysis could help to illuminate the possibilities and limitations of privatization in industrialized societies. While it is important to note that privatization is not new and that its scale of operation depends in part on definition, evidence reveals that the historical, political, and societal parameters of Western European states strongly influence those possibilities and limitations. It is beyond the main brief of this chapter to comment on the desirability or inevitability of private-sector involvement in health care provision. It does seem unrealistic, however, not to see a role (indeed, a continuing role) for the private sector. In the context of the United Kingdom, Maxwell (1987) argues that the private sector is indispensable in some areas of care and surgery. Further, just as Hindess (1987, 153) is surely correct when he contends that there can be no argument in favor of the market in all cases, "likewise, there are certainly cases where state services are costly, inefficient, and unresponsive to the needs of their clients." These are not inescapable effects of public provision; but just as there should be no idealization of the market, nor should there be one of state provision. State provision seems to work best where there is an ideological commitment to the welfare state. That in itself has required particular developmental conditions, particularly the power mobilization of the working class, which was (and is) itself aided by a divided Right.

Privatization is adopted as a solution to perceived cost-containment problems in societies that possess liberal distributional regimes. Health and welfare rights are more deeply entrenched, albeit for different reasons, in social democratic and conservative regimes. But all distributional systems have boundary problems in the sense that with slow economic growth and mature welfare states to finance, attempts are likely to be made to draw back from certain commitments. Withdrawal usually takes the form of reduced subsidization and increased cost sharing. But all cost-containment actions must be resonant with existing societal structures. As Mishra (1984) suggests, reform, however radical in rhetoric, must be incremental because it can proceed no faster than customary practice and statutory and constitutional responsibilities allow. Of course, statutes, constitutions, and minds can be changed, but such changes may be easier to accomplish in societies where there is weak loyalty to the state through citizenship or to the enterprise through occupation and status.

Variable loyalty (and therefore variable basis for legitimacy) means that what is contestable, what is considered the boundary, will vary from state to state. We saw further how committed most societies were to established practices, partly through inertia and custom, partly through vested interest. This means that the range of policy options applicable to any one society might be limited. Most Western European states have responded to cost containment by increasing state intervention through budgetary and personnel regulation. Further, this regulation, particularly of budgeting, is leading to the national health service model for health care delivery, allowing for national targeting, planning, and evolution (Abel-Smith 1985). Such models rely less on cost sharing to contain expenditures and, encouragingly, they also have at their base the provision of universal entitlement to all citizens—an equity consideration. Of course, the national health model does not preclude private provision or a very low level of entitlement (as in Greece), but it does allow for national control and regulation. And that is important because it should never be forgotten that health care delivery has to be paid for from finite resources. Shifting costs does not remove the need to pay. As Baker (1986, 235) says, "The burden—if that is what is—may depend more on the amount to be paid than on the way it is paid." That amount will itself depend on the commitment to welfare, which is in turn shaped by the nature and history of a welfare state.

Chapter 4

Restructuring the Welfare State

The Growth and Impact of Private Hospitals in New Zealand

J. ROSS BARNETT AND PAULINE BARNETT

Since the 1970s there have been many attempts to restructure the welfare state in capitalist industrial societies, especially those characterized by high rates of public expenditure, large budget deficits, and low rates of economic growth. Recession economies have forced governments to cut back social expenditure and to search for alternative means of funding the provision of essential social services (Gough and Steinberg 1981; Gough 1983; Navarro 1984; Therborn and Roebroek 1986). Attacks on, and attempts to restructure, the welfare state have, for the most part, been the preserve of the political Right, which has usually defended its actions on the grounds of questioning both the efficiency and the effectiveness of public expenditure. High rates of social expenditure are seen as having a negative impact upon rates of economic growth (Cameron 1982; Saunders 1985) and are also said to create social dependence and high levels of taxation, which act as disincentives to work and save. It is also argued that many public services are characterized by inefficiency and ineffectiveness (New Zealand Department of Health 1988). Perhaps nowhere is this more evident than in the health sector, where there has been a growing scepticism over the rising cost of medicine, especially in view of its relatively minor impact upon health outcomes in industrial societies (McKeown 1976; McKinlay and McKinlay 1977). Other criticisms of welfare spending frequently focus on its failure to achieve certain distributional objectives (Le Grand and Robinson 1984). Although equity has been an important goal of the postwar welfare state, it is clear that resources have frequently not been allocated on the basis of need and that, in some cases, allocation has intensified, rather than reduced, inequalities in access to social services (Friedman 1973; Barnett, Ward, and Tatchell 1980).

Whatever the validity of the above concerns we are nevertheless witnessing increasing attempts to roll back the welfare state and to reduce the level of public spending via a strategy that seeks to privatize the public sector. This is usually seen as a basic restructuring of social services away from collectivism and public funding and toward an increased reliance on the market and an emphasis on self-help. In this strategy, individuals and families, and not the state, are increasingly responsible for welfare (Klein 1984). Whatever the merits of this process, it has nevertheless resulted in healthy and vigorous policy debates over the future of the welfare state and about the appropriate public-private mix of social services (McLachlan and Maynard 1982; Weller and Manga 1983; Le Grand and Robinson 1984; Public Service Association 1985b; Day and Klein 1985; Health Benefits Review 1986).

The purpose of this chapter, therefore, is to analyze the significance and implications of recent moves to privatize the hospital sector in New Zealand, a small industrial society. Private medicine has boomed in New Zealand over the last few decades. Although primary health care has always been provided largely by private practitioners on a fee-for-service basis, this has not been true of the hospital sector. Public hospital services have been delivered at no cost to the user since 1938 and have been publicly funded via central government taxation since 1957. However, since the 1950s the hospital system has become increasingly privatized; over one-third of the population is now covered by private health insurance, and private institutions now contain over one-quarter of all hospital beds (Hay 1985; New Zealand Department of Health 1986a). Unlike the United States, which has always been highly privatized, or the United Kingdom, which has been highly socialized since 1948, the New Zealand health care system occupies a middle position with a strong, but declining, public sector and, until recently, a rapidly growing private sector. Such transitional systems are of interest since, with few exceptions (Scarpaci 1985b), most research on privatization has focused on contexts where private medicine is either strongly or weakly developed (Salmon 1985; Bergthold 1987; Whiteis and Salmon 1987; Mohan 1984a, 1985, Rayner 1987). However, while such research is of value in identifying the origins and eventual impacts of privatization once it has run its full course, it fails to capture important processes and stresses that are inevitably involved in the transition from one type of health care system to another.

This chapter has four objectives. First we examine the growth and extent of private hospital development in New Zealand in the post war period, when the state made its first moves to reprivatize health care. Second, we analyze the question Why privatization? to identify the major proponents of privatization in New Zealand and to examine their vested interests in encouraging the process and the policy objectives served by a return to private market arrangements. Third, we explore some of the implications of privatization for the pattern of financing and delivery of care in the surgical and geriatric sectors. The purpose here is to examine considerations of equity and efficiency with respect to the changing provision of care in both sectors. In the final section we explore some of the planning implications of privatization and the extent to which it should be encouraged in the future as a policy goal.

Growth and Present Status of the Private Hospital Sector

Before discussing the significance of privatization, it is necessary to gain some appreciation of the evolution of private hospital care in the context of the development of the welfare state and the wider political economy of New Zealand. Since the turn of the century, the balance between public and private responsibility for providing health care has changed from a system in which market arrangements were dominant to one of increasing public involvement in the development of the welfare state; and since the 1950s, market arrangements have increasingly been reemphasized (Fougere 1984). For instance, in the 1930s private hospitals accounted for approximately 25 to 30 percent of all hospital beds. With the development of the welfare state this soon fell to a low point of 14 percent in the early 1950s, but, since then, private provision has rebounded to pre–welfare state levels (fig. 4.1). Over the same period, the public hospital system has slowly lost ground. Although real cuts in health expenditure occurred for the first time in 1980, public bed availability peaked during the period of the 1957–1960 Labour government, after which the per capita provision (but not the actual number) of public beds declined.

The transition of the New Zealand health care system from private market to welfare state, followed by the resurgence of the market, is typical of many other industrial societies. State provision or subsidy of medical services occurred to serve the needs of the economy, to socialize the costs generated by the expansion of private enterprise,

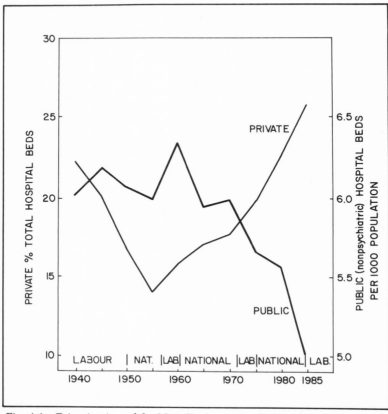

Fig. 4.1. Privatization of the New Zealand Hospital System, 1940–1985

and perhaps to preserve political stability by providing at least the illusion of equality. Thus, in the nineteenth century a rudimentary
system of public hospitals developed to cater to an increased population and a rapidly expanding agricultural and gold rush economy.
However, such developments were very modest. The absence of a
wealthy upper class meant that voluntary hospitals never developed
to any great extent; as a consequence, it was left to the state to fund
and provide health care (Fraser 1984). Public hospitals established in
the early years of the colony were basically places of last resort catering to the poor and medically indigent. However, they were not,
strictly speaking, public hospitals since a substantial portion of their
income was raised by fees paid by nondestitute patients. Thus, al-

though the distinction between public and private care was ambiguous, it was nevertheless apparent given the stigma attached to receiving public charity in public hospitals and the emphasis placed on self-help in providing medical care (Fraser 1984).

After 1870, urbanization and the expansion of the New Zealand economy placed increased pressures on the central government to expand the range and quality of medical services. Costs soon escalated, and by the 1880s the central government provided over 70 percent of the revenue to support the running of the nation's hospitals, with the balance coming mainly from voluntary contributions and patient fees (Fraser 1984). These increased pressures, accentuated by a recession economy, prompted a move in 1885 (somewhat reminiscent of revenue sharing in the United States in the 1970s) to devolve financial responsibility for providing hospital services from central to local government. The Hospital and Charitable Institutions Act (1885) reduced the proportion of funds contributed by the central government from 73 to 40 percent within two years while increasing local contributions from less than 5 percent to 35 percent. The rationale for the 1885 act was to limit public spending and at the same time encourage self-help in the provision of medical care (Fraser 1984).

Although free access to public hospitals was limited to the medically indigent and the indigenous Maori population, the act had the effect of increasing, rather than decreasing, social and geographical inequalities in access to medical care. By making central government subsidies dependent on the level of local spending, the system of local rating led to the development of an uneven distribution of hospital facilities as the wealthier and more populous rural areas inevitably spent more per capita on hospital services than urban ones. These inequalities were further intensified by the proliferation of small hospital boards from 1885 on, a fragmentation that limited a significant areal and interclass redistribution of funds. This system of local funding persisted, with little change, until 1957 and was only changed when the pressures on local government of funding an increasingly complex and expensive health care system became too great (Barnett, Ward, and Tatchell 1980; Fraser 1984; Hay 1985).

While the 1885 act determined the direction and pattern of public hospital funding over the next seventy years, it also perpetuated the dual health care system established in the early years of the colony. This was achieved by limiting the development of universal free access to health care and leaving those who were able to pay for it to find suitable care in the better class of private hospitals or in private wards in public hospitals (New Zealand House of Representatives 1907, 13). This two-tier system, which augmented market provision with charitable aid, was welcomed by the medical profession, who saw this type of government intervention as providing a stable income yet allowing the maintenance of professional autonomy (Hay 1985).

The dual health care system would have continued to grow in New Zealand had it not been for the depression and the election of a new Labour government in 1935. Since 1923, Labour party policy had advocated universally free medical services; but faced with united opposition from the country's doctors, the new administration was forced to compromise. Hospital care was to be provided free by state-salaried practitioners, but doctors were still able to supplement their incomes by other means. These included practicing part-time in private hospitals (on a fee-for-service basis) or in primary care, access to which was publicly subsidized, but which remained on a fee-for-service basis. The compromise between the state and the medical profession was enshrined in the 1938 Social Security Act, which institutionalized the dual hospital system that persists today.

The development of public hospitals to meet the demands of consumers, now eligible to receive health care as a right, rather than according to ability to pay, caused little stress to the system as long as economic growth continued and state revenues exceeded expenditures. However, since the 1950s, state expenditures increased more rapidly than the means of financing them, with the result that the 1970s saw a fiscal crisis emerge in New Zealand as in other developed countries. It became increasingly evident that the state could no longer satisfy demands for more and better health care. Since World War Two, New Zealand's economic growth has been among the lowest of all developed countries, and this naturally has had implications for the level of spending on social services. Thus, in recent years, especially 1975–1984, there has been reduced state involvement in the financing and provision of social consumption services such as housing and health, while social investment expenditure, aimed at stimulating and (until 1985) subsidizing economic development, generally increased (Davis 1984; Health Benefits Review 1986). As Taylor and Hadfield (1982, 244) observe, this contradiction between the requirements of private capital accumulation and the needs of consumers is an unequal battle. Since the state cannot usually satisfy both demands, the latter is inevitably sacrificed (O'Connor 1973).

The increased socialization of the health care system that followed the election of the 1935 Labour government was, therefore, a short-lived phenomenon. Although the extension of the welfare state caused an initial decline in the number of private hospitals, they soon expanded again following increased state support for their development. By the 1980s their share of total hospital beds exceeded pre–welfare state levels. In 1985 the private (for-profit and non-profit) hospital sector accounted for almost 27 percent of all hospital beds, a share that was considerably larger than in the United Kingdom (6 percent in 1985), about the same as in Australia (23 percent in 1984), but much smaller than in the United States (80 percent in 1984).[1] This share is likely to expand in the future. Although the newly elected Labour government imposed controls on all private hospital developments in 1985, this decision was partially reversed in 1987 with the deregulation of the surgical sector. Deregulation removed the requirement that the Health Department approve the establishment of additional surgical beds. This paved the way for the expansion of private surgical bed numbers in areas like Canterbury and Palmerston North (fig. 4.2) where, previously, additional beds would have exceeded Health Department bed guidelines (New Zealand Department of Health 1977).

Today, the majority of private hospitals in New Zealand are run on a non-profit basis by religous and church groups or voluntary and welfare agencies. However, the for-profit sector has grown rapidly in recent years, especially long-term private geriatric hospitals, where companies or small entrepreneurs now control 43 percent of all beds (table 4.1). Although New Zealand has no history of for-profit hospital chains, this organizational form may well grow in importance in the future. A multihospital chain is already present in the non-profit sector, and the first penetration of the New Zealand health system by a for-profit chain is already occurring. In 1987 a management contract was signed between the Hospital Corporation of Australia and the Wellcare Corporation of New Zealand to run and expand geriatric and other private health care facilities in the country's three major metropolitan areas (Beanland 1987).

The increased privatization of the hospital system coincided with an increased centralization of private hospital developments, although recent years have begun to see a reversal of this trend.[2] In 1945, private hospitals were present in all but two of the existing twenty-nine hospital boards, compared with only fifteen in 1985 (fig. 4.2). The increased concentration of beds was not only a response to

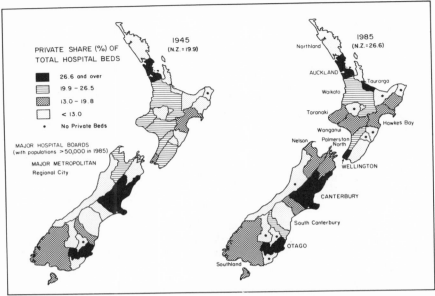

Fig. 4.2. Private Share of Total Hospital Beds in New Zealand, 1945–1985

market forces associated with the northward shift and continued urbanization of the population, but also reflected the changing composition of the private sector itself. Declining birth rates resulted in the
closure of many maternity hospitals, both public and private, especially in rural areas, while poorer access to public hospitals in the
larger cities encouraged a rapid expansion of the private geriatric and
surgical sectors in these areas. At first this expansion was largely
confined to the four main metropolitan centers, but increasing saturation of their health care markets has prompted a diffusion of privatization down the urban hierarchy (table 4.2).

Why Privatization?

The privatization of the New Zealand hospital system has evolved
in response to a number of pressures. Many of these have been
operating for a long time, but their significance has depended upon
the particular balance of political forces and conflict between those
who stand to gain and those who stand to lose from the extension of

Table 4.1. Change in Number and Private Share of Total Beds in New Zealand

	% Change in Number of Beds		Private Share of Total Beds (%)			%Private Beds Owned by For-Profit Organizations
	Public	Private	1978	1985	Change	1986
Geriatric	8.5	164.0	33.9	55.5	21.6	43.0
Surgical	-10.3	21.6	17.2	22.0	4.8	10.0
Medical	-7.5	-92.3	30.3	3.5	-26.8	--[a]
Pediatric	-13.4	-100.0	10.5	0	-10.5	--
Maternity	-20.4	-65.8	4.0	1.8	-2.2	34.2
Psychiatric	-11.4	- 18.2	0.1	0.1	0	91.7
TOTAL	-10.2	15.6	22.4	26.6	4.2	35.8

Source: New Zealand Department of Health 1978 and 1985a.

Note: No separate breakdown of public surgical beds was available prior to 1978.

[a]Included in geriatric and surgical.

Table 4.2. Rates of Privatization by Size of Hospital Board in New Zealand

SIMPLE CORRELATIONS BETWEEN

	Private Share (%) of Total Beds and Size of Board	Change in Share by Decade and Size of Board	% Change in Number of Private Beds and Size of Board
1945	.62		
1955	.59	-.09	.23
1965	.72	.56	.50
1975	.73	.45	.35
1985	.69	.23	.03

Source: Calculations based on unpublished data from the National Health Statistics Center, New Zealand Department of Health.

market arrangements. It is therefore important to identify the main proponents of privatization and their vested interests in encouraging the process.

One of the principal advocates for the privatization of health services has been the state, which has encouraged the process on both economic and ideological grounds. The state's ideological reaction against collectivism has been based on the now familiar argument that patients, rather than the state, should be primarily responsible for meeting the cost of health services. This stress on self-help has been based on two main philosophical assumptions. First, most social problems, including poor health, arise from individual rather than structural causes; there, responsibility for solving them should be an individual rather than a collective one. Second, it is frequently argued that patients should be made to feel the costs of health care so that they will act in a fiscally responsible manner. In other words, it is assumed that most of the escalation of health care costs is due to unnecessary consumer demand, stimulated by third-party insurance schemes, rather than the provider push (Weller and Manga 1983). We cannot explore both arguments in detail here, but it is important to note that both assumptions have been contradicted by the evidence. Individualistic explanations of social deprivation have been found wanting (Peet 1975). Also, it is clear that consumers have the least power within the health care sector compared with the monopoly power of the medical profession, which has been able to manipulate the quantity and cost of services provided (McKinlay 1980; McPherson et al. 1981). It is ironic, therefore, that most competitive privatization proposals are explicitly directed at changing consumer rather than provider behavior (Siminoff 1986).

Promoting the ideology of self-help has not been the only reaction on the part of the state to the rising cost of health services. Advocates of privatization also stress the economic benefits of deregulation and increased competition among health care providers. In theory such moves are seen as strategies for increasing efficiency and lowering health care costs as well as promoting greater choice for patients. It follows that patients will shop around and place pressure on providers to be more efficient. However, reality appears to be somewhat different. To begin with, there is no conclusive proof, despite all the rhetoric, that the private provision of health services is any more efficient than public provision (Relman 1983; Butler 1984; Maynard and Williams 1984). This is not surprising given that perverse incentives operate and escalate health care expenditure in both types of systems (McPherson et al. 1981). Similarly, the market model of cost-conscious consumers shopping around to get the best deal has been severely criticized by Maynard (1983, 1986) and Siminoff (1986), among others, who have clearly demonstrated that imperfections in health care markets produce outcomes inconsistent with the predictions of the market model.

Nevertheless, despite their weak theoretical foundations, it is interesting that these ideologies first started to be promoted in New Zealand in the 1950s when deliberate state support for privatization expressed itself in the form of private subsidies and capital-expenditure loan schemes to encourage the construction or expansion of private hospitals. Two factors encouraged such moves at that time: the lowest level of economic growth in the post war period prior to 1973 (Gould 1982) and the assumption in 1957 of total responsibility by central government for the financing of public hospital services. The new state posture ended the devolution of hospital funding established in 1885.

Since the 1950s the encouragement of privatization has taken various forms besides bed subsidies and capital loans. In 1967, private medical insurance became tax deductible, a move that stimulated the rapid expansion of such schemes (Hay 1985). Seven years later, private bed subsidies were extended to geriatric care for the first time, and this move, together with a further means-tested GHSAS (Geriatric Hospital Special Assistance Scheme) bed subsidy in 1977, had a dramatic effect on the privatization of this sector (see table 4.1). Finally, private hospital growth was also stimulated by the introduction, in 1982–1983 of a new system of financing public hospital services. Modeled after the British Resource Allocation Working party (RAWP) formula, the new system of population-based funding has resulted in a more equitable allocation of public hospital expenditure. However, unlike RAWP, the population-based funding formula assumes a complementarity of access to public and private care systems, and, as a result, public hospital board allocations are reduced in direct proportion to the level of use in the private sector (Barnett 1984). In reality such complementarity does not exist, and, ironically, this move has helped weaken the public sector by penalizing the larger metropolitan boards, which have traditionally been the focus of private hospital growth and have had the worst levels of access to public beds.

While the above policy initiatives suggest deliberate state support for privatization along the lines suggested by Marxist theory (O'Connor 1973), it is evident that the state has also inadvertently supported such moves. Nowhere is this more evident than in the impact of the

Accident Compensation Corporation (ACC). Introduced in 1974 and designed to provide comprehensive insurance against all forms of accidental injury, the ACC also provided an important stimulus to private hospital expansion. In responding to increased pressures on public hospitals the ACC introduced an approved procedures list in 1982. This list defined areas of treatment for which it was expected that there would be long public hospital waiting lists and, for these areas, gave doctors the power to refer patients directly to private hospitals without prior reference to ACC. This lack of control (which persisted until 1987) over the decision to opt for the private hospitalization of ACC patients meant, not surprisingly, that by 1986 almost one-fifth of the ACC's expenditure ended up in private hospitals, with other areas of care, particularly physiotherapy, privatizing rapidly, often at the expense of the public sector (Health Benefits Review 1986; McCallum 1986).

The privatization of health services has been supported not only by the state, but also by doctors. Ever since 1938 the medical profession has encouraged a return to private market arrangements mainly for reasons of greater professional autonomy and control over incomes and working conditions. Recently these have become even more important as a result of increased financial stringency in the public hospital system. In New Zealand it is noteworthy that the largest private health care insurance group, the Southern Cross Medical Care Society, was started by a group of forty-six surgeons in 1961 with the aim of expanding private hospitals and thus preserving the dual health care system (Hay 1985).

Privatization of social services is not only advantageous to the state and the medical profession but also has an important part to play in the recapitalization of capitalism, both in terms of freeing up public resources for private investment (O'Connor 1973; Elling 1981) and in providing ready-made markets for the private sector (Walker 1984). Thus, private investors have also been strong advocates of privatization because of higher returns on investment in health services, such as private rest homes (Phillips and Vincent 1986a), than in other parts of the economy. Employers also have favored private health care schemes, but often for other reasons. For example, in New Zealand the employer-funded group schemes, which are tax deductible, appear to encourage employee loyalty and minimize work disruption (Hay 1985). However, given such advantages, employer-funded group schemes do not appear to have been a major stimulus to privatization in New Zealand; Chetwynd and colleagues (1983) found that only 15 percent of a national sample was covered in this way.

Finally, privatization also inevitably reflects the influence of client-induced restructuring as a result of perceived or real dissatisfaction with the public hospital system. Although consumers of health services have never been a major force in the determination of health policy, their actions, by default, may cause a shift in the balance between public and private care. This is especially true where more affluent households opt for private care in areas where the public sector performs worst. Fougere (1978), relying on Hirschman's (1970) familiar conceptualization of "exit, voice and loyalty," sees this as a major factor in the growth of private hospitals in New Zealand. However, Fergusson, Horwood, and Shannon (1986) have questioned this explanation in a survey of Christchurch families whose private health insurance was not provided by an employer, concluding that the rapid rise of private health insurance has probably not been due to any major discontent with public hospital services. Instead they argue that it reflects the promotional activities of the insurance companies or the reaction of the population to the rapidly increasing costs of primary care. However, such conclusions are open to question. Only 23 percent of the sample felt that public health care services were inadequate, but 61 percent said that they had opted for private health insurance so as to avoid public hospital waiting lists and to obtain immediate care.

Another way of looking at the importance of public-sector deficiencies as a cause of privatization is to examine the correlation between these two variables over time. Table 4.3 lends support for Fougere's rather than Fergusson's interpretation in that it is evident that the correlation between the number of private beds per capita, or their share of total hospital beds, and the supply of public beds per capita has increased markedly since 1945. Much the same result is obtained when looking at patterns of change rather than cross-sectional data. Thus, we might infer that client-induced restructuring, due to deficiencies in the public sector, is becoming more important.

Implications of Privatization

Although the growth of private hospitals has undoubtedly provided greater choice for health care consumers and played its part in improving health care in New Zealand, it is important to assess the

Table 4.3. Correlations between Public and Private Beds Per Capita and
Private Share of Total Hospital Boards in New Zealand

	Private Share and Public Beds per capita	Private and Public Beds per capita
1945	-.32	.03
1955	-.50	-.32
1965	-.63	-.55
1975	-.70	-.58
1985	-.68	-.64

Source: Calculations based on unpublished data from National Health Statistics
Center, New Zealand Department of Health.

implications of such developments for the population as a whole.
Judgments on privatization ought to depend, not on ideologically
based beliefs, but on a careful evaluation of the process and its consequences. Based on the American experience, Torrens (1982) has
outlined four potential hazards of privatization: the creation of a dual
health care system, the diversion of scarce personnel out of the public sector and into the private sector, the fragmentation of social policy and planning, and a significant rise in health care costs, in part
resulting from an increased emphasis on technological responses to
medical problems. To Torrens's list we could also add the cream
skimming of more profitable patients with minor medical and surgical problems (Relman 1980), widening inequalities in the distribution
of resources and life chances (Walker 1984), and the monopolization
of health care markets at the expense of competition and public accountability (Bergstrand 1982). Although Torrens's warnings of the
potential hazards of privatization were directed at England, with its
small but expanding private sector, it is instructive to evaluate the extent to which such hazards have become a reality in New Zealand,
where private hospitals are more well established. In a more detailed
examination of surgical and geriatric sectors, the two main areas of
hospital care affected by privatization, the following discussion focuses on some of these concerns as they pertain to issues of equity
and efficiency.

Implications for Surgical Services

Privatization, by its very nature, limits access to care according to ability to pay, rather than need, and can be criticized on this basis. Two further consequences can be examined: first, the regional variation in the supply of all hospital beds and its effects on access to public hospital care; and second, whether or not privatization has necessarily resulted in a more efficient use of resources.

Privatization and Inequalities in Access to Hospital Services. Has privatization led to overcapacity problems in the hospital system? If one examines the British experience the answer is clearly yes (Mohan and Woods 1985). In England the basically unrestrained development of private hospitals has directly contradicted the National Health Service's (NHS) RAWP resource-allocation policy, which has sought to shift resources away from overbedded areas such as London (Eyles, Smith, and Woods 1982; Eyles 1987). In New Zealand, however, this has not been the case. Here private hospitals have mainly developed in the most urbanized hospital boards where the public sector is weakest (see table 4.3 and Figure 4.2). Despite an already well developed private surgical sector, the five largest boards (Auckland, Wellington, Canterbury, Otago, and Waikato) accounted for nearly half (47.4 percent) of the net increase in private surgical beds between 1977 and 1985.

While private hospital growth, in a crude distributional sense, seems to complement the pattern of public provision, it has also distorted access to public care. Private growth has led to the diversion of both public funds and professional staff away from public hospitals located in areas with a strong private sector, with a consequent impact upon public hospital surgical waiting lists. It could be argued that waiting lists represent a measure of unmet need; however, there is considerable disagreement over this issue. Salmond and O'Connor (1973) argued that the "so called waiting list problem" is not concerned with life-saving situations and instead is mainly a reflection of the demand for nonurgent routine surgery. While this view has some merit, it is also clear that, in many areas of New Zealand and for certain specialities, patients are now waiting much longer for surgery than before, that such patients include a higher proportion of more urgent cases, and that waiting times (after controlling for the supply of public surgical beds) also show some tendency to vary with the degree of privatization (table 4.4).

Table 4.4. Percentage of Public Hospital Patients Waiting More Than One Year for Surgery in New Zealand

Hospital Board[a]	General Surgery			Orthopedic Surgery			Total Surgery		
	1984	1986	Change	1984	1986	Change	1984	1986	Change
Palmerston North	20.4	33.7	13.3	40.3	60.9	20.6	19.9	47.4	27.5
Auckland	38.4	53.2	14.8	43.0	58.2	15.2	47.2	47.9	0.7
Wellington	9.7	12.8	3.1	10.8	7.6	-3.2	16.2	16.3	0.1
Canterbury	12.0	22.5	10.5	21.3	38.5	17.2	21.1	29.5	8.4
Otago	36.4	28.6	-7.8	6.6	19.4	12.8	13.2	14.5	1.3
Waikato	12.0	13.7	1.7	11.1	23.0	11.9	28.6	34.3	5.7
Southland	9.4	14.6	5.2	12.1	20.9	8.8	17.2	18.2	1.0
Taranaki	43.9	23.4	-20.5	29.4	39.4	10.0	32.9	36.9	4.0

Source: National Health Statistics Center, New Zealand Department of Health, unpublished reports.

[a]Hospital boards with <1.75 surgical beds per 1000 population. Boards ranked by degree of privatization of the surgical sector.

Taking into account some ambiguity in the interpretation of public hospital waiting lists, it is still necessary to ask whether privatization has had any impact upon these, for it is possible that private hospitals could reduce pressure on the public sector as well as diverting resources from it. In examining the British experience (Rathwell, Sics, and Williams 1985) the main conclusion drawn is that privatization, so far, has had only a relatively minor impact on NHS hospitals, particularly in the areas of staffing (and hence waiting lists, although these were not specifically examined) and lost revenue from NHS paybeds (public hospital beds that are set aside for fee-paying patients). However, in New Zealand, as in the United States (Kennedy 1984), the situation is somewhat different, for here a larger private sector has had a detrimental effect upon the public one. Public hospital surgical waiting lists have grown along with privatization (see fig. 4.3), despite increased public hospital admissions, increased public operation rates, and shorter lengths of stay.

Waiting lists tend to be longer in areas where the private sector is strongest, a trend first noticed by McKinlay (1980) and Davis (1981)

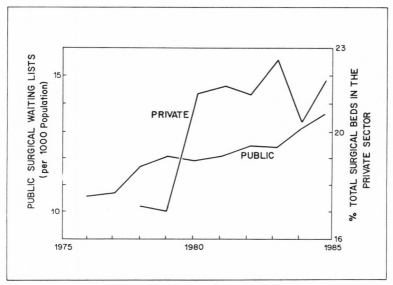

Fig. 4.3. Private Hospital Surgical Bed Share and Public Hospital Surgical
Waiting Lists, 1975–1985

and confirmed by Simpson (1986), who found that public operation
rates were generally lower where there had been an increase in the
share of operations being conducted privately. However, previous
research has failed to examine the independent effect of privatization
upon waiting lists, which are also long in areas without a strong private sector and where the supply of public surgical beds is relatively
low. Also, no attempt has been made to examine longer-term impacts of the growth of private surgical hospitals and whether their effects on public surgical waiting lists have increased over time. Tables
4.5 and 4.6 report partial correlations between two indicators of waiting lists and the proportion of surgical beds in the private sector after
controlling for variations in the supply of public hospital resources. It
is clear that the effect of privatization is hardly diminished once controls for public hospital resources are introduced (table 4.5) and that
this effect appears to have increased markedly over time (table 4.6).
Thus, while in a crude distributional sense the growth of private hospitals appears complementary to the pattern of public provision, this
growth has served to limit access to the public sector by diverting resources away from it. Most surgeons work in both sectors, salaried
in one and operating under fee-for-service in the other. Because

Table 4.5.   Privatization and Public Hospital Surgical Waiting Lists in New Zealand, 1984-1985

SIMPLE CORRELATIONS

Public hospital surgical waiting lists per capita and			Public hospital surgical waiting lists per average occupied surgical bed	
% Surgical beds in private sector	.72		.80	
Public surgical beds per capita	-.28		-.51	
Public surgical specialists per capita	-.38		-.44	
Public hospital nurses per capita	-.41		-.57	

PARTIALS   (F-ratio)

12.3	.70	(22.5)	.73	(25.9)
12.34	.65	(16.0)	.66	(16.7)
12.345	.62	(13.2)	.63	(13.7)

Source: Calculations based on information from New Zealand Department of Health 1985a and 1986a.

surgeons can increase their incomes by working in private hospitals, there is an incentive for them to spend an increasing proportion of their time working privately, and this appears to range from 15 to 40 percent of their work time depending upon the speciality (Smailes 1987). McPherson and colleagues (1981) have suggested that doctors may also manipulate demand via waiting lists, thus encouraging increased use, if not overuse of the private sector. Although the nature and extent of this process is unknown (Culyer 1983, 394), two pieces of information support this interpretation: hospitalization rates are more strongly related to the supply of beds in private, as opposed to public, hospital systems; and this difference also appears to be evident in the case of actual operation rates (Bunker 1970; McPherson et al. 1981).

The ability of surgeons to work in both sectors is, of course, depen-

Table 4.6. Privatization and Public Hospital Surgical Waiting Lists in New Zealand

CORRELATIONS BETWEEN

Public Hospital Surgical Waiting Lists per capita and

	% Surgical beds in private sector	Public surgical beds per capita	PARTIAL$_{12.3}$	R^2 $_{1.23}$
1978	.73	-.66	.47	.56
1979	.75	-.68	.50	.59
1980	.74	-.66	.56	.61
1981	.62	-.63	.35	.47
1982	.68	-.59	.47	.49
1983	.68	-.53	.52	.47
1984	.72	-.41	.65	.52
1985	.72	-.28	.70	.59

Source: Calculations based on information from New Zealand Department of Health, Hospital Management Data for 1978-1985.

dent upon the extent of any planning controls over the deployment of the surgical work force. In New Zealand few such controls exist; the balance between public and private care is largely a matter of personal choice. In marked contrast, the British NHS (despite the introduction of the 1980 Health Services Act, which gave consultants increased scope for private practice) allows surgeons to earn only 10 percent of their gross NHS salary from private practice (Rathwell, Sics, and Williams 1985). The absence of such controls in New Zealand is probably a reflection of the very small pool of surgical specialists, which, coupled with frequent shortages of their services, has meant that they have had considerable power in influencing the direction of health policy and the nature of their work patterns.

Privatization and Efficiency. Advocates of privatization have been strangely silent on the issue of equity, but not on the issue of efficiency. One of the main arguments in favor of privatization is that increased competition is seen as a means of improving the efficiency and quality of social services. This is not a new argument, having long been integral to public choice theory (Bish 1971), but only recently has it been applied to health services. There have been numerous claims, particularly in the United States, that private hospitals (especially those in investor-owned chains) must be more efficient than other types of organizations since they are out to maximize profits and have the advantage of corporate management and distribution structures. However, Arnold Relman (1983), among others (Roemer and Roemer 1982; Maynard and Williams 1984), has concluded that such claims cannot be substantiated based on the evidence available (see, for example, Larson 1980; Pattison and Katz 1983). Relman's view was based on the observation that for-profit hospitals within the United States do not necessarily have lower costs per unit of output (usually defined in terms of costs per inpatient day) than non-profit organizations, although nurses' salaries and maintenance expenses were lower. However, while operating expenses may have showed no significant difference between for-profit and non-profit institutions, this was hardly true of patient charges, which were 17 to 24 percent higher in the former (Relman 1983, 370–371).

Such comparisons may illustrate certain differences between these two organizational types, but they are of little use for making efficiency comparisons between public and private care. This is because, outside the United States, non-profit hospitals are frequently labeled as private, and even within the United States the distinction between these two types of organizations is becoming increasingly ambiguous (Salmon 1985).

Within New Zealand, despite recent moves to corporatize the public sector, there has been surprisingly little research on the relative efficiency of the public and private hospital systems. The main exception is a recent report produced by a business consulting firm and commissioned by the Southern Cross Medical Care Society, New Zealand's largest private health insurance group and owner of the country's major non-profit hospital chain (Southern Cross Medical Care Society 1986). Not surprisingly, the main conclusion of the report is that private hospitals are more efficient than their public counterparts and that substantial cost savings could be made by encouraging privatization. The basis of this conclusion is a comparison of average length of stay (ALOS) data in public and private institutions, for a sample of sixteen of the forty most frequently performed operations in which it is argued that patient age profiles and operating procedures are similar. As in England and Wales (Williams et al. 1985), in New Zealand it was found that ALOS was considerably shorter, in most cases (fifteen of sixteen), in private hospitals. Given this, the consulting firm estimated that if all sixteen operations were done entirely within the private sector, then a saving of 67 percent could be made in the number of bed days. Conversely, a 54 percent increase resulted when the corresponding group of private hospital operations were performed in the public sector.

Such findings, which suggest that private hospitals might be more efficient, are in reality highly questionable since a number of important clinical and patient population factors have been ignored in the analysis, although the authors discount these as influencing longer periods of public hospitalization. These factors include differences in the proportion of very elderly patients (over seventy-five years of age) in both sectors; differences in the severity of illness, which is usually higher for the lower-income groups who are more likely to use the public hospital system; differences in the degree of access to postoperative care, which is likely to be lower for public hospital patients either because of their lower socioeconomic status or because they are more likely to live in rural areas; and appreciation of the different functions of public and private hospitals in terms of the importance of the former as centers of medical training and how such differences affect average length of stay.

Thus, in view of the above discussion we must remain skeptical of economists and others who uphold market mechanisms as the solution to the problem of increased health care costs. The New Zealand evidence does not offer strong support for claims that private hospitals are more efficient than their counterparts in the public sector. Until researchers systematically compare the relative performance of public, voluntary non-profit and for-profit institutions we will continue to have a limited understanding of the economic implications of privatization.

Privatization and Geriatric Care

While the growth of private surgical hospitals has affected the capacity of the public sector to provide equal access to care, this has been less true of the geriatric sector. Due to increasing public control over the supply and use of private long-term beds, the effects of privatization have been less damaging than in the case of acute surgical care. Nevertheless, given the considerable growth in the supply of private geriatric beds over the last decade, it is necessary to consider the implications of both overall growth and the change in the public-private balance. The impact of these trends can be assessed in terms of the need for care, variations in access, and the achievement of public policy objectives.

The need for care is closely related to the age structure of the population. Since the early 1970s the "burden" of the elderly has become more apparent. Of particular significance is the increasing number of elderly over seventy-five years of age, the group most likely to need long-term institutional care (Fox 1983; King, Fletcher, and Main 1985). The supply of private and, to a lesser extent, public geriatric beds has kept pace with this growth; the overall bed supply has increased from 19.6 beds per 1000 population over sixty-five in 1981 to 22.8 in 1985, comparing favorably with recommended Department of Health guidelines of 18 per 1000 (New Zealand Department of Health 1985b). Although no guidelines exist for the population over seventy-five, the total supply of beds has also been maintained in relation to the growth of this group.

While the overall supply of geriatric long-term beds may be adequate, there nevertheless remains the question of access, which may vary regionally and according to patient dependence or ability to pay. Historically, there has been variation in the geographical distribution of private geriatric beds. Although there is an increasing urban bias in the private share of total geriatric beds (table 4.7), regional differences in the supply of all geriatric beds in relation to the population over sixty-five have become less significant over time (the index of dissimilarity between these two variables declined from 0.112 to 0.089 between 1978 and 1985). These trends are a reflection of increased public control over the allocation of GHSAS; geriatric bed subsidies; and the imposition of overall bed guidelines, which, if exceeded, mean that private hospitals licensed since 1981 are no longer eligible to receive GHSAS-subsidized patients.

Since the introduction of population-based funding in 1983, allocations to hospital boards with private beds in their area have been reduced in line with levels of private use. However, not all private use automatically reduces the resources available to the public (geriatric) sector; an exception is made for publicly subsidized GHSAS beds in private hospitals, which cater to means-tested elderly patients who are unable to gain access to public geriatric beds in their hospital board area. The funding formula compensates boards at a rate equivalent to the average national daily subsidy paid under the GHSAS.

Table 4.7. Geriatric Beds in the Largest Hospital Boards in New Zealand

Hospital Board	Geriatric Beds over 1000 Population over 65			Private Share of Total Geriatric Beds		
	1978	1985	Change	1978	1985	Change
Auckland	14.6	25.9	11.3	55.9	78.1	22.2
Canterbury	20.1	26.6	6.5	53.1	73.7	20.6
Wellington	17.1	27.7	10.6	27.0	52.3	25.3
Waikato	14.2	24.1	9.9	18.2	52.2	34.0
Otago	20.4	23.6	3.2	62.2	63.5	1.3
Southland	24.9	28.3	3.4	24.8	29.7	4.9
Palmerston North	15.1	20.7	5.6	--	37.7	37.7
Hawkes Bay	16.4	19.5	3.1	41.8	45.0	3.2
Tauranga	12.2	18.8	6.2	45.7	75.2	29.5
South Canterbury	21.2	29.1	7.9	14.9	16.2	1.3
Taranaki	14.4	17.1	2.7	17.4	45.0	27.6
Wanganui	18.7	19.2	0.5	--	11.5	11.5
Nelson	20.5	15.1	-5.4	27.8	36.0	8.2
Northland	9.5	7.6	-1.9	--	--	--

Source: New Zealand Department of Health 1978 and 1985a.

Note: Hospital boards with populations exceeding 50,000 (1985). These areas contained 88.9% of New Zealand's population over 65 years of age and 89.6% of all geriatric beds in 1985. Ranked according to the size of the geriatric sector (1985).

The result of this arrangement is that it is cheaper for hospital boards to subsidize private geriatric care than to provide it themselves. Such subsidies, therefore, mean that there is an incentive for private entrepreneurs to make up any shortfall in the supply of beds, at least to guideline levels.

Such policies have reduced geographic differences in the availability of all geriatric beds but accentuated regional variations in the privatization of this sector, yet the impact of this shift is not as great as it may first appear. Historically, public hospitals have given priority to more dependent patients. For example, while showing a similar range of patient dependence in the public and private sectors, Sainsbury, Fox, and Shelton (1986) have indicated a significantly

higher proportion of patients in private hospitals with lesser dependency levels. Similar trends have been found elsewhere (Campbell et
al. 1984; King, Fletcher, and Main 1985), although it appears that this
gap in dependency is narrowing since the introduction of GHSAS in
1977 and increased control exercised over medical criteria for access
to private care. Before the introduction of this more stringent assessment procedure, access to private geriatric care had been relatively
easy. The standard daily bed subsidy was readily available (on general practitioner referral) and, in the 1970s, formed a larger proportion of the total fee. Private institutions, therefore, attracted patients
who were both less dependent and more affluent than those who
were required to wait for a public bed.

The last few years have seen a gradual change in this pattern. C. S.
Higgins (1985) found that in 1982 only 33.8 percent of elderly people
then resident in long-term private hospitals in the Canterbury area
had been assessed by a geriatrician. By 1985 this had risen to 58 percent, an increase that is continuing. In Auckland, in 1986, nearly all
private hospital patients had been assessed by a geriatrician as being
in need of care (Sewell and Hawley 1987). This trend is due to the desire of hospital boards to exercise control over the use and level of
public subsidy of private beds and the increased availability of geri-
atricians to implement these policies. The management of a single
waiting list, based on clinically assessed need, for both public and
GHSAS-subsidized private beds is a common feature of areas where
there is a strong geriatric team.

Financial barriers to care seem more likely in areas where a large
proportion of beds are in the private sector. However, even here the
combined daily bed benefit and the GHSAS subsidy (which is subject to an income test and its availability dependent on bed guideline
levels) meet most of the costs of care. In 1985–1986 both subsidies accounted for two-thirds (68.6 percent) of total private health expenditure in the geriatric long-term sector, with the remainder mainly
coming from patients themselves (table 4.8). Thus, even where there
is a high proportion of private beds, it is likely that most patients will
be at least partly subsidized. In Auckland, for example, where 78.1
percent of all geriatric beds are private, all patients received the daily
bed benefit and 81.5 percent received the GHSAS at varying levels,
ranging up to 100 percent subsidy depending on income (Sewell and
Hawley 1987). Of those not receiving public subsidy, most met dependency criteria but failed to meet the income test for subsidy.

Joseph and Flynn (1988) have argued that where the private sector

Table 4.8. Relative Shares of Private Health Care Funding in New Zealand, 1985

	Total Expenditure	Public Purse	Insurance	ACC	Patients' Pockets
Long-stay geriatric	$94.06	68.6%	2.1%	0	29.3%
Acute surgical/medical sectors	$53.72	17.1%	46.6%	21.6%	14.5%

Source: Health Benefits Review 1986, 139.

is strong, elderly persons may be required to contribute their own resources to care, whereas in an area with a dominant public sector they will not. The idea of a means test for subsidy is not necessarily a contentious issue. However, the inconsistent occurrence of means testing based on regional variation in the balance of public and private beds creates inequity in access for people of similar medical conditions or financial circumstances. The extent to which this is acceptable probably depends on how well the situation and its implications are understood and the degree to which the management of health resources on a wider basis takes precedence over issues of personal equity.

In terms of public policy objectives the present structure of subsidies and controls in New Zealand is designed to maintain complementarity of public and private systems and to achieve an acceptable (or guideline) level of overall provision of geriatric beds while minimizing the level of public expenditure. The recommended levels of bed provision have largely been reached since 1978. However, efforts to contain expenditure by restraining both supply and use have not, so far, been particularly successful, at least in the larger population centers, where in all but three cases in 1985 the overall geriatric bed supply exceeded guideline levels (see table 4.2).

The impact of existing controls on overall levels of provision and use cannot be determined with any certainty because of the regular adjustments to which the system has been subjected. Even if the overall management objectives are achieved, there are important issues remaining. First, there is the regional variation, outlined above, in the requirement for means-tested access to long-term care, which seems to run counter to principles of entitlement inherent in social security legislation. Second, there is the possible impact on standards of care where the decision has been made to scale down the involvement of the public sector. We do not mean to suggest that private geriatric hospitals do not provide quality care; however, the public sector has traditionally been seen as a leader because of its wide range of services, its specialist medical work force, and its role in training and education and in exercising responsibility for the provision of a comprehensive range of services. A negligible involvement in long-term care, it is thought, will remove this visible focus of professional leadership and put overall standards at risk. Some hospital boards have recognized this and, while acknowledging the financial problem inherent in retaining a high level of participation, regard this as essential in order to achieve broader health care goals (Canterbury Hospital Board 1987). Third, there is the nature of the relationship between private geriatric hospital beds and private rest homes for the elderly and voluntary agency-funded residential care. Each sector represents differing levels of care, each is subsidized differently with varying criteria of access, subsidy provisions, guidelines, and controls. Effective management of public resources, applied to all forms of long-term care for the elderly, requires a more coordinated approach both centrally and regionally.

Summary

In New Zealand the privatization of hospital services has been going on for some time, in contrast to some other industrial societies, such as the United Kingdom, where it is a relatively recent development. The dual hospital system has remained an accepted part of health care policy, but attempts to strengthen the public sector have depended upon the particular political philosophy of the government in power at the time. Nevertheless, private hospital developments have been largely unregulated both fiscally and distributionally, in contrast to the more stringent controls recently imposed on health spending in the public sector. Ironically, privatization has been largely encouraged by public subsidies, which by 1986 accounted for half of the expenditure on private hospital services (Health Benefits Review 1986, 139). Although existing public subsidies for the use of private hospitals form only a small proportion of the total government expenditure on hospitals, both public and private (table 4.9), this proportion has grown steadily over the last few

Table 4.9. Public Expenditure on Private Hospital Services in New Zealand

Public Expenditure on Private Hospital Services	1978	1980	1982	1984	1986
In Millions of dollars	20.6	33.4	51.6	61.2	74.0
Percentage of hospital expenditures	3.6	4.1	4.4	4.7	4.7
Share by Sector (%)					
Geriatric	73.3	80.5	82.6	83.4	86.2
daily bed benefit	61.3	60.4	59.7	59.3	55.5
GHSAS	12.0	20.1	22.9	24.1	30.7
Surgical-Medical[a]	19.1	12.3	10.0	10.1	8.5
Psychiatric	6.2	5.4	5.6	5.2	4.2
Maternity	1.4	0.6	0.4	0.3	0.2
Nongeriatric long-term care	--	1.2	1.4	1.0	0.9

Source: New Zealand Department of Health 1986b.

[a]Discontinued in 1987.

years and may well be much higher once the variety of invisible subsidies (for example, for laboratory and radiological services) are taken into account.

The pattern of unregulated growth so evident in the past few decades now appears to be changing. Marked increases in the cost of private health insurance premiums, coupled with increasing market saturation, suggest that the growth potential of private hospitals in New Zealand may be limited. More significant, however, has been the gradual imposition of public controls over the distribution and use of private beds, first over publicly subsidized GHSAS geriatric beds (since 1981), and, more recently (1985–1987), over the supply of all private beds whether geriatric or surgical. However, locational controls over the expansion of private surgical beds were removed in 1987, when the surgical bed benefit was canceled (that is, the public subsidy for private surgery), although controls are still maintained for nonsurgical private beds that receive a subsidy. Since most of these are in the rapidly growing geriatric sector, removing controls on the expansion of surgical beds hardly amounts to massive deregulation.

Although the evidence is mixed, these developments suggest that the privatization of health services is entering a new phase. The state continues to withdraw from the financing but not the regulation of health services that are still publicly subsidized. Such moves do not necessarily entail a decline of the welfare state; rather, they involve its emergence in a new form.

The expansion of the postwar welfare state in New Zealand, as in other Western democracies, has been a mixed blessing. The main purpose of intervention, to improve access to health services for those in need, has largely been achieved, but only at the cost of increased fiscal stress and doubts about whether the services represent value for money in terms of improved health outcomes. However, although traditional forms of intervention may have fallen into disrepute, letting the market decide may not necessarily be the answer. As Maynard (1986) has indicated, because perverse incentives operate to produce inefficiencies in both public and private health care systems, privatization may leave us no better off with respect to efficiency, while compounding problems of equity. It would seem, therefore, that the key question is not simply one of assessing the merits of privatization, but of determining the appropriate public-private mix for health care and how the efficiency of both sectors can be improved. In New Zealand, changes in this direction could include limiting unnecessary hospitalization in areas where there is a more than adequate supply of public beds or minimizing the adverse effects of private hospital growth by regulating the deployment of surgeons in that sector.

Although the fiscal involvement of the state in encouraging privatization appears to have slowed, it is likely that alternative private-market health care arrangements will evolve in New Zealand given the commitment of the present Labour administration to corporatize and privatize the rest of the public sector. [3] However, before any such moves are made, what is needed in New Zealand (and in the privatization literature in general) is more empirical research on the costs and benefits of different degrees of privatization and alternative public-private sector interactions. On the policy side, such research would be useful in encouraging health policymakers to state formally what privatization is supposed to achieve. In New Zealand, at least, this is woefully lacking in the health care sector, but is clearly necessary for the future management of fiscally stressed health care systems.

Notes

[1] Data for Australia, the United Kingdom, and New Zealand refer to the private share of total (acute and long-term) hospital beds (Australia Bureau of Statistics 1986; Grant 1985; New Zealand Department of Health 1985b), while that for the United States includes acute nonfederal beds only (U. S. Bureau of the Census 1987). However, if total hospitals rather than beds are considered, 66 percent of American hospitals in 1984 were nongovernmental institutions. The Australian and British data also underestimate the importance of the private sector since they exclude private beds in public hospitals (Day and Klein 1985; Tatchell 1982; Wood and Thomas 1986).

[2] The index of dissimilarity between a hospital board's share of the total supply of private beds and national population increased from 0.14 to 0.21 (1945–1955) and peaked in 1965 (0.23). However, since then the index has declined slightly from 0.22 to 0.20 (1975–1985), reflecting the growth of private hospitals in selected regional cities outside the main metropolitan areas.

[3] In May 1988 a major review, commissioned by the government, was published (New Zealand Department of Health 1988). The report recommends the creation of a modified market with a proposed structure for health services that separates funder and provider and ensures competition among providers for service contracts. Whether these recommendations will be implemented by the present Labour Government is uncertain.

Chapter 5

Rolling Back the State?

Privatization of Health Services under the Thatcher Governments

JOHN MOHAN

A notable feature of ten years of Conservative government in Britain from 1979 is that only in early 1988 did the government institute a major review of the National Health Service's (NHS) funding and organization. Nevertheless, important changes had taken place in private-sector provision, and this paper considers the extent of health services privatization from 1979 to 1987. There are many different forms of privatization, as shown in chapter 1 (Hastings and Levie 1983; Le Grand and Robinson 1984). For this paper, the most relevant forms are the private funding and/or provision of services and the contracting-out of services from the NHS to private agencies. Some elements of privatization are not relevant to health care. The key question is the nature and delimitation of the boundary between public and private provision. Services can be provided in various ways, and there is considerable potential for substitution between private and public services (Gershuny and Pahl 1979; Pinch n.d.; Urry 1987). The criticisms of public service provision represent an attempt to redraw the boundary between public and private provision in favor of the latter. The notion of privatization represents an important break with the consensus on which the NHS was based. Hence the arguments for and against privatization in the British context must be examined.

Support for privatization has been mobilized around several claims for the virtues of private provision. The case for privatization rests on the arguments that private provision can supplement the state's finite resources, that the private sector is more efficient than public provision, that individuals should be free to choose private health care if they wish, and that public-sector trade unions are a source of inflexibility and inefficiency. On the other hand, privatization carries with it an implicit attack on the concept of the NHS. Although the government claims to be committed to the NHS, its conception of the organization and management of the service involves an emphasis, as never before, on performance, efficiency, and value for money. This has allowed opponents of government policy to raise questions about the merits of this more commercial approach to running the NHS. The government's encouragement of commercial health care has likewise raised questions about priorities and the ethics of for-profit health care.

In addition to these technical arguments, privatization accords well with the wider "two nations" political strategy that the Conservative governments have pursued. Briefly, this strategy involves the protection and consolidation of support from a "first nation" comprising the "productive" members of society—in general, those engaged in profit-making private-sector activity. At the same time, the "second nation" becomes more marginalized. This second nation is held to comprise, among others, those working in the "unproductive" state sector, those dependent on state benefits, those living in depressed regions or inner cities, and so on (see Jessop et al. 1984 for a full discussion of this interpretation of Conservative political strategy). Crucially, the productive members of the first nation are to be rewarded through the market for their contribution to production. This could involve encouragement of private health care or education or the expansion of private provision of ancillary services, thus creating new material interests in the private provision of services. This, in turn, strengthens the political lobby favoring private over public provision. It may be that privatization has been pursued more because of its political significance in consolidating electoral support than because of its technical advantages.

Privatization has also had important spatial and social consequences. Spatially, the balance between NHS and privately provided services has been altered dramatically in some areas, leading to talk of a dual or even a two-tier health care system (Hunter 1983; Day and Klein 1985). In social terms, possession of private medical insurance may lead some individuals to reconsider their attitudes toward the NHS. Privatization can also have direct material effects, especially for those ancillary workers whose jobs are affected by competitive tendering. Finally, privatization means important changes in the relationship between private capital and the state. Not all requests from representatives of the private sector for greater state intervention have been granted by the government; conversely, in some respects the government has gone further than private-sector representatives have sought.

This chapter examines four key aspects of privatization under the Conservative administrations since 1979: the private finance and provision of health care, the public finance and private provision of health care, the subcontracting of NHS services to the private sector, and the commercialization of the activities of health authorities. We examine policy initiatives and their social and spatial impacts for all four aspects. In the concluding section we discuss the wider political implications of these developments.

Private Funding and Provision of Acute Hospital Care

Because of the extent of public support for the NHS, there has been no attempt to replace it with an insurance-based system. Instead, the government has created a climate favorable to the private sector, encouraging its growth on the grounds that public resources are necessarily finite. Arguments for private provision usually counterpose the private sector's supposed virtues of efficiency, responsiveness to demand, and consumer sovereignty to the alleged shortcomings of the NHS (Adam Smith Institute 1981; 1984; Bow Group 1983; Forsyth 1983; Minford 1984). This is part of the New Right's attack on collectivism and is part of an attempt to set the agenda for a society where individual preference and choice replace the dead hand of the state, thus releasing more resources and creating a climate of enterprise (Bosanquet 1983). Private-sector advertising has attempted to exploit public dissatisfaction with the NHS by stressing the advantages (notably, avoiding waiting lists) of going private (Griffith, Iliffe, and Rayner 1987).

However, the prime minister's claim that "the NHS is safe with us" has so far precluded any overt attack on the NHS, so the steps taken to expand private health care have been indirect. For example, there has been a relaxation of controls on new private hospital developments and NHS consultants may carry out more private practice than hitherto, but the government has not introduced tax concessions for those taking out private medical insurance (Griffith, Rayner, and Mohan 1985). The private sector is seen by the government as supplementing, not supplanting, the NHS. It increases the total volume of health care provision at a time when the state's resources are limited. Undoubtedly, the limited growth in NHS funding and the general public perception of a crisis in the NHS have also encouraged individuals to contemplate insuring against the cost of private treatment.

Hence, there has been a steady expansion in insurance coverage. There are now over two million subscribers to private health insurance schemes, representing an insured population of some five million (just under 10 percent of the population). Much recent growth has been in company-paid schemes, under which all or part of the subscription is paid by employers. These now account for over half the insured population (BUPA 1986). Although peak rates of growth were experienced in the postelection years of 1979 and 1980, expansion had started in the mid-1970s in response to restrictive incomes policies; many firms offered insurance as part of recruitment packages for senior employees (Incomes Data Services 1984). Insurance coverage is skewed towards prosperous southeast England and toward the professional and managerial classes. For instance, 23 percent of all professional and managerial socioeconomic groups are covered for private health care (U.K. OPCS 1985).

Reflecting this growth there has been rapid expansion in the acute hospital sector. There are now over ten thousand beds in some two hundred independent hospitals. The key feature of this expansion has been commercialization and the entry of multinational capital (Griffith, Rayner, and Mohan 1985; Mohan 1985; Rayner 1986, 1987). Prior to the 1970s the indigenous private sector comprised mainly charitable or religious institutions. These could not generate the capital for new developments, so market leadership quickly passed to the commercial sector. In particular there has been greater market penetration by multinational hospital chains, including United States–based corporations (e.g., Hospital Corporation of America [HCA] and American Medical International [AMI] and Middle East–backed organizations. The United States–based chains had targeted England because, as the 1983 edition of the *Directory of U.S. Investor-Owned Hospitals* put it, "opportunities for expansion are especially bright in countries with ailing health care systems, such as England" (quoted in Griffith, Rayner, and Mohan 1985, 37). England was also a target because of the lack of organization in the indigenous hospital sector and because of the reluctance of the city of London to invest in private health care (Mohan 1985).

As a result, there has been a selective expansion of the private acute hospital sector. In total, 3,488 new beds opened in the United

Kingdom between 1979 and 1986, an increase of 52 percent. The great majority of new beds were owned by profit-making organizations, and, as a result, the charitable sector owned 46 percent of acute hospital beds in 1986, compared with 71 percent in 1979. Of the sixty-four hospitals opened since 1982, 90 percent were owned by for-profit groups. American-owned beds accounted for 23 percent of the 1986 total, compared with 6 percent in 1979 (AIH 1987). Increased competition has produced excess capacity, leading to hospital closures and mergers. This has principally affected small, under-capitalized single-hospital units run by charities, though small commercial hospitals have not been exempt. Thirty-four hospitals closed between 1979 and 1987, and in 1985 there was a net loss of 112 beds (AIH 1987).

Heightened competition has exposed divisions within the private health care sector. Senior executives, schooled in the British tradition of non-profit health care, have attacked the profit motive as being in-imical to British traditions and for generating inflationary pressure. In response, United States chains have pointed to their role as market leaders, the quality of their facilities, and the scale of their investments in Great Britain (Griffith, Iliffe, and Rayner 1987, chapter 4). There have also been suggestions (see Mohan 1986b) that the government could and should do more to stimulate private-sector expansion, such as by granting tax relief on medical insurance premiums. However, this would involve a subsidy to the private sector from the public purse, and so it seems unlikely at present. The possibility of taking account of private-sector provision or work load in the calculations of NHS regional resource allocations in England has been suggested (Klein 1982; Williams et al. 1984a, 1984b), but this poses technical and political problems. The technical problems concern the precise relationship between private and NHS provision: whether it is a complementary or a substitute service, whether to take provision or work load into account, and the pace at which any change would be introduced. Politically, taking account of private facilities in these calculations would be an acceptance that part of the nation's health care resources should be provided privately, thus exposing the government to the charge of producing a two-tier health care system. The most likely option seems to be an expansion of contractual arrangements between the NHS and the private sector, perhaps in-volving some degree of private finance for new NHS capital developments, as has already been proposed in the South East Thames Regional Health Authority (RHA) (Rayner 1986).

There are two main implications of this, one relating to the future geography of health care and the other, more generally, to public attitudes toward the welfare state. Although the private sector has grown rapidly, England is still far from having a two-tier health care system. However, in some localities private health care plays a substantial role. In the South West Thames RHA, 25 percent of elective surgery is carried out privately (Williams et al. 1984b). The private hospital sector also has a substantial presence in major cities, not only in central London but also in Birmingham and Manchester. As Hunter (1983) forecast, on a local scale a two-tier system may develop.

Concerning public attitudes toward welfare, in certain areas, such as the outer metropolitan area around London, some 15 percent of the population has private medical insurance (U.K. OPCS 1985), and this proportion may rise to 20 percent locally (Mohan 1984a). This creates a substantial constituency who do not need the NHS except in emergencies. It may have an important ideological effect: "Many people will become accustomed to building up for themselves mixed bundles of public and private welfare . . . without seeing any great ideological implications in this" (Crouch 1985, 14). This may prepare the ground for the introduction of much more commercialization in the management and planning of the NHS. In such a scenario, the private sector will play a much greater role.

Public Finance, Private Provision: Nursing Homes for the Elderly

The previous section was a discussion of an area of privatization in which both funding and provision are the responsibility of the private sector. In numbers of clients, however, the private provision of long-term accommodations for the elderly is of much greater significance. This type of care is much closer to the United States model in that it relies to a large and increasing extent upon public funds.

The provision of long-term care for the elderly population is a major social-policy challenge for all societies and is a localized problem because of the concentration of the elderly in areas of retirement migration. In England these are concentrated on the south coast (Law and Warnes 1984); in some communities in Devon, 60 percent or more of their population is of retirement age (Maguire and Mohan 1986). The Conservative government has permitted the cost of accommodating elderly people in private nursing homes to be met by the social security budget in cases where no suitable public-sector accommodation is available (Godber 1984). No assessment of individual needs is made. Andrews (1984, 1520) has argued that residents may be selected on the grounds of their docility rather than their disability. Initially, there was no limit on the amount of money that could be paid to cover the costs of private accommodation, but, subsequently, upper limits have been set. The principal effect of this policy has been to stimulate rapid expansion of the nursing home industry. In total there were 41,570 beds in private nursing homes for the elderly in 1985, representing an increase of 134 percent on the 1982 figure of 17,728. To put this in context, the average number of available beds in all NHS hospitals in England in 1985 was 325,000. Hence the private sector is around 15 percent of the size of the NHS. In the District Health Authorities (DHAs) of Brighton, Hastings, and Worthing, there are now more beds available in private institutions than in the NHS (U.K. Hansard 1987). There are exceptional concentrations of such homes within health authorities (Blacksell, Phillips, and Vincent 1987).

There are three main implications of this growth in private nursing home beds. First, the growth of private nursing homes is a response to the needs of localities that have a high proportion of elderly people as a result of retirement migration. However, the very availability of accommodation is stimulating additional migration, which increases demands on local health and social services. Consequently, some local government authorities have limited the amount of nursing home accommodation (Phillips and Vincent 1986b; Ray 1987).

Second, there is the issue of the regulation and monitoring of standards in private nursing homes. There is anecdotal evidence that standards of provision can leave much to be desired. A report on nursing homes in the West Midlands, for example, found evidence of "a pattern of bad practice" in a sample of nursing homes. It noted that many homes "fall well below any acceptable standards of decency and are a disgrace. . . . Ill treatment, indignity and abuse are a daily occurrence" (West Midlands County Council 1986, 1). Such practice is not confined to private homes, of course, but what this points to is the need for strict regulation of all providers of welfare services (Day and Klein 1987; Higgins 1984). This poses an interesting ideological dilemma: private nursing homes symbolize the archetypical small business so favored by the Conservatives, yet they depend on public money. Further regulation would compromise still further the independence of these businesses (Phillips and Vincent 1986a).

Finally, social security payments to residents of private nursing homes are geographically concentrated in areas of retirement migration. The sums are considerable; Harman (1987, 2) reports that over £200 million per annum is being spent in this way. Given the distribution of private nursing homes, it is clear that even on a pro rata basis the bulk of this money will be spent in the south of England. This represents a revenue transfer back into precisely those areas from which NHS resources are being transferred under the RAWP (Resource Allocation Working party) scheme (U.K. DHSS 1976).

The other principal form of privatization in this context is the transfer of former patients of long-stay psychiatric hospitals out of institutions into the community. The aims of this policy are to help patients lead autonomous lives and to avoid the stigma and institutionalization associated with long-stay hospitals. Community care has a long history, but actually "making a reality of community care" has proved elusive. Since 1981, however, a policy of community care has been officially endorsed by central government (U.K. DHSS 1981). This policy has recently been evaluated by government agencies (U.K. House of Commons 1985a), and these evaluations are summarized here.

A key problem in managing the transition to community care is ensuring that resources are available to provide replacement facilities when long-stay hospitals are closed. The House of Commons Social Services Committee emphasized that genuine community-care policies were achievable only in the context of a real increase in resources over a period of several years. There were important obstacles to building up community-based services. It was difficult to provide such services without closing down long-stay institutions in order to release the necessary resources. Equally, the closure of long-stay institutions was problematic without alternative facilities being available. Health authorities were thus caught in a vicious circle. There was also pressure from central government for health authorities to close down what were regarded as underused facilities, in order to realize the value of these assets, but there was no parallel pressure to develop the kind of facilities that could replace hospitals (U.K. House of Commons 1985a, xxi). Local social services departments were often reluctant to take over responsibilities for the care of ex-NHS patients, especially the mentally handicapped, while central government restrictions on local-authority expenditure severely constrained their ability to provide suitable services (Phillips and Radford 1985).

The effects of this have been that many patients have been discharged into a community that is simply unable to care for them.

Many former patients have ended up on the streets, in doss-houses (flop-houses), or in prison (Haynes 1986, 227). Others have found private-sector accommodation. Some of this is inadequate rented or bed-and-breakfast accommodation where the discharged patients are often vulnerable to exploitation by landlords. This type of accommodation is not conducive to leading autonomous lives (Eyles 1986). Others obtain places in private nursing homes, which poses questions about the regulation of such facilities and the training of suitable proprietors for them. A more general problem is that private hostels become available in unplanned locations and unplanned quantities. This imposes additional and unpredictable demands on statutory services, and it can mean that services are not always planned in relation to the needs of patients (U.K. House of Commons 1985, 1x–1xiii). Thus, the private sector is being asked to shoulder an important new role of caring for former patients of long-stay psychiatric hospitals, but this is posing questions about regulation, the appropriateness of facilities to need, and possible exploitation of patients. Finally, the ideological underpinnings of the notion of community care must be noted. A persistent theme of Conservative government rhetoric has been that there exists in the community an untapped "pool of carers" (like Bush's "thousand points of light") who are able and willing to provide informal care (Walker 1982). These carers are, by and large, women, and the community-care program thus assumes that women's roles should be confined to the "private" sphere of the family and the home. This dimension of privatization has been neglected by many geographical studies of service provision (Kofman and Lethbridge 1987). The notion of privatization can thus be extended beyond a simple classification of the provision of formal health services in the public domain to include consideration of the roles of men and women in the private sphere of the family and the home.

Subcontracting Ancillary Services

In addition to the direct provision of health care, privatization encompasses the private provision of ancillary services such as cleaning and catering. Subcontracting ancillary services in England began in several Conservative-controlled local authorities in the early 1980s. Following the 1983 election, all health authorities in England were required to expose their services to competitive tendering. The timing of this initiative reflected the government's increased confidence after being returned to office with an enlarged majority and its desire to weaken NHS trade unions following their involvement in major NHS industrial disputes in 1978–1979 and 1982. The move toward competitive tendering fit well with other managerial initiatives pursued after the 1983 election, notably the drive toward greater efficiency in the NHS embodied in the Griffiths Report on NHS management (U.K. DHSS 1983b).

Health authorities were instructed to submit their main support services (laundry, cleaning, and catering) to competitive tender to discover "whether savings can be made and resources released for improved patient care" (U.K. DHSS 1983a). The standard NHS terms and conditions of service, which stipulated wage rates, holidays, sickness benefits, and bonus entitlements, could be ignored because local market forces were to be responsible for setting wage rates. Thus, the policy accorded well with other strands of Conservative thinking on the labor market, which stressed the importance of removing labor market inflexibilities.

The implementation of the policy was marked by considerable conflict. Resistance was to be expected from the work force—after all, some two-hundred-thousand jobs were potentially affected— but many DHAs had built up good relations with their work forces, which they were reluctant to disrupt. Hence there was conflict between DHAs and central government and between trade unions and DHAs. The extent of contracting-out of services has been uneven. As of September 1986, the target date for completion of tendering, health authorities had sought tenders for 68 percent by value of their ancillary services, with values for individual RHAs ranging from 46 percent in North East Thames to 88 percent in the North Western and Wessex RHAs. Although there was no obvious pattern to the proportions of services put out to tender, it was notable that private contractors had been considerably more successful in the Thames RHAs than elsewhere. Private contractors had won over 50 percent of all contracts in North West Thames, and between 30 and 49 percent in the other five RHAs in the southeast (fig. 5.1; National Audit Office 1987, 13). An analysis of competitive tendering to the end of the 1984–1985 financial year showed that progress had been more rapid in rural than in urban DHAs and that, within London, several inner London DHAs had initially been slow to put services out to

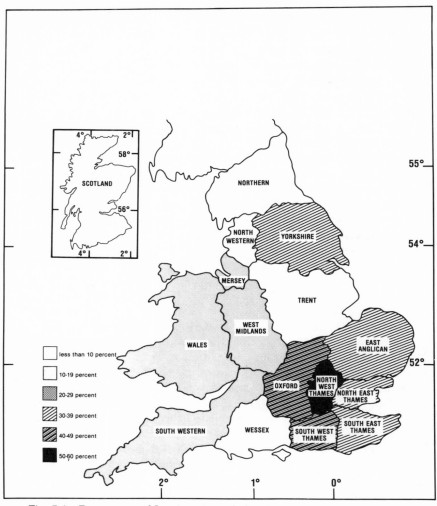

Fig. 5.1. Percentage of Services Awarded to Contractors in Great Britain
to September 1986

Data source: National Audit Office 1987. Crown copyright. Reproduced
by permission of the Controller of Her Majesty's Stationery
Office.

tender, whereas in suburban DHAs, tendering had proceeded much more quickly (Mohan 1986a).

There are technical and political reasons for variations in contracting-out. The cost of capital equipment can be a barrier to entry for laundry and catering industries. Economies of scale mean that it may not be worthwhile for a private contractor to tender for a catering contract if the hospital has less than four-hundred beds. Likewise, in rural areas the volume of work to be done and the logistics of collecting and delivering laundry and meals imply that catering and laundry contracts will be less attractive to contractors (Sherman 1985, 806). Capital developments in NHS hospitals in the past two decades have meant that a large proportion of laundry and catering plants are now modern and efficient, so contractors have struggled to break into the market (Ascher 1987, 171–181). It is also likely that established laundry and catering firms with reputations to lose will be reluctant to push their contract prices too low for fear that they will be unable to maintain their customary quality. This may help account for the private sector's relative lack of success in laundry and catering. Private contractors, have, therefore, been most active in tendering for cleaning services. Barriers to entry are very low for cleaning services, and a large proportion of the cost of the tender is accounted for by wages. Private contractors are able to undercut NHS tenders substantially by cutting down on the wages bill, and the scope for doing so is much greater in cleaning (Griffith, Iliffe, and Rayner 1987).

Several political factors, including union resistance, health authority reluctance, and government interference, have also influenced the process of subcontracting ancillary services. Government ministers have overruled several decisions reached by health authorities. For example, some health authorities have been compelled to put contracts out to a private contractor, rather than accept to tender from their own employees, even though the private contract has not always been the cheapest option (Ascher 1987, 186). Many health authorities initially refused to comply with government instructions on competitive tendering, but few have maintained their opposition. Trade union resistance has been generally confined to well-publicized disputes at individual hospitals such as those at the Barking and Hammersmith hospitals in London (Huws and de Groot 1985). More extensive opposition was mounted in the northeast of England. There, hospital staff and non-NHS unions mounted demonstrations and stoppages. In a region where unemployment was approaching 20 percent, campaigners were able to stress the social costs of unemployment and the importance of NHS jobs. These campaigns achieved their short-term objective of dissuading health authorities from pursuing competitive tendering, but their long-term impact remains to be seen (Mohan 1986a).

The impact of contracting-out in the NHS has, therefore, been uneven, reflecting a complex mix of technical and political factors. In considering its wider implications we should examine whether the declared aim of releasing resources for patient care has been achieved. Cash savings of some £103 million have been claimed by the government (U.K. H.M. Treasury 1988). Against this must be set several unquantified costs, including redundancy (unemployment) payments to former NHS employees, social security payments to those forced to accept lower wages, and the considerable costs in staff time and effort of preparing specifications for contract tender documents. Bearing in mind that the total gross savings amounted to less than 0.5 percent of the NHS budget, one can sympathize with the view of the House of Commons Social Services Committee that the competitive tendering initiative had "not brought home the bacon" (U.K. House of Commons 1985b, xx).

Contracting-out also has very important implications for the work force. NHS contracts have to be offered to the lowest tender, and the main source of financial savings is to reduce the costs of labor. This has been done, in general, by cutting back on nonwage costs. For example, holiday and sickness benefits and bonus payments are reduced, and a higher proportion of part-time workers are employed, thus circumventing the need for the employer to pay national insurance contributions for workers employed for less than sixteen hours a week. Private contractors typically also seek higher work loads from their employees (there are parallels here with the intensification of labor that has characterized recent developments in manufacturing industry [Massey and Meegan 1982; Mohan 1988; Pinch n.d.; Urry 1987]). Cost savings are, therefore, being generated at the expense of the worst-paid section of the NHS work force by increasing the rate of exploitation of labor and passing on some of the (formerly socialized) costs of reproducing the labor force—a classic capitalist solution to economic problems. The process is divisive, and its worst effects are felt by the part-time, predominantly female, work force in the NHS ancillary services (Coyle 1985; Paul 1986). The process has important parallels with the casualization of the peripheral sectors of the labor force—those whose labor is marginal to the goals of their organization (Atkinson and Meager 1986).

Blurring the Boundaries: Public-Private Sector Collaboration

When the NHS was founded, all but some three-hundred hospitals were taken into state ownership. The remaining private hospitals often collaborated with the NHS by taking NHS patients on a contractual basis. This helped the NHS considerably in cases where new hospitals could not be built in the early postwar years due to public expenditure restraint. More recently, there has been evidence both of greater government encouragement for collaboration and of increased private-sector confidence in its ability to assist the NHS. Three examples are cited: the encouragement of charitable fundraising for hospitals, a proposal for joint planning between a DHA and the private sector, and the possibility of commercial involvement in the running of parts of some hospitals in London.

Government ministers have frequently stressed the desirability of supplementing public funds with private finance. Charitable support for hospitals is something no one, presumably, would discourage. However, at least one hospital was saved from closure in 1983 only because a charitable trust agreed to provide funds when the health authority responsible was unable to do so (Sherman 1984). More recently the government has made it clear that its financial commitment to the NHS is finite, for it has refused fully to fund the £50 million capital cost of redeveloping the Great Ormond Street Children's Hospital in central London. Hence, a national appeal has been launched for the balance—some £20 million. This appeal for a national specialist children's hospital has attracted considerable support, but it will make it harder for local appeals to succeed, backed as it has been by enormous media coverage.

The second example of government encouragement of private-sector collaboration is one DHA's proposal to investigate options for keeping open a small hospital with private finance. The DHA concerned (Brighton) had originally planned to close the hospital as part of its longer-term strategic plan, but it recognized the value of small hospitals to the local community. Therefore, it was worthwhile to seek alternative sources of supplemental funds in order to confine health authority funding to a level consistent with wider priorities (S.E. Thames RHA 1985, 1). This seemed to imply that the public funds made available to the DHA were insufficient to keep the hospital open. The proposal was to set the hospital up as a charitable trust financed by private funds and the DHA, who would contract out private health care. NHS funds would underwrite the hospital's running costs so that private care could be offered at a lower price than in private acute hospitals. Thus, the proposal would expand choice for those able to afford private treatment, and, to the extent that the numbers of local people choosing private care increased, it would reduce NHS waiting lists. However, the proposal rested on the assumptions that NHS funds were necessarily limited and that the only way to keep this hospital open was to rely on private funds.

Commercial hospital chains have also sought greater collaboration with the NHS. Some examples include the proposal by AMI to build a private hospital within the grounds of Addenbrooke's Hospital, Cambridge (*Guardian,* September 27, 1986, 3); the London Independent Hospital's suggestion that it share skilled staff with nearby London Hospital (*Guardian,* November 9, 1986, 4); Charter Medical's statement that it was prepared to provide funds for a joint development with the Institute of Psychiatry, London (*Guardian,* December 11, 1985, 4); and bids by commercial organizations for the management of private wings in NHS hospitals. These developments can be seen as giving the private sector a foothold in NHS hospitals and as a logical extension of the private sector's policy of locating as close as possible to NHS facilities. Opponents, however, have pointed to the dangers of split loyalties on the part of staff and potential abuse of NHS facilities (Griffith, Iliffe, and Rayner 1987).

At present, there are few of these initiatives. While they could be welcomed as sources of additional funds for health care, their impact will be uneven. Opportunities for businesses to make profits will be greatest in the private wings of NHS teaching hospitals but nonexistent in small, peripheral hospitals and in geriatric and psychiatric services. Charitable and voluntary support may be much more forthcoming in the prosperous southeast than in the relatively depressed north of England, revealing important parallels with the pre-NHS situation. Finally, it can be argued that such initiatives will lead to a much more commercial approach to NHS planning and management in which considerations of profit and efficiency become dominant. Whether this is appropriate to the NHS is a theme taken up in the conclusion.

Conclusion

In evaluating the impact of privatization, the British experience is considered in terms of the claims made for privatization. These claims are that privatization generates additional resources for health care provision; that the discipline of competition leads to greater efficiency and to innovation, thus saving money; and that private provision is in some way superior to public provision since it rolls back the state and reduces the tax burden imposed by public expenditure. Following this, current attempts to review the basis of NHS funding are examined.

Privatization has generated additional resources—as evidenced by sums of money spent on private health care (some £1,000 million) or saved by competitive tendering for ancillary services (£100 million). Nonetheless, there are costs that are less easily quantified. Thus, the independence of the commercial health sector is questionable because it does not contribute to training nurses and doctors; many private hospitals have charitable status, conferring certain tax concessions; private hospitals draw staff from the NHS, contributing to NHS recruitment problems; and private hospitals often use NHS facilities for pathology and radiography (Griffith, Iliffe, and Rayner 1987, 243–251). Contracting-out ancillary services, likewise, has the hidden costs of making individuals redundant or forcing them to work shorter hours. Competitive tendering forces these workers to claim social security to compensate for their reduced income. There are also reduced contributions to the social security budget as a result of this (Paul 1986). Finally, the community-care program implicitly relies on unpaid sources of care in the family and community.

These hidden costs should be properly accounted for if the true financial impact of privatization is to be assessed. How these resources are used is another important question, which is bound up with considerations of efficiency. If one takes as evidence of efficiency the total absence of waiting lists for private treatment and the low average length of stay in private acute hospitals (around five days), then one might make a case for the superiority of private care. Yet, there are problems of comparability (Judge and Knapp 1985). The private acute sector only deals with a small proportion of total demand for health care, namely, nonurgent procedures performed, in general, on middleclass patients (Williams et al. 1984a, 1984b). Whether the private sector would be so efficient if it dealt with a full range of demands is a matter of speculation. The private sector's concentration on a limited market also suggests that competition does not necessarily breed innovation. Only one company, AMI, has attempted much diversification beyond acute medical and surgical treatment. There is also the question of priorities: the private sector makes little contribution to geriatric and psychiatric services, with the exception of private nursing homes, which are largely financed publicly.

Whether the state has been rolled back is also debatable. Obviously there has been an expansion of private-sector finance and provision, and the way the NHS is being run suggests growing private involvement. If the state has been rolled back in one sense, in another sense the state's regulatory role is greater: the growth in private provision of publicly funded care requires closer monitoring of private-sector activities. Likewise, the contracting-out of ancillary services requires close scrutiny of the services delivered by contractors (Day and Klein 1987). There has also been a qualitative change in the relationship between central and local government in the NHS, especially in relation to contracting-out. The available evidence suggests a considerable restriction of local autonomy in decision making (Ascher 1987). Thus, in health care, as in other areas of society, there have been attempts to roll back the state in some respects but to roll it forward in others (Gamble 1979; Hall and Jacques 1983).

Thus, the recent expansion of private-sector activity has clearly not been without problems. Further expansion of the private sector's role seems certain. The present crisis of underfunding in the NHS has certainly been a political problem for the Thatcher government, but it has given the government its opportunity to date of attempting to introduce a much greater degree of private finance into health care provision. The prime minister's review of the NHS was launched in January 1988 against a background of rising public discontent with developments in the NHS. Government thinking seems to be moving on two related paths. First, there is concern about the efficiency with which resources are deployed in the NHS. Government spokespersons have regularly pointed to variations in costs among DHAs, hinting strongly that these must reflect inefficiencies in the NHS (while ignoring the possibility that they reflect geographical variations in case mix, severity of conditions, social factors, or the cost of inputs). Hence, we can expect some variant of an internal-market scheme, under which health authorities would seek out low-cost providers of care (whether public or private) while keeping their costs low to attract trade. This would certainly involve a higher level of mobility of patients, and the competitive logic underpinning such a scheme would probably bankrupt older hospitals whose outdated physical plant would make it difficult for them to compete. Because hospital provision in the NHS is still heavily dependent on an uneven prewar legacy, NHS hospitals would be disadvantaged, and the most likely result would be a boost to the commercial-hospital sector, which has spare capacity and generally modern, efficient hospitals.

Second, Great Britain's poor record on health care spending (expressed as a percentage of GNP) is now being explained away as a result of its relatively low expenditure on private health care, so steps will be taken to expand spending on health care. We can probably rule out, for the moment, an insurance-based system because of evidence from the United States that it fails to provide comprehensive coverage (see, for instance, Cohodes 1986) and because of the massive transitional problems of moving to such a system. However, the 1987 Health and Medicines Act now empowers health authorities to raise funds from various commercial and charitable sources. Estimates suggest up to £70 million (some 0.3 percent of NHS expenditures) could be raised. The sums involved are thus marginal to the total cost of the service. More far-reaching possibilities seem to be on the agenda; right-wing analysts are increasingly calling for tax concessions to those taking out private health insurance or for experiments with Health Maintenance Organizations (HMOs). In particular, the possibility of individuals actually contracting out of the NHS and into private schemes is now being actively examined. All such schemes seem to contradict two fundamental principles of the NHS: that the healthy subsidize the sick and the rich subsidize the poor. The more the healthy and wealthy contract out of the NHS, the weaker the political lobby in its defense and the higher its unit costs of treating what it will be left with: the elderly, chronically sick, and working-class patients. For these reasons, such initiatives are to be resisted.

In conclusion, the problems with the limited privatization introduced in Great Britain in the last ten years are twofold. First, the measures described here are being introduced less for their technical superiority than as part of an ad hoc strategy to supplement the politically constrained budget of the NHS. Second, because these measures depend upon commercialization and competition, they will inevitably exclude some people and geographical areas from their benefits. The more the British NHS moves in this direction, the more closely it will approximate a two-tier system.

The financial support of a postdoctoral research fellowship (grant no. A23320036) from the Economic and Social Research Council (ESRC) is gratefully acknowledged.

Chapter 6

The Politics of Privatization

*State and Local Politics
and the Restructuring of
Hospitals in New York City*

SARA L. McLAFFERTY

The past two decades have witnessed increased privatization of hospital services in the United States. For-profit hospital chains have grown rapidly and have emerged as major providers of hospital care in many regions of the United States. At the same time, non-profit institutions, faced with increased competition and limited reimbursement, are adopting the diverse corporate strategies of profit-making firms. The growing financial and competitive concerns of both non-profit and for-profit hospitals are having important effects on the spatial organization of hospital services. Some communities are being left with few essential services, whereas others, targeted for investment, are receiving an array of new facilities and services.

These changes in the delivery, structure, and location of hospital services are generating some of the most important political conflicts over health service delivery since the 1960s. While much of this conflict is national in scope, significant debates are also occurring at the state and local levels, where the impacts of privatization are most visible and the tension between community and health care provider interests is most evident. Faced with significant service cutbacks, many community groups are organizing to preserve and improve health services in their local areas. What is the scope for community opposition to hospital restructuring and how can community groups confront the greater economic and political clout of health care institutions?

The privatization of health services is also raising important questions for state and local governments: should they allow competitive forces to determine the distribution of hospital services, or should they intervene to ensure minimum levels of access to services? I argue that in making such choices the state must confront the ever-present tension between supporting health care as an entitlement—that is, as a service that should be available at certain basic levels to all people—and supporting health care as an industry. The former favors government intervention to promote community health and maintain adequate access to services, whereas the latter favors allowing privatization to continue and competitive forces to determine the delivery and spatial organization of hospital services.

The purpose of this chapter is to examine the privatization of hospital services in New York City and the political controversies that have emerged as a consequence. The discussion focuses on the geographical changes in hospital service delivery brought about by privatization, the community opposition to such changes, and the role of the state in the privatization process. The political activities and power of hospital institutions, business organizations, local communities, and the state are considered. Particular attention is given to the conflicts between community and institutional interests and to the scope of community opposition to hospital restructuring.

The chapter is divided into three sections. The first consists of a brief discussion of the politics of health care and the main interest groups involved in making health policy. The next section considers the privatization of hospitals in the United States and the political and economic forces behind privatization. The final section examines the privatization of hospitals in New York City and analyzes in detail one hospital's corporate restructuring plan. The politics of the state's approval of the plan are discussed, along with the implications for community struggles over health care in other parts of the United States.

Politics of Privatization

The perspective adopted here is that the politics of privatization in the United States reflect the interplay between the interests of capital (businesses), the state, and local communities (Alford 1975; Mohan 1984b; McKinlay 1984). In understanding the nature of privatization in local areas, we have to consider the interests and demands of each of these groups, their political power and expertise, and their influence on state and institutional decision making.

Capital is not a homogeneous group, but consists, for our purposes, of two broad segments. First, it includes health care providers (hospitals, physicians, administrators) and the industries that produce and distribute medical equipment and supplies (pharmaceuticals, medical instruments). With health care accounting for more than 10 percent of the GNP, this group now constitutes one of the nation's largest industries (Relman 1980; Starr 1982). A broad range of economic and social concerns affect the behavior of firms and institutions in this group. Like all firms in a market economy, they are concerned with profitability while striving for enhanced prestige by providing specialized services and conducting advanced medical research (Ehrenreich and Ehrenreich 1970). These interests are strongly interrelated; profits provide the means to enhance prestige, and prestige in turn increases profits.

The second segment of capital consists of businesses not directly involved in health service provision. Their interest in health care relates primarily to the provision of employee health benefits. Such benefits are a significant expense; hence, businesses are concerned with the overall cost of health care and the level and quality of services available. Businesses also have a strong interest in the scope of government-financed health insurance programs. If such programs exist and eligibility criteria are generous, businesses may be able to shift the costs of employee health benefits onto the state.

The interests of the two segments of capital are often in conflict. The first group, health-related business, generally supports policies that increase demand for health care, such as increased government health expenditures and expansion of employee health benefits. In contrast, the latter group favors controlling health expenditures by reducing employee benefits and regulating health facilities. Each group puts pressure on the state in order to promote its interests (Marmor and Morone 1980; Bergthold 1987).

In addition to these pressures, the state has its own, often contradictory, interests. The first is the state's interest in controlling public expenditures for health care under Medicare, Medicaid, and other public health programs. In effect, the state is one of the largest purchasers of health care and therefore is legitimately interested in cost-control issues. The second is the need to support health care as an industry and as an essential component of the local economic base. Both nationally and locally, health care accounts for significant levels of employment and income generation and is closely linked with, for example, high-technology industries such as biotechnology and pharmaceuticals (Erickson, Gavin, and Cordes 1986). As a consequence, the state must be responsive to, and support, the more powerful and economically important interests in the health care industry. The result is a contradictory pressure to limit health expenditures while supporting the expansion of the health care industry (O'Connor 1973).

The politics of health care also concern community interests in obtaining adequate health services. Community, consumer, and labor groups have a long history of involvement in health affairs in the United States (Hatch and Eng 1984). Their political efforts address the most basic health care issues—for example, the accessibility and quality of health services, public health, and occupational health and safety. According to Alford (1975), community interests are often repressed because no social or political institutions ensure that such interests are met. Not only do communities lack the power, resources, and information needed to articulate their demands to the state, but also the state's response is often biased toward the more powerful interests of capital (Alford 1975). Communities are likely to become a more vocal force in health care politics, however, as service cutbacks increase and as the social costs of privatization become visible and politicized.

Political and Economic Context of Privatization

The term *privatization* has a somewhat different meaning in the United States than in other countries. Because so few health services have ever been provided publicly in the United States, privatization rarely entails the direct transfer of health service provision from public to private control. Instead, I use the term *privatization* to refer to two separate but related trends in the hospital industry. The first is *corporatization*—the increased role of large profit-making firms, such as hospital chains and hospital suppliers, in the delivery of hospital services (Starr 1982). *Corporatization* describes the transformation of hospitals, and health care in general, from an industry dominated by small, independent providers into an industry increasingly dominated by large national and multinational firms (Zuckerman 1983). The second trend is *proprietarization*, which refers to the increased tendency for non-profit hospitals to behave like profit-making firms (Kennedy 1985; Salmon 1985). The growth of marketing and advertising by non-profits, their diversification into profit-making businesses, and their increased business orientation provide vivid evidence of proprietarization. Thus, *privatization* refers here to changes in the behavior of health care institutions and the structure of the health care industry.

As noted in greater detail in chapter 2, the origins of privatization of hospitals in the United States lie in changes in health care financing that occurred during the 1950s and 1960s. Critically important was the enactment of Medicare and Medicaid in 1965. Under these programs the federal government assumed responsibility for paying for the health care of millions of elderly and poor Americans. By removing financial barriers to service use, Medicare and Medicaid made possible the use of health services that were previously unaffordable. The result was a sharp increase in hospital use and a corresponding increase in public expenditures for hospital services (Davis and Schoen 1978; Vladeck 1985). Just as important as Medicare and Medicaid to the emergence of privatization was the rapid growth of private health insurance coverage in the postwar period. This occurred as workers won improved health benefits during this period of low inflation and rapid economic growth. As with Medicare and Medicaid, the expansion of employee health benefits fueled the demand for hospital services, poured billions of dollars into local health systems, and began what has been called the "monetarization" of health care (Ginzberg 1984).

The effect of all this was to make health care a highly profitable area for corporate investment (Ehrenreich and Ehrenreich 1970). It is no mere coincidence that the first hospital chains appeared in 1968, just after the enactment of Medicare and Medicaid (Light 1986). Firms providing the entire array of medical products, technology, and services also grew rapidly (Whiteis and Salmon 1987); and by the early 1980s, health expenditures had risen to over 10 percent of the nation's GNP.

The rapid rise of health costs during the 1970s made cost control the dominant health policy concern of the 1980s. Pressure for cost control came from two principal sources. First, it came from businesses who had seen their outlays for employee health benefits increase much more rapidly than the rate of inflation. As early as 1970, businesses began calling for a basic restructuring of the health care industry as a way of controlling health costs (Bergthold 1987). Pressure mounted through the 1970s and became particularly intense during the recession of the early 1980s as businesses searched for ways to reduce costs and restore profitability. Health care fringe-benefits costs, which had risen so rapidly, were a logical target. At this time businesses began forming partnerships with the state around the issue of cost control. In many states, business groups actively lobbied for reimbursement controls, health facilities regulation, and other forms of cost containment (Bergthold 1987). Businesses also took direct steps to control their outlays for health benefits. These included reducing insurance coverage, increasing deductibles, and requiring second opinions for surgical procedures (Demkovitch 1986). These measures reduced reimbursement for hospitals and worsened competitive conditions in the hospital industry.

The state faced a similar crisis over health care costs. By the early 1970s, state, federal, and local governments were paying for a substantial portion of all health care under Medicare and Medicaid, and those expenditures had risen more rapidly than the rate of inflation. Faced with fiscal crises and large budget deficits, governments began searching for ways to reduce health care expenditures (Brown 1984). The economic necessity of reducing costs was reinforced by right-wing political ideology and public sentiment against the welfare state. Consequently, cost control emerged as the foremost health policy issue of the 1980s.

Initially, cost-control efforts focused on regulating the supply of health services and creating a "more rational" service delivery system (Altman 1983; Starr and Marmor 1984). Federally funded Health Systems Agencies (HSAs) were established in 1974 to coordinate regional planning of health services, certificate-of-need (CON) laws were enacted to regulate facilities' expansion and acquisition of new technology, and policies to encourage competition were adopted (Ginzberg 1983). But these programs had relatively little impact on health costs (Salkever and Bice 1976; Sloan and Steinwald 1980), and, by the late 1970s, attention turned to more direct cost-containment policies. The most important of these was the prospective payment system (PPS) for Medicare enacted in 1983. Under this system, hospitals are reimbursed a fixed amount for each diagnosis (DRG, or diagnosis-related group) regardless of the amount of resources used in patient treatment (Scarpaci 1988a). Although originally established for Medicare, PPS has been extended in many states to cover other third-party payers, such as Medicaid and Blue Shield.

What is emerging out of PPS and other cost-control initiatives is a new system of health care based on minimizing the costs of treatment and maximizing profitability. Its main feature is a shift of patient care away from the hospital and into less expensive settings (Ermann and Gabel 1985). The results are a shrinking market for hospital care and worsening competitive conditions for the hospital industry (Ginzberg 1983; Goldsmith 1980). While these forces are undermining hospitals' traditional role as providers of inpatient services, many hospitals have responded by moving into nontraditional service areas like ambulatory surgery, medical labs, and home care (Zuckerman 1983; Coddington, Palmquist, and Trollinger 1985). Hospitals unable to respond successfully have closed their doors (Hernández and Kaluzny 1983).

Other economic and social forces have exacerbated the effects noted above, especially for hospitals in urban areas. One important factor has been population change. During the 1970s, many cities in the Northeast and Midwest experienced population decline and a corresponding reduction in the demand for hospital services. Some urban neighborhoods lost more than half their population during the 1970s, and others changed dramatically in terms of economic and social status. For some hospitals, these local population changes have had a significant effect on the level and type of services needed within their catchment areas (Pleines 1980). Even more important than demographic change is the growth of population lacking health insurance. This is a diverse group comprising the working poor, the unemployed, illegal aliens, and the homeless (Vladeck 1985). It consists of people unable to qualify for Medicaid, lacking employer-sponsored insurance, and too poor to afford their own health insurance. The number of uninsured has grown in recent years as a result of reductions in Medicaid eligibility and the shift in employment from manufacturing to low-wage service industries. The latter often provide little, if any, employee health benefits (Cohodes 1986). Because most uninsured ultimately seek medical treatment at hospitals, and few can pay the full costs of care out-of-pocket, treating the uninsured represents a direct financial loss to hospitals. For public hospitals and non-profit facilities located in low-income areas, the losses may be substantial (Cohodes 1983).

These forces of economic and demographic change, coupled with government regulatory and cost-control policies, have dramatically altered competitive conditions for the hospital industry. The effects are evident locally, in the shifting geographic patterns of hospital facilities, in changes in health care employment and the structure of the hospital industry, and in changes in the mix and intensity of services provided. In some instances, these changes have prompted local opposition and debate, and in general it is at the local scale that issues of access to health care have been raised most effectively (Kirby 1984).

At the same time, hospital restructuring and community opposition to it have raised broader questions concerning the government's role in health care delivery and the limits and extent of state intervention: What is an appropriate balance between community and institutional interests, and can the state ever achieve such a balance in policy-making? These questions are played out in local community struggles to improve health conditions and obtain or maintain adequate health services.

These issues are explored in an analysis of privatization in New York City and the tension between community and institutional interests. I begin by discussing the privatization of hospitals in New York during the 1970s and 1980s. I then examine one hospital's corporate restructuring plan and the political response at the local and state levels. I analyze the hospital's planned relocation of services, community opposition to the plan, and the state's final decision in favor of the plan. The study is by nature a case study, limited in generality in both time and space. However, I will argue that the case study illustrates some of the fundamental health care issues facing local communities, governments, and hospitals, now and in the decades to come.

Privatization of Hospitals in New York City

The hospital industry in New York consists of three independent, but interrelated, systems: the municipal, voluntary (non-profit), and private (for-profit) systems. Municipal hospitals, which account for 20 percent of all hospital beds, are publicly funded facilities operated by a quasi-independent organization, the Health and Hospitals Corporation. Voluntary hospitals, the largest group, are operated by charitable institutions and include most of the city's teaching hospitals and many other large, prominent institutions. Finally, investor-owned, private hospitals constitute a small and shrinking share of the local market. Although the three hospital systems are functionally independent, they are linked by affiliation contracts, patient referrals, and other formal and informal arrangements. Moreover, all are affected by changes in government policy and by competitive forces in the health care industry.

Before discussing the privatization of hospitals in New York City, it is necessary to explain several factors that distinguish hospitals in

New York from those in many other parts of the United States. The first concerns the level and scope of state regulation of the hospital industry. Unlike many other states, New York has a long history of hospital regulation (Ginzberg and Ostow 1985). In 1969, New York adopted the nation's first prospective payment system (PPS) for hospitals (Bulgaro and Webb 1980). Under the original system, each hospital was reimbursed at a fixed rate per patient day, regardless of services rendered. Recently, however, New York shifted to the federally mandated, diagnosis-based PPS. Because rate setting bears so directly on hospital finances, rate setting has been the state's most powerful weapon for regulating hospital behavior and containing costs. In addition to limiting reimbursement, New York State has actively regulated hospital expansion and attempted to control acquisition of new technology by hospitals (Hillman 1985). New York has certificate-of-need laws requiring that hospitals obtain state approval for all new capital expenditures. The state has used this power aggressively in shaping the distribution of hospital services. For example, in 1982 the state imposed a freeze on $2 billion in capital-improvement plans by the major teaching hospitals. Since then, the state has approved some of those plans, but only after extracting concessions from the hospitals to increase their levels of community service (Wessler 1986).

A second factor that distinguishes the hospital industry in New York City from that in many other places is the presence of a substantial number of large teaching hospitals. Aptly termed "medical empires" (Ehrenreich and Ehrenreich 1970), these hospitals dominate the industry not just in size, but also in power, prestige, research, and service provision. They have extensive political and economic clout, and their actions greatly influence the nature of hospital care in the city (Vladeck 1981). The third distinguishing factor is the presence of the nation's largest municipal hospital system comprising eight acute-care hospitals and numerous clinics that service many of the city's neediest communities (Bellush 1979). During the fiscal crisis of the 1970s, municipal health facilities were cut significantly; today, however, the system's hospitals are so linked to teaching hospitals through affiliation contracts and so critical in service delivery to low-income areas that additional cutbacks are unlikely (Ginzberg and Ostow 1985).

The 1970s and 1980s were a tumultuous period for hospitals in New York City. The forces affecting the hospital industry cannot be discussed here in depth, but several deserve mention. Important changes in New York's hospital reimbursement policies were made in this period. The first occurred in the early 1970s when the state adopted its first PPS covering Medicaid and Blue Cross. In the early 1980s, the state shifted to a new reimbursement system, the New York Prospective Hospital Reimbursement Methodology, covering all third-party payers (Thorpe 1987). Finally, in 1986 the federally mandated DRG system was adopted. Compounding these events, certain long-term demographic trends have greatly affected the demand for hospital services. These include the presence of a large uninsured population (estimated at 1.4 million) whose numbers are expected to increase as the city's economic base shifts from manufacturing to services; localized patterns of population growth and decline; the increased numbers of poor, homeless, and elderly; and the recent AIDS crisis (McLafferty 1982; Ginzberg and Ostow 1985).

These forces produced hospital closures and excess capacity in the hospital industry in the city. Since 1970, more than forty hospitals have closed, representing a loss of 30 percent of all hospital facilities and 15 percent of all hospital beds. Most of the closed hospitals were small facilities with less than three-hundred beds (McLafferty 1982). A large percentage have been investor-owned, proprietary hospitals, though voluntary hospitals also make up a large share of all closures (table 6.1). Additional closures are likely in the near future because of falling occupancy rates and substantial excess capacity in the industry. Recent estimates place excess capacity in the hospital industry at 25 percent (*New York Times*, July 14, 1986, A-4), and achieving capacity reductions even close to that level will involve additional closures.

As a result of hospital closures, the hospital industry has become substantially more concentrated. The median bed size of hospitals in New York increased from 220 in 1970 to 409 in 1986, and large hospitals (those with more than 500 beds) increased their share of total patient days from 39 percent in 1970 to almost 50 percent in 1986.

Table 6.1. Number of New York City Hospital Closures, 1966-1986, by Hospital Type

Type	Number of Closures	Percentage
Proprietary	21	48
Voluntary	18	41
Municipal	5[a]	11

[a]Net change (7 closed, 2 opened)

Thus, with the closure of small hospitals, patient care has become more concentrated in the city's large, tertiary-care facilities, whose dominance in health care delivery has increased through the past two decades.

The worsening competitive health care environment has affected large hospitals as well as small. The shrinking size of the market for inpatient hospital care has set off intense competition among hospitals to preserve and enhance market share. To increase market share, hospitals have adopted a diverse array of corporate strategies analogous to those used by private firms. Advertising and marketing, once unheard of among hospitals, have become commonplace as hospitals compete for scarce patients. Hospitals are also diversifying into profit-making activities such as long-term care, medical laboratories, and real estate development. Changes in tax laws made these activities possible by permitting non-profit hospitals to maintain their tax-exempt status while operating for-profit subsidiaries (Roach 1982). The profits generated can be used to offset losses from inpatient care. Finally, financial constraints have made hospitals acutely aware of the images and profitability of the market areas in which they are located. To achieve entry into more favorable areas, hospitals have merged, established satellite facilities and doctors' offices for admitting patients, and bought up hospitals in profitable suburban locations (McLafferty 1986). The result is the erosion of services in unprofitable neighborhoods and concentration of facilities in more lucrative market areas.

The following discussion focuses on one hospital's geographical corporate strategy and the political conflict that ensued. The hospital is Saint Luke's–Roosevelt Hospital Center (SLRHC), a large voluntary institution, which in 1982 proposed an ambitious half-billion-dollar capital-investment plan. Certificate-of-need laws require that New York State approve such plans and obtain community input in the process prior to implementation. The politics of the implementation process in this case provides a useful illustration of the scope for community opposition to hospital restructuring and the conflicts inherent in the state's response.

Saint Luke's–Roosevelt Case Study

Formed by the merger in 1979 of 780-bed Saint Luke's Hospital and 535-bed Roosevelt Hospital, SLRHC is currently the largest voluntary hospital in New York City. The institution's two separate hospitals are located three miles apart on the West Side of Manhattan (fig. 6.1), at both ends of the rapidly gentrifying Upper West Side (Schaeffer and Smith 1986). The hospital's service area, as defined by the institution for planning purposes, runs from 34th Street to 134th Street and encompasses 40 percent of the hospital's inpatients and 60 percent of outpatients (SLRHC 1986). The population of the service area is socially, racially, and economically diverse. There are signifi-

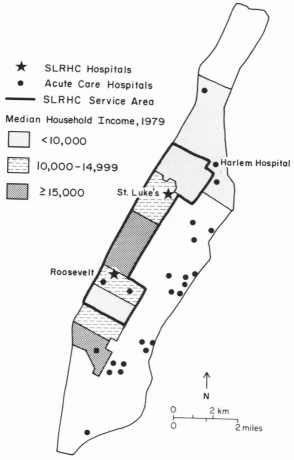

Fig. 6.1. Median Income Levels in and near the SLRHC Service Area, 1979

Data source: U.S. Bureau of the Census. 1980. *Census of population.* Washington, D.C.: GPO.

cant concentrations of high-need groups, including the elderly, the poor, and ethnic minorities. With the exception of the elderly, these high-need groups are most heavily concentrated in the northern part of the service area. On the other hand, the central and southern parts of the area contain a wealthier population and are experiencing rapid gentrification and new real estate development (SLRHC 1986).

When the two hospitals merged, both faced serious financial problems, though Roosevelt's problems were more severe. Merger provided a way to pool financial resources, consolidate services, and improve the institutions' access to capital markets (A. Choolfaian of SLRHC, letter to R. Gumbs of HSA of New York, January 14, 1987). It also helped to establish the hospitals' tie to the increasingly profitable, high-income market area of the Upper West Side and create a barrier to entry by other hospitals. In effect, with the merger the hospitals' orientation turned inward, rather than outward toward the lower-income communities to the north and south.

Though the merger did much to stabilize the financial condition of SLRHC, the institution still had seriously outdated facilities and services at both sites. These capital needs became the subject of a $434 million rebuilding plan, which the hospital submitted for state approval in 1982. The aim of the plan was to modernize facilities at both sites and consolidate and rationalize services. To achieve this, the hospital proposed a major reallocation of beds, resources, and services between the two sites. Each site was to offer a full complement of emergency, ambulatory, and basic medical-surgical services; however, the majority of specialized services and the bulk of inpatient capacity were to be shifted to Roosevelt (table 6.2). A new thirteen-story, 628-bed hospital was to be built at Roosevelt to serve as the new center of inpatient care. In contrast, the plan called for reducing the number of general-care inpatient beds from 728 to 348 at the Saint Luke's site, with more space devoted to research and administrative functions.

With reference to specific services, the plan proposed shifting all obstetric and pediatric beds to the Roosevelt site and concentrating drug detoxification, psychiatric, and AIDS cases at the Saint Luke's facility. Thus, Saint Luke's was to have a much smaller share of general inpatient beds, but a much greater share of beds for treating drug, alcoholism, psychiatric, and AIDS patients (127 beds versus 52 at Roosevelt). Viewing these disparities, community groups opposed to the plan charged the hospital with attempting to ghettoize the Saint Luke's facility by withdrawing essential services such as obstet-

Table 6.2. Distributions of Beds, St. Luke's-Roosevelt Hospital Center, New York City

Service	Existing in 1986		Proposed	
	Roosevelt	St. Luke's	Roosevelt	St. Luke's
Med/Surg	408	578	374	310
ICU/CCU	25	29	42	38
AIDS	0	0	19	37
Pediatrics	0	47	33	0
Neonatal ICU	0	16	22	0
Maternity	40	58	82	0
Alcohol detox	0	16	17	16
Drug detox	0	0	0	15
Psychiatric	39	36	16	59
Physical rehab	23	0	23	0
TOTAL	535	780	628	475

Source: SLRHC 1986, 6.

rics and emphasizing services stereotypical of poorer communities (Manhattan Health Working Group 1987).

SLRHC presented several arguments to justify shifting inpatient services from Saint Luke's to Roosevelt. The first centered around a demographic analysis of the hospital's service area. Based on an assessment of population trends and new housing construction, the hospital argued that population growth was concentrated in the southern part of the area, nearer the Roosevelt facility. However, in making its calculations the hospital failed to take into account the sharp disparities in need for services between the north and south. These issues later became the focus of community opposition to the plan.

A second reason given was the superior public transportation at the Roosevelt site. Roosevelt Hospital is located in midtown Manhattan at the hub of many major bus and subway lines. It is more accessible than Saint Luke's to New York City residents; however, accessibility within the SLRHC service area is not necessarily superior at the Roosevelt site, particularly for the low-income population residing in the northern section of the service area. The additional travel time from there to Roosevelt by public transit is between twenty-five and forty-five minutes depending on the mode of transit used and time of day. Such additional travel times could cause residents of the northern section to use alternative hospitals or forgo care altogether.

The third reason for shifting resources was financial. The buildings at Roosevelt were older and more dilapidated than those at Saint Luke's. As a result, the plan proposed replacing the Roosevelt facilities with a new and more economical multistory structure, while retaining some of the existing buildings at Saint Luke's. These architectural changes in turn affected decisions about the location of specific services. For example, a major argument in favor of concentrating all obstetric and pediatric services at Roosevelt was that the new Roosevelt facility could accommodate all nursing units on a single story, whereas the Saint Luke's site would require two storys. Single-story units generate significantly lower capital and operating costs than multistory units (Choolfaian to Gumbs, January 14, 1987).

While SLRHC insisted that the main motive for the plan was service consolidation and that the hospital maintained its commitment to community service, the plan clearly represented an attempt to reposition the hospital both geographically and socially. Underlying the plan was a marketing study conducted for the hospital in 1981. The study described data on consumer preferences and demographic, economic, and social trends within various parts of the hospital's service area. Strategies for improving market penetration, particularly among higher-income consumers, were discussed in detail. For example, the report concluded that

> consumers with low income levels are more likely . . . to prefer Saint Luke's hospital. . . . While preference for Roosevelt hospital is similar throughout the range of household incomes, preference for Saint Luke's is lower among respondents with incomes greater than $30,000 than among those in other income levels. . . . The need for SLRHC to improve its image among higher income households and those with more complete insurance coverage is clear. (SLRHC 1981, 64–65)

Although one can only guess at the exact role of the marketing study in plan formulation, the final plan is consistent with the marketing objectives stated above. By concentrating general-care services at Roosevelt, the hospital hoped to attract a higher-income clientele and thus improve its financial position and image among better-insured patients. Services at the Saint Luke's facility, on the other hand, would be more oriented toward Medicaid, psychiatric, and drug treatment patients, while deemphasizing general inpatient care. The result was an institution comprising two separate and unequal facilities.

Local Opposition

SLRHC's plan received relatively little public attention until September 1986, when the Health Systems Agency of New York called for a public hearing as part of its review of the hospital's CON application. At that time a coalition of local health activists, hospital workers, politicians, and representatives of community organizations formed to oppose the plan. The group called itself the Committee to Save Saint Luke's (CSSL). While strongly supporting SLRHC's need to modernize facilities, CSSL opposed the proposed redistribution of services from Saint Luke's to Roosevelt because it went against the pattern of community health needs in the service area.

Much opposition centered around the proposal to move all inpatient obstetric and pediatric services to Roosevelt. CSSL pointed out the plan's failure to take into account the large concentration of medically high-risk, underserved, childbearing populations in the northern part of the service area. Over half the babies born at SLRHC are to mothers who reside in areas north of the Saint Luke's site, areas that have some of the highest rates of infant mortality and low birth weight in the city (New York City Department of Health 1984). In fact, in 1985, just one year earlier, the state had designated that region as a "high-risk perinatal area" because of its exceptionally high incidence of perinatal problems. CSSL noted the irony of the situation, commenting on the hospital's "dereliction of responsibility to a high risk perinatal area" (CSSL 1986). In addition, CSSL emphasized that eliminating obstetrics at Saint Luke's would increase use of the already overcrowded services at nearby Harlem Hospital (see fig. 6.1). This, they suggested, could lead to significantly lower quality of care for the needy residents of northern Manhattan.

Similar arguments were expressed concerning the proposed shift of general medical-surgical beds to Roosevelt. CSSL noted that such beds were more heavily used at Saint Luke's than at Roosevelt and that shifting beds to Roosevelt would increase crowding at Saint Luke's. Finally, the CSSL questioned why the hospital had failed to include zip code 10031, directly north of the service area, within its service-area boundaries. The hospital's market penetration in that zip code (i.e., the percentage of the zip code's total hospital discharges to SLRHC) actually exceeded that for another zip code, the southernmost one in the service area, which had been included in the service area (fig. 6.2). Adding zip code 10031 to the service area would favor expanding services at Saint Luke's because far more patients from that zip code used Saint Luke's than Roosevelt.

These issues were raised at several public meetings during the fall of 1986 and expressed in letters to state and local health officials.

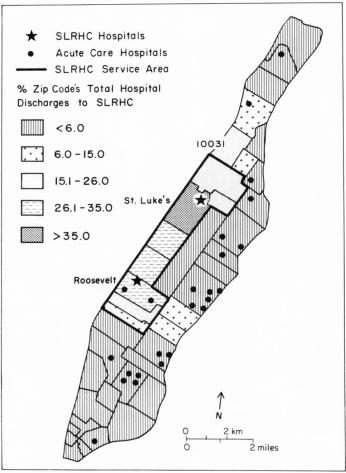

Fig. 6.2. SLRHC Market Penetration by Zip Code
Data source: United Hospital Fund of New York. 1982. *Inpatient hospital use in New York City, 1982.* Vol. 3 of *Community profiles.* New York: United Hospital Fund.

Other community groups, representing west Harlem and northern Manhattan, also joined in opposing the plan. Opposition was not universal, however. Community boards from the central and southern parts of SLRHC's service area came out in favor of the plan while recognizing CSSL's concerns about the relocation of obstetric services. In this context, with the community divided, the Health Systems Agency of New York approved the plan and forwarded its recommendation to the state. However, R. Sweeny of the New York State Department of Health, which must grant final approval, wrote to G. Gambuti of SLRHC asking the hospital to respond in detail to community objections, particularly concerning the relocation of obstetric services (December 30, 1986).

In its response, SLRHC emphasized the financial and architectural advantages of consolidating obstetric and pediatric services at Roosevelt. A detailed analysis was presented of the costs of three alternative service configurations: (1) providing all obstetric and pediatric services at Roosevelt, (2) providing all services at Saint Luke's, and (3) providing separate obstetric services at each site. An independent accounting firm estimated the costs of each alternative based on data provided by the hospital.

The analysis showed the first alternative to be substantially cheaper than the others due to both higher revenues and lower operating and capital costs (Choolfaian to Gumbs, January 14, 1987). Higher revenues were projected because of the facility's ability to bring in more patients covered by Blue Shield insurance (as opposed to Medicaid or uninsured patients). Presumably, SLRHC would attract such patients away from other tertiary hospitals in Manhattan. It is unclear, however, why more Blue Cross patients would be attracted under the first option than under the third option, which also included a full range of services at Roosevelt. The cost savings under the first option were more clearly spelled out. They stemmed from architectural considerations related to the smaller size of the floor plate at the Saint Luke's site. Providing all, or even some, obstetric services at Saint Luke's would require several floors, rather than the single floor that would be possible at the new Roosevelt facility. This would generate savings in labor and capital costs while enhancing coordination of services.

State Response

State health officials found SLRHC's cost and architectural arguments compelling and in early March 1987 approved the hospital's rebuilding plan. In response to state and community concerns, however, the hospital did agree to minor changes in the distribution of beds between the two sites: sixteen psychiatric beds were shifted from Saint Luke's to Roosevelt, and twenty medical/surgical beds from Roosevelt to Saint Luke's. In addition, the state and the Health Systems Agency called for continual monitoring of the impact of the relocation of obstetric and pediatric services, although the details and nature of the monitoring process were left vague (D. McGowan of HSA, letter to R. Sweeny, February 25, 1987). Finally, the state asked SLRHC to ensure that "any patient have access to the whole of SLRHC services regardless of which site they enter" (McGowan to Sweeny, February 25, 1987, 9). Here again, the state extracted an important promise from the hospital, but did not set up a mechanism for monitoring compliance.

What do the reactions of the New York State Health Department and Health Systems Agency to the SLRHC plan reveal about the politics of privatization? Although the state responded to community demands, it was not a fully objective arbitrator. Especially revealing is the way the state addressed the proposed relocation of obstetric services. To a large extent, the state's vision was limited from the start: it simply reacted to the three alternative proposals as put forth by the hospital (with input from the HSA), rather than devising and considering a full range of options. If, for example, obstetric services were to be provided at both sites, as in the third option, why must the two obstetrics units be approximately equal in size? Could not the floor plate at Saint Luke's accommodate a small unit for routine deliveries? By defining the set of alternatives, the hospital channeled political discussion in its favor.

In addition, the state and HSA were not highly critical in their analyses of the hospital's proposals. For example, in its proposals to the state, the hospital assumed that its service area would remain constant regardless of the configuration of services between the two sites. Yet any redistribution of services affects patient travel patterns, thus altering the hospital's service area and the relative need for beds at the two sites. The HSA recognized this possibility when it predicted that the consolidation of obstetric services at Roosevelt would cause some patients from the northern part of the service area to shift to other nearby hospitals. However, SLRHC was not asked to adjust either its revenue calculations or its bed-need proposals to reflect the patient shift.

Finally, and perhaps most important, is the way community

health care needs were considered during the planning and approval process. Both the state and HSA are responsible for ensuring that changes in the spatial organization of services are consistent with community health care needs. Yet it is unclear how needs figured in the final approval decision. Concerning the relocation of obstetric services, both the state and HSA recognized that needs were greater in the northern part of the service area. But neither organization attempted to predict how the relocation plan would affect that high-risk population's ability to use essential services. In the end, the HSA did call for "these changes to be monitored by local perinatal providers . . . as to impact on local residents" (McGowan to Sweeny, February 25, 1987, 4), but it made no attempt to forecast the likely impact and incorporate it in service planning. In approving SLRHC's plan, the state was implying that the cost advantages of relocation outweighed any adverse impacts on perinatal health. Thus, while paying lip service to community needs, the HSA and the state ultimately ruled in favor of the institution, supporting its right to relocate obstetric services according to its own financial imperative.

Conclusion

The privatization of hospital services is having profound effects on health care delivery in local areas. Although privatization is a national, and even international, process, its effects are uneven and highly localized. It involves the simultaneous expansion of services in some communities and withdrawal of services and investment from others, as health care providers seek out new and profitable market areas. Ironically, the communities most vulnerable to service cutbacks are often those with the greatest health care needs: low-income, underserviced communities in urban and rural areas. Only through local political action and state intervention can such communities oppose the privatization process.

This study has pointed out the limits of community struggles against privatization and the conflicts inherent in the state response. Community groups face many difficulties in organizing around health care issues and opposing market-based restructuring of health services. These difficulties stem in part from the basic nature of community interests. As Marmor and Morone (1980) have argued, community interests in health care issues are often diffuse and poorly defined. It is difficult for individuals to evaluate the effects of cutbacks on the quality and accessibility of services, and therefore to assess the costs and benefits of political action (Klarman 1978). As noted earlier, many of the communities adversely affected by service restructuring are, as in the SLRHC case, underserved communities where health is but one of a larger set of social and economic problems. Individuals in such communities lack the resources and political clout needed for successful political action and have many different issues that require their political attention. It is no surprise, then, that in the case study described here the most active members of the Committee to Save Saint Luke's were local health care activists and health workers rather than members of the larger community. Finally, the community itself often has disparate interests. In cases where the restructuring involves a shift of services from one location to another, the adverse effects on one community are offset by beneficial effects on another. With community interests so polarized, any decision appears to be a decision in favor of community interests.

The factors just described dilute the power of community groups in opposing service restructuring and decrease their chances of success. Their powerlessness stems not just from the characteristics of community groups, but more importantly from the political and economic dominance of the major health care institutions. The dominance of major institutions stems from their prestige in the medical industry, their strong representation on health planning organizations, and, increasingly, from their importance in local economies. The power of such institutions includes the power to define the agenda, to generate proposals for state aproval, and thus to control the direction of public debate. In the SLRHC case, the hospital set the agenda within which the state pursued its own goal of cost containment; community concerns were addressed only as an afterthought. Thus, communities are forced into a reactive stance and are left with no control over the nature and direction of discussion.

The difficulties inherent in community opposition to hospital restructuring reflect more fundamental issues in the privatization of health services. If health services are privatized and thus commodified, how can the health care needs of underserviced communities be protected? Maintaining adequate service levels in such communities clearly requires state intervention. The state, however, faces the near-impossible task of simultaneously ensuring that community needs are met and supporting the economic viability of health care institutions. If the state does not approve institutional requests, it risks losing the institution, either through closure or relocation, and losing the associated services, jobs, and income. Thus, the very fact that hospital care is provided by private or non-profit firms under market conditions requires that the state support the structure of the hospital industry and the position of the dominant institutions.

What, then, is the potential for community struggles to improve access to health services? Like many previous studies this one illustrates the difficulties community groups face in organizing around health care issues (Alford 1975; Ehrenreich and Ehrenreich 1970). The political and economic dominance of health care institutions, businesses, and the state makes communities relatively powerless. However, in this and several other cases, community groups have won minor modifications to hospitals' corporate plans (Gallagher 1986; Wessler 1986). This suggests that in states with responsive regulatory postures, community groups can win some local victories as long as they do not seriously compromise the interests of major health care providers and the state. Such victories will most likely be small and local in character, however, and it is only by linking struggles over health care to struggles over other social, economic, and health-related issues that communities can hope to achieve major changes in the structure of health care delivery in the United States.

PART TWO

Mental Health Services

Chapter 7

The Restructuring of Mental Health Care in the United States

CHRISTOPHER J. SMITH

Statistics about mental health care are enlightening, both for what they reveal and for what they conceal. A look at the recent data suggests that the delivery of mental health services in the United States has changed significantly in the last two decades. The system is now much larger and more complex organizationally, and it is increasingly dominated by privately operated services. In New York State alone, for example, 21 million units of inpatient and outpatient mental health service were provided in 1985 (table 7.1). In addition to the size of this operation and what it tells us about the mental health of New Yorkers, the cost to the taxpayer is enormous. It has been estimated that inpatient and outpatient treatment for mental illness in New York State cost more than $1.5 billion in 1985 (New York State Office of Mental Health 1986, 23). On the other side of the balance sheet, $1.5 billion was used to create jobs and generate incomes for New Yorkers, an activity that helped establish and solidify a vast range of constituencies whose self-interests have increasingly come to dominate the delivery system.

As this chapter will illustrate, changes in the mental health delivery system at the state level are much more likely to result from economic and political forces than from a concern about the quality and effectiveness of the treatment that is provided. Unfortunately, the primacy of these forces has had some disastrous consequences for those who receive the services. In New York State, for example, the cost of providing 11.4 million inpatient days of care was $1.6 billion in 1985, compared with only $400 million for 9.6 million units of outpatient care. The conclusion reached by policymakers who review such data is that tax dollars can be saved by changing the locus of care for the mentally ill through a policy of deinstitutionalization (Talbott 1983).

Table 7.1. Mental Health Services Provided in New York State, 1985

Units of Service (millions)	All Facilities	State-Operated Facilities	Local Providers
Residential days	11.4	8.6	2.8
Inpatient	9.5	7.8	1.7
Community residence	1.1	0[a]	1.1
Family care	.8	.8	0
Nonresidential visits	9.6	2.3	7.3
Clinic treatment	5.0	1.0	4.0
Day or continuing treatment	2.5	0.7	1.8
Other nonresidential programs	2.1	.6	1.5

Source: New York State Office of Mental Health 1986, 23, table 7.

[a] Fewer than 50,000 days.

In subsequent years the wisdom of this policy has been seriously questioned (Brown 1985) because, although patients no longer had to be supported in hospitals, they still needed extensive care in the community. The major costs incurred by shifting the burden of care onto the community are not borne by the state mental health systems, but by the federal government and the individual communities. The federal government has opted to phase out big government's role in the provision of human services, and many cities and states have chosen to avoid the expense of providing a comprehensive set of alternative services in the community (C. Smith 1986). The net effect of neglect by the federal government and the inability or unwillingness of the cities to care for the mentally ill is that the deinstitutionalized and the never-institutionalized have been forced onto the streets in the 1980s (Morrissey and Gounis 1987; Dear and Wolch 1987).

The Transfer of Care: A Case Study of New York State

The provision of mental health care in a state like New York is a vast and complex business. In general, New Yorkers want to have a system that provides easy access to high-quality mental health care

(Governor's Health Advisory Council, 1984). It is no surprise to find that New York State has more psychiatrists, clinical psychologists, psychiatric social workers, and psychiatric nurses per capita than any other state and that the state spends almost twice as much on each mental health client as the national average (NIMH 1983). A traditionally liberal philosophy toward the provision of services has resulted in a delivery system that is based on "conscience," to use Rothman's (1983) term. In the area of program development this conscience has been manifested in the following principles:

1. It is incumbent on the mental health system to provide a comprehensive array and a full continuum of services necessary to meet the needs of persons who are mentally ill.
2. It is essential that public mental health services be available and accessible to individuals of all cultures and be responsive to their special needs.
3. Public mental health services must be equitably distributed to address population need and reflect geographic variations.
4. It is essential that there be integration between the public mental health system and necessary generic health, housing, and social service systems to link the various providers into a total human service system. (Governor's Select Commission 1984, 18–19).

In spite of these high-minded principles, New York's delivery system has lurched through a series of violent and often contradictory changes within a relatively short time span. The changes are the result of what can be described as various forms of "transfer of care" (Brown 1985, 1988). The most visible of these has been the geographical transfer of patients from a centralized to a dispersed delivery system (from the asylum to the streets). Accompanying this has been a transfer of responsibility from the mental health to the public welfare sector, a transfer of financing from public to private sources, and a transfer of quality from professional care-givers to amateurs. Instead of having a system that is shaped by the public's conscience, New York is in danger of ending up with one that is shaped largely by convenience (Rothman 1983).

In New York State there has been a fiftyfold increase in the use of mental health services since the early 1950s (New York Medical and Health Research Association 1983). In spite of this, there is no evidence that the actual prevalence of mental disorder has increased significantly; in fact, most indicators suggest that the rates have stayed about the same (Ashbaugh et al. 1983). It appears, therefore, that the major changes in the pattern of mental health care are occurring in response to changes within the mental health system itself, particularly within the institutions and agencies providing care and between the cared-for and the not-cared-for. In the 1950s the mental health care system was the essence of simplicity. The poor went to public mental hospitals, while those who could afford to went either to individual psychiatrists or to private hospitals. Today, in New York and in many other states, we find an allied public-private sector that has resulted from the introduction of both public and private sources of funds into the delivery system.

Some of the changes that have occurred nationwide are illustrated in table 7.2. In spite of the sharp growth in outpatient mental health

Table 7.2.   Geography of Mental Health Care in the United States

	% of total mental health facilities		Inpatient Admissions (per 100,000)		Outpatient Admissions (per 100,000)	
	1970	1980	1970	1980	1970	1980
Public mental hospitals	10.7	7.5	244.4	172.0	82.5	36.8
Private mental hospitals	5.0	4.9	46.2	63.2	12.8	13.5
General hospitals	26.5	24.8	240.1	256.7	85.7	104.5
VA hospitals	3.8	3.6	67.9	84.0	8.4	5.6
CMHCs	6.5	18.5	30.0	110.6	88.7	548.6
Residential treatment centers for children	8.7	9.9	3.8	6.9	4.0	8.8
Freestanding outpatient clinics	36.9	28.3	--	--	270.4	370.3
All other facilities	2.3	2.5	11.8	10.8	23.4	49.9
TOTAL			644.2	704.2	575.9	1,188.4

Source: National Institute of Mental Health. 1983. *Mental Health, United States, 1983.* Edited by C. A. Taube and S. A. Barrett. DHSS Pub. no. (ADM) 83-1275. Rockville, Md., tables 2.3 and 2.8.

care from 1970 to 1980 (more than double the rate of admissions) and the much-publicized trend toward deinstitutionalization, institutional care still dominates the system and its budget (Deiker 1986). Inpatient admissions to all institutions increased from 644.2 per 100,000 in 1970 to 704.2 in 1980, although most of the increases were in general and private hospitals rather than public mental hospitals.

In New York State the trend toward private institutional care has been even more pronounced. Inpatient services in public mental hospitals fell from 23.2 million days in 1970 to 10.8 million in 1980, while the number of psychiatric beds in general hospitals and private mental hospitals more than doubled in the same period (Levenson 1985). Not shown in table 7.2 are three other largely private service categories, which now provide a major portion of the delivery system. A major concern about these new care providers is that they are largely staffed by people who are not mental health professionals, which has raised some important questions about the quality of care provided. The first category is the skilled nursing home (skilled nursing facilities, or SNFs). Since the population of state mental hospitals began to decline sharply in 1955, nursing homes have become the largest single provider of institutional services for the mentally ill; in fact, in statistical terms the proportion of individuals living in mental hospitals and nursing homes essentially replaced each other between 1950 and 1970 (New York State Communities Aid Association, 1983, 29). In New York State a recent study estimated that, of a total of 64,371 individuals living in nursing homes, 68.1 percent had significant mental disorders (Governor's Health Advisory Council 1984, 20).

A second group of nonprofessioinal providers to enter the mental health care scene in New York has been domiciliary care facilities (private proprietary homes for adults, or PPHAs). Of the nearly twenty-three thousand residents in such facilities in 1979, 30 percent had formerly been in state mental hospitals and another 15 percent were judged to be in need of mental health services (Welfare Research Inc. 1979). A third group of service providers that has recently emerged is the wide array of shelters for the poor and homeless. Although this remains a controversial issue, many have argued that the shelters are dominated by the deinstitutionalized and never-institutionalized mentally ill (Lamb 1984).

Looking beyond these statistics we can see an ever-expanding system of care in which clients are constantly moving from one facility to another. The quality of the psychiatric care they receive, if they receive any at all, is questionable. The net effect is that the policy of

deinstitutionalization has degenerated into one of transinstitutionalization as former public hospital patients have been admitted to the
psychiatric wards of general hospitals (Schoonover and Bassuk 1983)
and as many of those released to the community have ended up in
the new institutions such as SNFs, PPHAs, and shelters for the
homeless (Brown 1985). The image of clients in constant motion,
shuffling from the streets to the new institutions and then back onto
the streets, is reinforced by the news media in New York City. The
case of Sylvia Frumkin (a pseudonym) illustrates the plight of the
mentally ill; she spent a lifetime checking into and out of a variety of
inpatient, outpatient, and residential settings (fig. 7.1; see Moran,
Freedman, and Sharfstein 1984).

Two other observations are important in assessing changes in the
delivery of mental health services in New York State. One of these is
the marked geographic variability in the pattern of delivery from one
part of the state to another. In New York City itself, for example,
there is a chronic shortage of acute adult psychiatric beds, even
though the city has a much higher bed capacity per capita than almost all other areas of the state (table 7.3), and at most times these
hospitals are kept fully occupied (New York State Office of Health
Systems Management 1982). The shortage of beds has been attrib-
uted in part to the overall lack of mental health facilities, especially of
community-based services, which means that many discharged and
never-admitted patients have to be admitted to institutions. By 1981
this revolving-door phenomenon reached a crisis point, and over 40
percent of all Medicaid acute psychiatric inpatient days were accounted for by only 8 percent of the inpatients. New York City lags
behind the rest of the state in the number of beds provided in community residences, particularly in family care homes (including room
and board facilities), which suggests that there is a continual imbal-
ance between the demand for and the supply of services. This results
in a squeeze on other facilities within the system, which pushes out
needy clients who would otherwise have been served.

Another possible explanation for the shortage of psychiatric beds
in New York City is that there is an unusually large proportion of residents in high-risk categories for mental disorder, and this creates a
high level of demand for services. In New York State as a whole the
inpatient psychiatric population has changed considerably in the last
two decades. The most recent data show that the inpatient census
fell by 12.5 percent between 1980 and 1986 (New York State Office of
Mental Health 1986). This reduction can be interpreted in two ways.
In the first place, New York has traditionally had higher rates of

institutionalization than all other states, so the large-scale exodus represents a convergence with the nationwide trend toward deinstitutionalization (Smith and Hanham 1981). In other words, New York State is now actively doing what other states did in the 1970s. A second interpretation of the trend toward smaller institutional populations involves the changing age structure of the inpatient population; specifically, New York's institutions are beginning to house a much younger population than ever before. The discharge and admission rates among patients older than sixty-five have changed significantly in the 1980s, resulting in a 25 percent reduction in the resident population in that age group between 1980 and 1986 (table 7.4). Again it is important to point out that because New York has traditionally hospitalized more older people than most other states, a reduction of this magnitude (caused by lower admission rates and the transinstitutionalization of the elderly into nursing homes and domiciliary care facilities) has significantly affected the entire inpatient population (fig. 7.2).

Among the younger age groups the 1980s have witnessed a growth in resident patients in spite of the overall decline. This is particularly the case for the patients in the eighteen to thirty-four and thirty-five to forty-four age groups, which increased by 17.5 percent and 21.6 percent respectively. In these two age groups, often referred to as the "young chronics," it is also clear that admissions (and readmissions) are significantly higher among men than women. It appears that, since 1980, young adult male admissions to state hospitals have increased, and that once admitted they are staying longer. In a recent survey of these patients in New York State institutions it was noted that they are "sicker, more hostile, and less predictable than previous groups of young adult chronic patients" (Weinstein and Cohen 1984, 600). The fiscal and policy significance of this trend is that the young chronics will probably need extensive and often lifetime care within the institutions. The average length of stay for these patients is now increasing for the first time in nearly two decades. The longer they stay, the less likely it is that they will ever be able to live independently in the community.

Factors Influencing the Provision and Use of Mental Health Services

There is no doubt that demand factors are creating pressure on the mental health care system in states like New York. A combination of

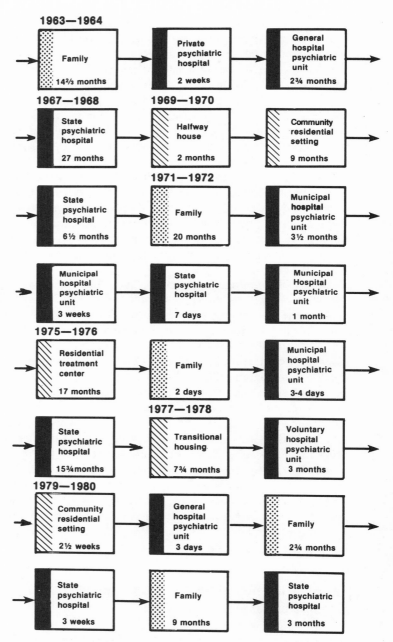

Fig. 7.1. Treatment Settings Used by Sylvia Frumkin during Her Career as a Chronic Mental Patient, 1963–1980
Source: Moran, Freedman, and Sharfstein 1984.

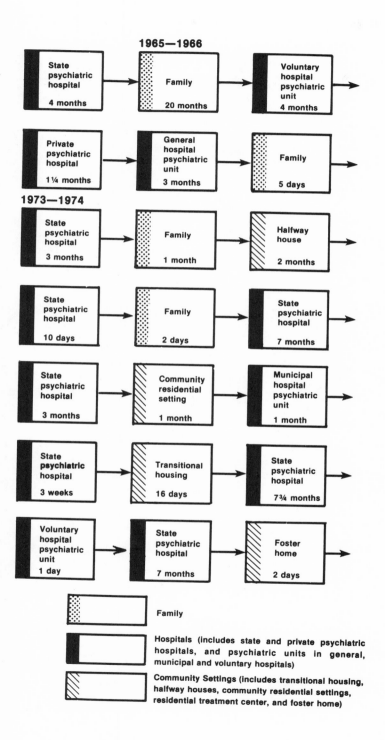

1965—1966

State psychiatric hospital — 4 months → Family — 20 months → Voluntary hospital psychiatric unit — 4 months →

Private psychiatric hospital — 1¼ months → General hospital psychiatric unit — 3 months → Family — 5 days →

1973—1974

State psychiatric hospital — 3 months → Family — 1 month → Halfway house — 2 months →

State psychiatric hospital — 10 days → Family — 2 days → State psychiatric hospital — 7 months →

State psychiatric hospital — 3 months → Community residential setting — 1 month → Municipal hospital psychiatric unit — 1 month →

State psychiatric hospital — 3 weeks → Transitional housing — 16 days → State psychiatric hospital — 7¾ months →

Voluntary hospital psychiatric unit — 1 day → State psychiatric hospital — 7 months → Foster home — 2 days →

Family

Hospitals (includes state and private psychiatric hospitals, and psychiatric units in general, municipal and voluntary hospitals)

Community Settings (includes transitional housing, halfway houses, community residential settings, residential treatment center, and foster home)

Table 7.3. Mental Health Service Availability in New York State, 1980

| | Service Type | | | | | |
| | Acute Inpatient[a] | | Community Residence[b] | | Family Care[c] | |
OMH Region	Beds	Rate	Beds	Rate	Beds	Rate
Western	513	2.05	603	2.94	1,356	6.61
Central	410	2.01	384	1.89	1,182	5.82
Hudson River	1,258	4.32	1,057	3.63	847	2.91
New York City	2,514	3.56	1,159	1.64	199	.28
Long Island	831	3.20	222	.85	237	.91
State Total	5,526	3.31	3,425	2.05	3,821	2.29

Source: Governor's Health Advisory Council 1984, 10, table 1-D.

Note: Rates per 10,000 general population.

[a]Includes beds only in general hospitals and proprietary mental hospitals.

[b]A residence in the community with 10 or fewer beds providing partial or 24-hour on-site mental health professional supervision.

[c]Includes room and board and limited supervision to 1-4 mentally ill persons in the personal residence of a homeowner.

Table 7.4. Percentage Change in Inpatient Population in New York State's Psychiatric Facilities, 1980-1986

| | Residents | Admissions | | |
		Total	Men	Women
All ages	-12.5	+ 7.8	+13.3	+ 0.2
<18 years	- 8.8	+33.8	+36.9	+28.4
18-34	+17.5	+ 9.2	11.4	+ 4.5
35-44	+21.6	+18.4	+26.9	+ 9.2
45-64	- 21.8	- 8.3	+ 0.5	-14.6
65+	- 25.5	-10.7	-12.0	- 9.8

Source: New York State Office of Mental Health 1986, table 9.

NEW YORK   **REST OF U.S.**

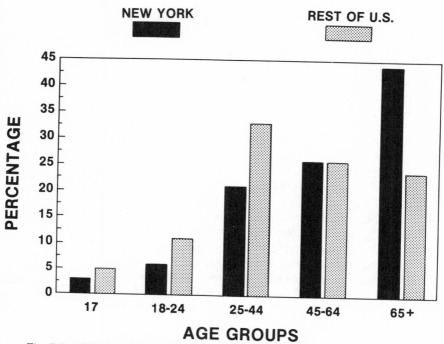

Fig. 7.2. 1980 State Hospital Census
Source: New York State Office of Mental Health 1982.

economic, demographic, and geographical factors have resulted in
more clients presenting themselves for services. In New York City,
for example, a combination of high unemployment rates among minority groups, a shortage of cheap and adequate housing, and a relative increase in the population of young adult males (eighteen to
forty-four years old) appears to have contributed to the rising admission rates in this age group. In the 1970s, a decade in which New
York's population dropped sharply, the percentage of individuals living in poverty in New York City increased from 15 to 20 percent. The
only age cohort that did not decline significantly in numbers was the
eighteen to forty-four group and nonwhite males made up 47 percent of this group in 1980, compared with 23 percent in 1970 (Alba
and Batutis 1983). The population of young, poor, minority males in
New York City is increasing, and this tends to increase the demand
for mental health care, bearing in mind that the eighteen to forty-four
age group accounts for more than half (56 percent) of all acute psychi-

atric admissions, as compared with 32 percent for those forty-five
and over (Governor's Select Commission 1984, appendix F).

One of the most significant changes in the pattern of service delivery in recent years has been the growth of outpatient (ambulatory)
services. In New York only 2 percent of the total mental health expenditures in 1950 was allocated to outpatient services (of a total of
$101.5 million). This increased to 3.6 percent in 1960, 16.8 percent in
1970, and 25.9 percent in 1980, or $369.7 million out of a total of more
than $1.4 billion (Governor's Health Advisory Council 1984). A large
part of this change represents a shifting pattern of supply, most notably the growth in outpatient services provided by community mental
health centers and freestanding outpatient mental health clinics (see
table 7.2).

Another important contributor to the rising level of demand has
been the increased availability of insurance as health insurance policies have been amended to cover outpatient mental health care. It is
generally believed that increases in insurance coverage produce a
greater use of mental health services than is the case for medical care.
One study reported that the demand for mental health care is relatively elastic and that a one percent increase in the charges paid by insurance companies produces an increase in the number of visits by
an average of 0.4 percent, with significantly greater effects for lower-
income clients (McGuire 1981). This suggests that insurance has
helped to democratize access to mental health care by making it more
available to poorer people, although it is important to point out that
the overall expenditure on mental health care remains low; in fact,
less than one-twentieth of total health expenditures in the United
States (Manning et al. 1984). It is not clear whether the demand for
mental health care will grow over time even as coverage remains stable, but McGuire (1981) has suggested the presence of a bandwagon
effect, in which social and cultural prejudices against the use of mental health services may be broken down as individuals witness others
in their social networks and workplaces making use of mental health
services (Brady, Sharfstein, and Moszynski 1986).

One of the reasons for the growth in availability of private insurance coverage for mental health care has been the observation of an
"offset effect" on overall health care costs. After a lag period of at
least six months, clients who receive mental health services make
significantly less use of medical services (Brown 1988). This is particularly the case for illnesses that respond to positive health behavior,
presumably because the mental health care helps to improve such

coping skills (Schlesinger et al. 1983). As a result, it makes good economic sense for an employer to add mental health coverage to the insurance package, and it is beneficial in cost terms to add outpatient mental health care to both fee-for-service and fixed-charge medical care systems. It is important to point out, however, that this suggestion appears to be relevant only for less seriously ill clients because the overall cost of care for more serious complaints more than offsets the offset effect (Borus et al. 1985).

As this discussion illustrates, the use of mental health services is increasingly falling within the domain of consumer behavior, especially for those clients with less serious disorders. It appears that mental health care has been targeted as an area of service delivery where high profits can be enjoyed, partly because supply continues to lag far behind the potential level of demand. It is reasonably well known, for example, that only a minority of the people suffering from clinical disorders have ever sought treatment at official service agencies (President's Commission on Mental Health 1978; Regier, Goldberg, and Taube 1978). Most of their complaints either go untreated or are treated by a non–mental health professional. There is, in other words, a vast area of potential growth in the demand for mental health care, although it is obvious that the decision to seek mental health care is probably very different from and affected by many more factors than the decision to seek health care services (Joseph and Phillips 1984).

In spite of the changes in the pattern of demand, there is no doubt that mental health care is still dominated by the providers and their wishes, and this explains why most private care-givers generally provide services to clients with the least-serious diagnoses and the most resources (Horwitz 1982). It is also true that the collective demands made by mental health clients are far less strong and pervasive than in the general health area. The mental illness lobby has grown significantly in recent years, but it remains relatively small and poorly organized (Levine 1981; Foley and Sharfstein 1983). The reasons for this are obvious: very few people who are currently well expect to encounter mental disorder, so it remains something one chooses not to think about or draw attention to. There is an effective network of constituencies that work diligently to protect their own and their clients' interests (including state and local mental health associations), but the bulk of demand-side forces operating on the mental health care system represent either the providers themselves or groups of individuals who are already within the system and receiving care.

There is little evidence of a significant grassroots movement acting in the interests of potential mental health care consumers. It is reasonable, therefore, to focus the remaining discussion on the supply-side factors that have produced changes in the mental health care delivery system.

Arena Building and the Politics of Mental Health

As the pattern of mental health care delivery has expanded, a variety of new constituencies has emerged, including government at the federal, state, county, and city levels; independent community mental health centers; and a number of private concerns ranging from psychiatric hospitals and clinics to community halfway houses, sheltered workshops, nursing homes, room-and-board facilities, single-resident-occupancy (SRO) hotels, homeless shelters, and hostels. In addition, there are thousands of individual practitioners in the fields of psychiatry, clinical and counseling psychology, and social work operating in both private and public settings, all represented by powerful professional organizations.

In theoretical terms, the current situation in the field of mental health care delivery can best be interpreted from a social constructivist view of social problems (Smith 1987; Gusfield 1984). According to this view, the way a society deals with a social problem has much less to do with the facts of the problem than with the processes involved in interpreting the facts. In a pluralist society a wide array of constituencies compete with each other to make sure their claims are heard in the public arena (Spector and Kitsuse 1977). In many cases .these groups include individuals who have encountered the problem in question, and their claims-making activities require a response from existing institutions and policymakers. Mental-patient groups, for example, have been quite successful in this regard and have helped to bring about improved conditions in institutions (Brown 1985). It is clear, however, that their success has often resulted from the input of lawyers and mental health providers whose interests were largely economic or professional (Brown and Smith 1988).

With the growing emphasis on community-based psychiatric services beginning in the 1970s, a large portion of the responsibility for care was transferred into the hands of two groups of providers. The first of these was a group of professional service providers who received a shot in the arm from new federal and state mental health financing sources such as Medicaid, Medicare, and Supplemental Security Income. This group included professionals who worked for social welfare programs, mental health centers, and family service agencies. The second group included a large number of relatively unsupervised and untrained private service providers operating in nursing homes, hostels, hotels, shelters, and boarding homes. All of these providers, working both as individuals and as members of professional groups, have been concerned that their collective voice be heard in the public realm. To achieve their goals they are willing and increasingly able to make demands on legislatures and other decision-making bodies. In doing so they effectively build up an arena around their specific problem by protesting and continually drawing attention to the issue in question in addition to fund raising, lobbying, and creating alliances with other organizations. In this sense the issues they represent become political constructions because the protagonists have to fight continually in a resource-scarce environment to renew their mandate (Wiener 1981).

In a hostile environment such as this, political fighting often produces some unplanned and unwanted effects in the delivery of mental health services. To illustrate this, it is useful to describe briefly two different areas of conflict: one operating between different levels of government and the other between different professional groups in the delivery system.

Conflicts Between Administrative Levels. The recent history of mental health care has involved a complex web of interactions between planning bodies and funding mechanisms at the federal, state, and local levels. To most onlookers these relationships are stupifying in their complexity, and it is no surprise to find that an entirely new constituent group of budget and finance experts has emerged in the mental health field. The relative contributions of federal, state, and local authorities to mental health care differ across space. At the state level, for example, there are dramatic differences in the proportions of state and local contributions. The shift toward local responsibility for mental health programs and the resulting development of a locally based, integrated system of services have produced a unique service system in such states as California (Barter 1983). In New York State, however, the service-delivery system is much more centralized, and only sporadic attempts have been made to provide integrated local mental health programs at the county level (Pepper and Ryglewicz 1983).

An additional complication entering the sphere of state and local relationships in the area of mental health has been the operation of the federal and state Medicaid programs (Sharfstein 1982). Medicaid provides federal reimbursement for inpatient and outpatient services for clients who meet income eligibility standards (because they are poor). The federal contribution to this program has helped to reduce the financial burden on the individual states and has also resulted in a significant expansion of outpatient services (Sharfstein, Frank, and Kessler 1984). Most mental patients in the public system are eligible for Medicaid, but the regulations prohibit those between the ages of twenty-two and sixty-four (which includes the young chronics) from using Medicaid funds for inpatient state mental hospital care. This regulation has contributed significantly to lowering the resident population of state mental hospitals and raising the population of general hospitals, where Medicaid funds can be used (New York State Communities Aid Association 1983). In New York State this has made a dramatic difference in the delivery system; by 1981, general hospitals had admission rates for psychiatric patients that were five times higher than those for public mental hospitals. The net effect is that in New York more than a third (37 percent) of the psychiatric days in general hospitals are now supported by Medicaid funds, which is only slightly less than the figure for public mental hospitals (table 7.5).

Table 7.5. Psychiatric Inpatients in Public, General, and Private Hospitals in New York State, 1981

	Public Mental Hospitals	Psychiatric Units or Beds in General Hospitals	Private Psychiatric Hospitals
Number of hospitals	31	300	12
Census (population on given day)	23,000	5,500	1,000
Admissions per year	25,000	2,000,000	350,000
Average length of stay	12 years	15 days	38 days
% older than 65	40	20	25
% Medicare days	2	23	30
% Medicaid days	45	37	8

Source: New York State Communities Aid Association 1983, 57, table 4.

The complexities in Medicaid regulations have produced some unfortunate conflicts between the state of New York and local mental health planners. It is obvious that the New York Office of Mental Health, facing a huge annual budget request (now in excess of $2 billion a year), would prefer that clients in need of inpatient services (between the ages of twenty-two and sixty-four) be admitted to general hospitals, most of which are organized and financed at the local level. The localities, on the other hand, want as many clients as possible to be admitted to the state psychiatric centers and hospitals, which are funded totally by the state.

Conflicts at the Professional Level. Throughout the three decades in which significant changes have been occurring in the delivery of mental health services, there has been a running battle for ascendancy between the various professional groups claiming mental health as their unique territory. The traditionally two-tiered system of care, with the public hospitals serving the poor and private psychiatrists serving the rich, was dominated by the medical profession (Brown 1985). With the advent and growth of community mental health care (CMH) in the 1960s, the stranglehold of psychiatry was weakened. This was particularly the case in the new community mental health centers (CMHCs), where the mean number of full-time equivalent psychiatrists in the centers dropped form 6.8 in 1970 to 3.8 in 1981 (Biegel 1984), a trend that was also reflected in executive directors (55 percent of all centers were directed by psychiatrists in 1971, but only 10 percent in 1982).

Naturally the psychiatric profession has expressed considerable concern about this trend, and by the end of the 1970s there was a strong push to redefine the goals of the CMH movement to make the psychiatric (medical) profession more central (Sabshin 1977). The original drive to provide mental health care in the community was based largely on a series of assumptions about how to provide a preventive milieu in the community. In essence this involved a social/ public health model of mental health care in which the role of the expert psychiatrist was diminished. With the apparent failure of such optimistic strategies to make a significant dent in the mental health problem and the obvious presence of serious medical problems among the long-term chronically mentally ill, community mental health has to some extent been "remedicalized" in recent years (Pasnau 1987). Many of the young chronic clients will need to be maintained on medication for years, and, obviously, psychiatrists will be needed to administer the drugs and to monitor their long-term effects.

These changes have caused many community mental health centers to conduct vigorous searches for psychiatrists, either in a full-time or a consulting capacity (Biegel 1984), and these arrangements have proved lucrative to psychiatrists, many of whom were afraid that their incomes would dry up as a result of a projected decline in the availability of insurance coverage for mental health care (Brady, Sharfstein, and Moszynski 1986). This fear has been particularly prominent since the federal government reduced the Federal Employees' Health Plan (FEHP) between 1980 and 1988 (Hustead et al 1985). Mental health care insurance coverage was cut back much more than that for physical illness. Blue Cross and Blue Shield reduced their coverage to sixty days of inpatient care (high-option plan) and to 70 percent reimbursement for up to fifty outpatient visits (Hustead et al. 1985).

Psychiatrists are being drawn back into community mental health in other ways, largely as a result of attempts to increase competition or to reduce overall costs. A popular strategy has been for mental health care programs to affiliate themselves with primary health care settings such as health maintenance organizations (HMOs). In such settings, reimbursement of the client may depend on the authorization of a primary-care physician. As one psychiatrist predicts with obvious relish, "If psychiatrists can position themselves as the major referral source for these . . . physicians, their collaboration will also help to remedicalize community mental health" (Biegel 1984, 1116).

The remedicalization of community mental health has not affected some of the administrative and fiscal changes that emerged in the 1970s. As psychiatrists became less dominant in outpatient mental health programs, their places were often taken by persons trained as managers or in the business field who may have had only a secondary interest in mental health care. In this sense, mental health care has followed general health care in the direction of cost consciousness. As mental health professionals have been replaced by business administration specialists, we have entered a new era in which the concern with economic survival has dominated all program development strategies. In a recent series of articles dealing with the future of CMHCs, for example, there was serious discussion about how best to "sell the product," "penetrate the market," develop a "community image," and improve "worker productivity" (Zelman et al. 1985). In the words of one observer, "A failure to serve new market segments with greater ability to pay for services may mean retrenchment and a failure to serve an expanded mission for the entire community" (Sorenson 1985, 224).

Economic Determinism and the Industrialization of Mental Health Care

The vast increase in the cost of health care in the United States has been well documented (Gibson and Waldo 1982; Relman 1983; Starr 1982). Between 1965 and 1985, the consumer price index rose 250 percent, but health care costs increased by more than 900 percent (hospital costs by 1,135 percent, and physicians' fees by 870 percent; see Califano 1986). Total annual expenditures in 1987 are expected to be in excess of $500 billion, which will consume 12 percent of the gross national product (Bittker 1985). In the 1980s the average person is spending twice as much on health care as in 1965, and the situation is deteriorating rapidly. In 1982, health care costs rose three times faster than the annual inflation rate; health insurance costs rose by 16 percent, which was the biggest increase ever; and the average cost of a hospital stay, adjusted for inflation, rose from $316 in 1965 to $1,844 in 1980 (Sharfstein and Biegel 1985).

Although the rising cost of mental health care has been less dramatic than this, it has nevertheless become a major concern in the late 1980s. In the 1960s, most decisions about resource allocation in the mental health area were made by government, and most of the care was provided in the public sector. Resources were distributed according to the assessed need for services, tempered by such factors as a particular locality's concern with welfare issues and the interplay of political interest groups (C. Smith 1986). Since the 1960s, many changes have taken place, and mental health care has moved increasingly toward resource-allocation decisions made in the marketplace. Choices increased, and potential clients could select from a variety of providers who were offering a number of different packages of care. The major culprit in the rising costs of health care, and this also goes for mental health care, has been the virtual insulation of the consumer from the escalating prices of modern medicine. The introduction of third-party insurance and federal programs like Medicare has inadvertently provided an incentive for greater use and greater provision. Because the costs of expensive care are often fully insured, price considerations do not enter into either consumer or provider decision making. In this sense it is a cruel irony that the egalitarian demands of the 1960s for equal access to high-quality mental health care have probably contributed to this process by establishing the concept of rights to mental health care. The development of the federal support programs in the 1960s that were part of the Great Society program (for example, Medicare for the elderly and Medicaid for the poor) and an expansion of low-cost insurance programs helped to increase the demand for mental health care. Treatment was now considered to be an entitlement, regardless of the costs involved. As the use of mental health services rose and costs skyrocketed, a new pro-competition approach was adopted that would ultimately have an adverse effect on the clients who were most in need of services.

In the old system of open-ended reimbursements, there was no need for the consumer to be frugal and little incentive for the provider to be cost conscious. What arose in response was a variety of strategies to reduce costs either by increasing out-of-pocket consumer payments (through higher deductibles and increased premiums) or by instituting a system where services were paid for in advance, either based on a specific diagnosis (English et al. 1985) or as part of a group fee-for-service situation like an HMO (Sharfstein and Biegel 1985). A number of trends have been significant in the 1980s:

1. Preferred provider organizations (PPOs) have been established that are intended to reward patients who use lower-cost providers (Altman and Frisman 1987). This is a group of independent providers who agree to provide care to an insured group at a negotiated, often discounted, rate. Clients receive the discount only if they use the so-called preferred providers. This combines consumer and provider cost consciousness (Levin and Glasser 1984).

2. Investor-owned hospitals have increased in number (Levenson 1985). The economic advantages of these hospitals, resulting from their size and efficiency and the ease with which they have been able to obtain capital, helps to explain their phenomenal recent growth (see chapter 2). By the early 1980s, private psychiatry provided about one quarter of all inpatient beds— more than twice the proportion they controlled a decade earlier (Eisenberg 1986). The most significant change has been in the pattern of ownership. In 1985 psychiatric hospital chains owned 86 of the 130 proprietary hospitals in the United States, an increase of over 100 percent from the situation two years earlier.

Of these 86, the four giants in the field owned 71 in 1982 (Eisenberg 1986). The four were the Hospital Corporation of America (HCA), American Medical International (AMI), National Medical Enterprises (NME), and Community Psychiatric Centers (CPC). In 1983, HCA, with revenues of $3.2 billion and seventy-one thousand employees ranked thirteen in *Fortune's* list of the largest service companies. HCA owns and operates 339 facilities in forty-one states and five foreign countries (Eisenberg 1984). In addition, it owns a substantial portion of an independent company, Beverly Enterprises, which is the nation's largest operator of nursing homes (Levenson 1985).

3. Privatization has occurred in noninstitutional care, particularly as community-based services financed indirectly by public (welfare) sources are shifting over to private management (for example, nursing homes, community residences, and halfway houses).

4. There is a shift to a reimbursement system that, instead of being retrospective and provider determined (and therefore inherently inflationary), is prospective and payer determined (Scarpaci 1988a; Widem et al. 1984).

In spite of the magnitude of these changes, cost-control strategies in the psychiatric field have been much less severe than in the area of general medicine, and there are a number of reasons for this (Gaylin 1985). In the first place, the majority of mental health service planning is focused on chronic mental disorders, whereas chronic care is rarely a concern for planning in general medicine. The public sector of mental health care today is rarely allowed the luxury of dealing with the mental health needs of the "normal" population, as was the case during the more idealistic years of the Great Society, when the CMH movement was launched. In the late 1980s the bulk of planning and public funding is oriented in the direction of the chronically mentally ill (U.S. DHHS 1980; Group for the Advancement of Psychiatry 1978). One of the implications of this is an economic one, as noted earlier. The rising prevalence of chronic mental disorders among young adults who will probably spend many years in inpatient care, will place an increasing fiscal burden on the state.

There is also a difference in the size and structure of the mental health care system in comparison with general health care. Because the delivery of services to the mentally ill is less subject to capital-intensive, high-technology innovations, there has traditionally been less incentive for investment from the private sector. In addition, the medical sector has always had far more surplus wealth than the mental health system, which made it easier to institute cost rationalization such as prospective payments (Brown 1988). Because of the tendency toward full occupancy in psychiatric inpatient units (which is especially the case in New York City), there has until recently been relatively little to gain from the competitive marketing strategies that have been witnessed in voluntary (general) hospitals. The trend toward hospital closures and reductions in bed capacity that has been typical in the general health sector has not occurred in the mental health sector—in fact, remarkably few hospitals have closed, and new psychiatric and alcoholism beds have been added in many hospitals as a trade-off for reducing the number of medical and surgical beds (New York State Office of Mental Health 1986).

The mental health care system is also much more decentralized than the general medical care system both geographically and organizationally. Mental health services are offered in a wide range of locations, and they are administered by a variety of different agencies and levels of government. Clients move between a number of medical, psychiatric, social service, and criminal justice agencies; and the funding for their care comes from a baffling assortment of public and private sources. The result is that government at both federal and state levels, has typically had a much more active role in funding and planning mental health care than in general health care, where the major government responsibility is more likely to be at the local (city or county) level. All of these factors result in rather poorly developed planning for mental health service delivery (Morrissey 1982).

Although the privatization and corporatization trends in the mental health field are still in their infancy, the rate of change is startling. Thus, for example, the annual growth rate for chain-owned psychiatric hospitals between 1978 and 1982 was 25 percent (Ermann and Gabel 1984); and the chains are now making threatening advances toward the relatively few psychiatric hospitals that remain in the voluntary sector (Eisenberg 1986). The immense size, diversity, and economic power of the chains could well put them in a highly competitive position if psychiatric care does shift to a system of prospective payment. When (or if) this happens, each hospital will need to develop a fully computerized patient information system and an entirely new accounting system. The chains, as a result of their economies of scale, may have a natural advantage in responding to such costly innovations: "Rather than each of its hospitals having to develop its own computerized systems, a chain can do the necessary development work in its central corporate offices and then provide the system for all affiliated hospitals. While the independent hospitals must hire consultants to work on these new requirements, a chain can provide centralized expertise at a much lower cost per hospital" (Levenson 1985, 161). Another important advantage the chains will have is that they can provide a wide range of services in addition to inpatient beds. If DRGs shorten hospital stays, the demand for community placement will increase (Light et al. 1986). Most of the chains have their own facilities offering general health care or residential services in the community, including nursing homes, so they will be able to respond to the extra demand for community-based care.

The mental health care system is now offering an extremely lucrative window of opportunity for investors, partly because the demand for services is far greater than the supply. More than a few investors have noticed the system is ripe for the introduction of new services. In a recent book entitled *The New Economics and Psychiatric Care*, the editors noted that the epidemiological data on the prevalence of mental illness "suggest the possibility of expanding the 'market-share' of patients in need of treatment who could benefit from one or another of the forms of psychiatric treatment. . . . The potential of the untapped pool of patients . . . will lead to innovative organizational responses and open new opportunities for psychiatrists and others to deliver cost-effective care" (Sharfstein and Biegel 1985, 7).

All of this suggests that the current trends toward privatization are partly the result of attempts to hold down ever-rising costs and partly an attempt to make the most of what appears to be an excellent investment opportunity. A Wall Street brokerage firm advised its clients of such an opportunity in 1985. The company noted that from October 1984 to January 1985 the price of shares for companies catering to psychiatric inpatients rose by 23 percent compared with a 9 percent rise for general acute-care hospitals and a 6 percent rise in the Dow-Jones average (Maidenberg 1985). Unfortunately, the reasons investors are interested in psychiatric care are precisely the reasons why there is concern about the quality of such care (Nadelson 1986). Mental health care is still basically a two-class system: high-quality care is provided in private facilities, where good profits can be made; while lower-quality care continues to be provided in a variety of public facilities. In addition, it will probably always be difficult to implement cost-control strategies in psychiatric care because of the imprecision in diagnosis and the difficulty of predicting the extent of recovery. As Eisenberg (1986) has observed, "The very features of current psychiatric care that trouble (or at least should trouble) psychiatrists enchant stockbrokers. . . . It appears that what is bad for patients is good for investors" (1016).

At the present time it is difficult to predict the outcome of these trends toward corporatization and privatization in the provision of psychiatric care. There is a continual fear that costs will rise, as they have done as a result of similar trends in general hospitals (Pattison and Katz 1983). What is more likely to happen is that economic considerations will produce some unfortunate changes in the way mental health services are provided. One example of such a change is the tendency (generally referred to as cream skimming) for facilities to cater only to paying patients, leaving the more costly services and the care of medically indigent patients to public hospitals. Hospitals operating on a for-profit basis are also much less likely to involve themselves in community services that are beneficial to their local community but are difficult to reimburse, such as emergency telephone services, suicide prevention units, and the provision of home care.

Recent developments in corporate psychiatry have followed fairly closely the trends that have been observed in general hospital care (Starr 1982; Ginzberg 1984). They can be summarized as follows: (1) horizontal developments—consolidation of hospitals (including closures) until they reach a size that makes economies of scale possible; (2) vertical developments—chains acquire other types of psychiatric facilities, including outpatient programs, nursing homes, and halfway houses; and (3) realignments—general hospital chains acquire psychiatric facilities, and corporations acquire HMOs and public health clinics. These trends serve to reduce the separateness of psychiatric care and bring it once again more fully under the aegis of medical care, thus effectively ending the more than two decades of experimentation with community mental health care based on a social and public health model of mental disorder (Brown 1985).

Conclusion

Modern psychiatry has been corporatized to such an extent that it is now reasonable to interpret the services provided as a group of commodities. Although this has come as a shock to some observers, it is simply part of a series of changes that began in the 1960s with the community mental health movement. At that time a bold new approach to mental health care was introduced, with the public funding of community-based services to provide equal access to quality care for all Americans, regardless of income, age, race, or sex (Smith 1983). It was hoped that the newly funded centers would become the ambulatory-care version of the older state mental hospitals, focusing on the problems of minorities, the poor, the elderly, and the chronically mentally ill. As we now know, this did not happen—in fact, fewer than half of the centers were built, and in 1981 the federal funding for the program was abandoned (M. Levine 1981). As we have seen in this chapter, public institutions remained the largest service sector in the mental health systems of most states; in the last decade, however, the share of public inpatient services has declined sharply, and there has been rapid growth in the provision of private psychiatric beds in both specialized psychiatric hospitals and psychiatric wards of general hospitals.

In addition to the failure of community mental health centers to replace public inpatient facilities, the movement has been criticized for its failure to fulfill its early promises to launch a significant attack on the underlying structural causes of mental disorder in American society. Although this promise was always more a matter of faith than a reality (Smith 1983), the early enthusiasm of the center directors has not been matched by their subsequent achievements. In spite of this, some of the central tenets of community mental health are still intact today, although they are now being pursued most vigorously in the private sector. For example, the focus on preventive mental health services and early detection, community-based services, programs in the workplace, team care with case-manager services, and ambulatory care will continue (Panzetta 1985). The major difference will be that, instead of being provided by CMHCs, they will become the responsibility of corporate medical systems and will be based in preferred provider organizations (PPOs), health maintenance organizations (HMOs), and employee assistance programs (EAPs).

At the same time, some of the features of community mental health will not be reproduced in the new corporate psychiatry. Most importantly, the idea of community involvement and participation will be replaced by the stockholder. Also missing will be the attempt to deal with problems within a geographically defined concept of community, which will be replaced by the ability to pay for services and the need to have work-based insurance coverage. In other words, mental health care will increasingly adopt a new concept of the community, one that is dominated by the workplace. As

Panzetta (1985, 1178) observes, "Accountability is (or will be) determined not by geographic boundaries but by inclusion in a mental
health benefits package."

Public funds that were used to launch the community mental
health movement will become a thing of the past and will increasingly be channeled into programs for the poor, the chronically
mentally ill, and the homeless populations (Lamb 1984). This will
essentially leave the corporate sector of psychiatry free to focus
on the employed and insured middle classes. The wealthy will continue to have access to private psychiatrists, so the new development will bring about a three-level system of mental health care, with
community mental health now redefined as the system of care for
the middle-class employed person. In this regard, not much has
changed in the delivery of mental health care during the last three
decades. The system has become much larger, and its organizational
structure and financing mechanisms have changed, but it is still characterized by a class-based segregation of its clients.

Delving deeper into the possible motives behind the corporate
takeover of the community mental health movement, it is possible to
interpret some recent developments as attempts to anticipate, plan
for, and control some of the side effects of alienation in the workplace that can damage productivity. From this perspective both the
demand-side and the supply-side arguments developed in this
chapter to account for the restructuring of mental health care are secondary to the economic and political priorities of the business community. In developing an argument along these lines, Ralph (1983)
contends that community mental health has been largely based on
methods that were developed in industrial psychology, where the
goal has been to help workers and their families adjust to increasingly alienated, degraded, and pressured conditions in the workplace, thus preventing or rechanneling potential labor unrest. To
support this argument Ralph notes that many of the innovators of
community psychiatry techniques developed their methods with
generous corporate funding and used them in industry long before
they were applied in community settings. This was the case with the
use of the mental health team, testing, nonprofessional counselors,
family and group involvement in therapy, and preventive psychiatry. Industrial psychologists also conducted much of the research
that was instrumental in developing tranquilizers and other drugs
that could help workers to function adequately under stress, and
much of this research was funded by the major corporations. This
can be interpreted as a possible forerunner to the drug maintenance

of former psychiatric patients, which was later to transform the way mental illness was treated in the community (Scull 1977).

In 1967 the director of the newly formed National Institute of Mental Health recognized the intimate link between industry and mental health. In a speech to the National Association of Manufacturers he noted: "Since we live in a working society, in the largest sense, all our mental health is 'occupational' mental health. It is to our mutual advantage (business and government) to promote the mental health of our population. . . . Our motives may stem from compassion or from a need for human productivity, but our success will profit all of us" (Yolles 1967, 47).

The definitions of what are considered to be symptoms of mental disorders have expanded considerably in recent years, and this has contributed to the growing number of episodes of treated mental illness. From the corporate perspective, mental disorder can be interpreted as one of the nation's costliest health problems, threatening the economy through low productivity, absenteeism, and the skyrocketing costs of insurance coverage. Although it may be too farfetched to argue that there is widespread alienation in the workplace that could result in organized resistance to the corporate world, there is a widespread array of unwanted and deviant behaviors that threaten to interrupt the smooth operation of production of a service organization. As Ralph (1983, 49) observed, workers "get ulcers, headaches, and insomnia; they have accidents; stay home, drink, get irritable, daydream, and sometimes go raving mad, all of which is very costly to management."

To deal with these disorders, corporate-sponsored community mental health services have appeared and have been the most rapidly growing sector of a restructured delivery system. The services are oriented largely toward the employed, and their goals are to increase worker tolerance to the demands of the workplace and to reduce the potential for alienation. A subsidiary goal is to help pacify displaced and potential workers, a category that includes disproportionately large numbers of unemployed adolescents, minorities, and women working in the home. It follows, of course, that community mental health services for people in these categories will only be available to those who still have access to benefit packages that include mental health coverage. The long-term and permanently unemployed will probably remain outside the sphere of the new community mental health sector, relegated as ever to the public mental hospitals or to the streets of the public city.

Chapter 8

Deinstitutionalization and Privatization

Community-based Residential Care Facilities in Ontario

GLENDA LAWS

   The two objectives of this chapter are to outline the links between the policies of deinstitutionalization and privatization and to explore the implications of these two policy directions for local urban places. The empirical discussion will draw on recent experiences from Ontario, Canada, where deinstitutionalization has been an explicit policy for several decades. Privatization has more often been an implicit policy in Ontario—an unstated consequence of deinstitutionalization as well as of more explicit policy objectives. These policies aim to promote private-sector activity in the delivery of social services, and their outcomes for urban areas have important political and planning implications. As the empirical discussion of Ontario will show, in most North American cities there has emerged a concentration of housing for special-needs populations in the inner-city core, which also contains many of the services on which these populations depend. As these concentrations have grown there have been attempts to disperse them, but resistance has arisen in potential host communities (Dear and Laws 1986). There is, therefore, a clear need to understand the processes that produce these problematic outcomes if policies to rectify the situation are to be formulated and if insights into the processes of deinstitutionalization and privatization are to be gained.

   Four sections follow this brief introduction. In section 1, I make some general comments about the processes of deinstitutionalization and privatization, two forms of restructuring that have been adopted by many Western welfare states over the last two decades or so. I argue that deinstitutionalization and privatization are state policy responses to a range of internal and external pressures, not policies that the state simply decides to impose upon its constituents. I further note some of the problems in generalizing about the process of privatization—problems stemming from the different forms privatization may take, each of which may have different origins and consequences. In section 2, I focus on how these policies have evolved in Ontario over the last two decades. One critical component of deinstitutionalization in Ontario has been the privatization of residential care facilities; in section 3, I discuss this process as it has occurred in Hamilton, Ontario. This case study provides an opportunity to explore the ways in which local conditions are influenced by state policy and how these local conditions influence the form of state policy in local places. Some conclusions regarding the possibility that privatization actually marks an extension of the state's control function (rather than a necessary erosion of the welfare state, as is popularly argued) and about the effects of this process upon local social and built environments are presented in the final part of the chapter.

Privatization and Deinstitutionalization

The concomitant processes of privatization and deinstitutionalization can only be understood as specific historical forms of the restructuring of the welfare state. Three features characterize the welfare state. First, there is a commitment by the state to provide some level of social security, broadly defined, for constituents. Second, this commitment has witnessed the development of a formal state apparatus charged exclusively with dealing with welfare issues. Third, the growth of the welfare state has been accompanied by a rapid injection of public monies into social-welfare expenditure. Too often, studies of the welfare state have argued that policies developed within the state apparatus are little more than a means of reproducing the capitalist mode of production and therefore afford little opportunity for social change. Thus, health services are conceived of as a means by which a healthy (and thus potentially productive) labor force is reproduced. Such analyses have rightly been criticized for their functionalism. They imply that state policy has predetermined outcomes and ignore the various forces with competing interests calling upon the state to redistribute these resources. Central to my argument is the idea that restructuring cannot be conceived unproblematically as a "top-down" process whereby the state imposes particular policies. Rather, internal and external pressures on the state both influence and are influenced by the form of these policies. Internal pressures, for instance, include the fiscal crises experienced by many contemporary states (O'Connor 1973). External pressures include calls by both business and community groups for a greater share of the state's resources. These external pressures might take the form of class struggle (Fincher and Ruddick 1983), conflicts organized around issues of gender, ethnic-based groups lobbying the state, or neighborhood-based conflicts (see Castells 1983). Such pressures result in the restructuring of welfare-state policies, the process of rationalization and reorganization undertaken by the state in response to demands made upon its resources.

The Move to Community-based Care

During the 1960s many welfare states adopted deinstitutionalization as one means of restructuring social service programs. Deinstitutionalization involves transferring the treatment of various client groups from an institutional model of care to a community-based approach. Deinstitutionalization has been particularly widespread in the field of psychiatric care (see also chapter 7). Between 1955 and 1977 the population of mental hospitals in the United States, for example, declined by about 60 percent, from 500,000 to 190,000 (Ashbaugh and Bradley 1979). In Ontario, Canada, the number of psychiatric beds fell from 15,141 in 1960 to 4,831 in 1986, a drop of around 75 percent. Accompanying this decline in the inpatient population has been a significant drop in the average length of stay (ALOS) in hospitals. Canadian statistics show that today about two-thirds of the ALOSs are less than two weeks, and 90 percent are less than a month. This contrasts with the situation twenty-five years ago when more than 50 percent of Canada's psychiatric inpatients were interned for more than seven years (Ontario Ministry of Health 1986, 2). Other institutionalized groups, including alcoholics, orphans, juvenile delinquents and offenders, have also been subject to this shift in treatment philosophy (Otto and Orford 1978; Simmons 1982; Scull 1977; Chan and Ericson 1981).

Deinstitutionalization gained momentum during the 1960s when it received unilateral support from politicians, medical professionals, social workers, and the community at large. By removing people from the isolation of an institution it was felt a more humane and nurturing environment could be created within smaller facilities

(Mamula and Newman 1973). This would, in theory, also allow more "normal" social relationships to develop between special-needs clients and members of the neighboring community, a fundamental objective of the principle of normalization underscoring many policy initiatives (Wolfensburger 1972). At the same time, developments were being made in the use of psychotropic drugs to control the behavior of some chronically psychiatrically disabled persons (Ontario Department of Public Health 1954, 1961).

It has frequently been argued that deinstitutionalization was introduced by welfare states as a means of curbing public expenditures (Bassuk and Gerson 1978; Klermen 1977; Scull 1977). However, there is mounting evidence that questions the accuracy of these arguments. First, as we will note in the discussion of the Ontario case, deinstitutionalization as policy and practice began prior to the onset of the so-called fiscal crisis of the state. Second, the shift toward community-based care has not been accompanied by a reduction in costs. In fact, costs have increased, (Goldman, Adams, and Taube 1983; Lerman 1982; Borus 1981). This is because community-based care must include a network of community centers for successful implementation. Other factors are that some kinds of institutions need to remain in place (and at smaller operating scales, per capita costs are likely to increase), and expensive drugs must be used.

Obviously it is not enough to argue that deinstitutionalization arose simply from a state decision to curb expenditures nor that state policies are simply imposed from above. To explore this idea further it is instructive to consider the case of privatization briefly. We will note in the following section that there are very strong links between privatization and deinstitutionalization in Ontario; in fact, the shift from institutional models of care to community-based services has been paralleled by a shift from the public to the private sector.

Pressures to Privatize

Privatization is one of the most conspicuous forms of restructuring; and, as the essays in this collection highlight, it is a process employed by welfare states worldwide. At the most general level, privatization involves a shift from public-sector responsibility for service provision to increased levels of responsibility by the private sector. Thus, privatization is sometimes equated with a withdrawal from or erosion of the welfare state. But it can be argued that privatization is one way the state extends its sphere of influence over the private sector as the state contracts with various agencies and thus places regulations upon their activities (Laws 1987).

Three general sets of forces are at work to promote privatization. Again it is useful to think of internal and external pressures so that we move away from the notion of state policy as something that is imposed. First, there is little doubt that the fiscal crises of contemporary welfare states have resulted in policy options that attempt to reduce mounting debts. Moreover, privatization appears to be one means of doing so, primarily because (theoretically) the public-sector wage bill will be reduced. This is illustrated by the Ontario experience. In 1971 the provincial government announced that "the province has moved out of a period when funds were relatively plentiful and when demand for new programs was not as great as it is today. For the foreseeable future, the problem will be how to allocate limited resources to existing and new program demands. This means setting new priorities, which, in turn, could involve the termination of some programs" (COGP 1971, 3:11). Privatization was explicitly identified as one mechanism by which the state could use community resources and thus shift some of the burden for service provision from the welfare apparatus: "In future, selective reprivatization of program delivery could tap community skills and resources needed to meet policy objectives. These skills may be found in non-profit organizations, in private, profit-oriented corporations, or in community corporations organised by special interest groups" (COGP 1971, 3:751).

Second, neoconservative interests within civil society are calling for a reduction in the welfare state because of its erosion of the incentive to work and its inefficiencies (Mishra 1984). Business interests argue that they can perform the same functions as the state sector at substantially reduced costs and that competition will provide more choice for consumers.

Third, the public is calling for a lessening of state intervention so that social service consumers might have greater control over the services that they use. Consumer groups have often expressed dissatisfaction about the dependency created by professionals and the service network in which they operate, and calls to lessen this form of control are, in fact, calls for one form of privatization.

Given these various pressures for the privatization of social services it is not surprising that privatization takes many forms (cf. Knowles 1985). That is, privatization is not a singular process with one set of predictable outcomes. There are a variety of forces calling for privatization, and they suggest a variety of possible outcomes. Privatization includes the promotion of commercial activities, the development of the non-profit and cooperative sectors (including voluntary organizations), and the return of the responsibility for care to the domestic sphere as households are asked to assume greater responsibility for the well-being of their members. Deinstitutionalization in Ontario provides a case study for examining the outcomes of these various calls for, and forms of, privatization and their impacts on local communities.

The Case of Ontario

Almost without exception, legislation passed during the 1960s and 1970s that promoted community-based alternatives to the institutional model of care (which had dominated Ontario's welfare state since the nineteenth century) also encouraged the participation of private service providers. The private sector has entered the field of community-based care via a number of routes. During the 1960s and 1970s, concern was expressed about the environments in which Ontario's dependent groups were being cared for (Roberts 1963; Anglin and Braaten 1978; OAMR 1972). Both professional and patient advocate groups called for a reconsideration of the institutional model. They argued that the alienation and stigma experienced by residents in large institutions served only to impede their rehabilitation and that this could be avoided in community settings. The principle of normalization was first adopted by Ontario's mental retardation professionals, but was soon adopted, and adapted, by various other groups including those working in the areas of children's services, corrections, care for the elderly, treatment for the mentally ill, and care for the handicapped (Simmons 1982; Chan and Ericson 1981).

At the same time, an increasingly conservative political climate set in as the recession of the early 1970s was felt in the Ontario economy. This encouraged a concern for minimizing public expenditures, a concern that has continued through the mid-1980s. Deinstitutionalization promised savings through the lower per diem rates charged by private, community-based services. The data in table 8.1 suggest on first examination that it is cheaper to house people in the community than in institutions. However, it must be recalled that institutions offer a variety of ancillary services. The costs of these support

Table 8.1. Comparative Costs of Institutional and Community-based Care in
Ontario, circa 1985

	dollars
Community-based facilities	
Lodging home (Hamilton, 1986)[1]	25.00
Home for special care[2]	
residential	20.88
nursing	49.16
Group home (Hamilton, 1984)[3]	45.00
Nursing home[4]	49.16
Institutions	
Prisons[5]	60.00
Hamilton Psychiatric Hospital (December 1985)[2]	239.13
General Hospital (1984)[6]	
Chedoke-McMaster	439.40
Provincial average	289.52

Sources: [1]Hamilton-Wentworth Regional Social Services Department 1986, Personal communication; [2]Hamilton Psychiatric Hospital 1986, Personal communication; [3]Elliott 1985; [4]Ministry of Health 1986, Personal communication; [5]Hamilton Detention Center 1986, Personal communication; [6]Ontario 1985.

services are taken into account in the institutional per diem rate. This is not the case in the community-based services, where ancillary services are provided elsewhere or not at all. In either case, they usually go unaccounted. Reporting on the Ontario situation, Heseltine (1983, 22) notes that "while the number of psychiatric hospital beds has been reduced, the size of psychiatric hospitals' budgets has not." This is not a particularly surprising conclusion given the much higher rates of admissions, particularly readmissions, that now characterize the province's mental hospitals (table 8.2). Total mental health expenditures actually increased significantly throughout the 1970s, and the anticipated cost savings were not realized. In the early 1980s there was some decline in expenditures, which may have been a function of the restraint policies introduced during the recession of 1981 (table 8.3). It appears, then, that deinstitutionalization may have contributed to the expansion of welfare expenditures, rather than amounting to any significant savings.

Political conservatism fostered other pressures for the deinstitu-

Table 8.2. Admissions and Discharges in Ontario Psychiatric Facilities

	Public Mental Hospitals		Public Hospital Psychiatric Units	
	1960	1976	1960	1976
First admissions	4,575	5,433	3,041	16,670
Readmissions	3,664	8,886	1,396	13,332
Total admissions	8,239	14,319	4,437	30,002
Discharges	6,426	14,319	4,386	28,920
Deaths	1,629	341	19	32
Total separations	8,055	14,660	4,405	28,952
Bed capacity	15,141	5,314	431	1,946

Source: Heseltine 1983, tables 2.1 and 2.2.

tionalization of certain groups. Growing demands to lessen the role of government and promote the role of the private sector involved both commercial and non-profit organizations, which felt they could more efficiently provide care in smaller facilities. Pressure to alter policies was exerted by groups external to the government such as the commercial nursing-home lobby, operators of lodging homes, and voluntary organizations such as the Elizabeth Fry and John Howard societies (in the field of correctional service). Taken as a whole, such demands amounted to calls for the privatization of social services because the role of the welfare state was rolled back.

Table 8.3. Mental Health Expenditures by the Department of Family Services and the Ministry of Community and Social Services, Ontario, Selected Years

Years	Amount
1970/71	281.6
1978/79	411.2
1980/81	421.1
1981/82	415.7

Source: After Heseltine 1983, table 3.1.

Note: In 1971 millions of dollars.

The Homes for Special Care Act and the Homes for Retarded Persons Act had been passed in 1964, resulting in the first major transfers of psychiatric inpatients from hospitals to community-based residences, including nursing homes and private homes. This was the beginning of a process of reprivatization, returning the responsibility of caring for dependent groups to the private sector. However, the mentally ill and retarded were not returned to the charitable institutions that had cared for them in the nineteenth and early twentieth centuries. Patients were placed in commercially operated homes, the owners of which received a per diem payment from the Ontario Department of Health. These homes received fifteen thousand patients between 1965 and 1981 (Heseltine 1983, 22–23). The innovations in deinstitutionalization began in the Ministry of Health (formerly the Department of Public Health; the name was changed in the 1960s) during the early 1960s, but it was not until 1972 that the provincial Ministry of Community and Social Services was created with an explicit mandate to promote community-based care. Policymakers and those responsible for the internal reorganization of the provincial government saw this new ministry as the rightful administrator of services for the mentally ill and retarded who had been returned to the community (Simmons 1982; Williams 1984). The transfer of patient care to the community occurred largely after 1974 with the passage of the Developmental Services Act. Table 8.4 shows the growth in the budget of Community and Social Services as greater emphasis was put on community-based programs. There was a noticeable increase in expenditure after the 1966 introduction of the Canada Assistance Plan (a federal cost-sharing program), and again in 1972 when the Ministry of Community and Family Services was reorganized into the Ministry of Community and Social Services.

Some organizations, such as nursing homes, have had a long history of involvement in the operation of residential care facilities. That their infrastructure was in place meant that they were prime candidates for government contracts when programs like the Homes for Special Care were introduced, and, in this case, it was largely commercial operators who benefited. As more and more community-based programs were developed, the provincial government increasingly awarded purchase-of-service contracts to both commercial and voluntary agencies. For example, the Ministry of Health contracts with voluntary and, to a lesser extent, commercial agencies for the delivery of nursing and homemaker services under its Homecare program. This particular program has grown rapidly over the last decade as more and more elderly people are cared for in their homes (a

Table 8.4. Expenditures by the Ontario Department of Family Services and
Ministry of Community and Social Services, Selected Years

Year	Expenditures
1966	103.7
1968	115.5
1970	133.3
1972	366.2
1974	389.0
1976	613.4
1978	674.7
1980	676.4
1982	727.5

Source: Ontario, various years.

Note: In 1971 millions of dollars.

domestic form of privatization) rather than being placed in institutions. Such contracts have stimulated the private sector. At the same time, however, the increasing reliance on government financing has resulted in some loss of autonomy for these private organizations because they are obliged to meet certain regulations governing the receipt of funds. Privatization in this form extends the scope of the welfare state into previously independent areas; it is not causing the dismantling of the welfare state.

The private sector has also become a more active participant in social services by default. Changes in Ontario's social policy have resulted in demands for new types of services, but the state has not responded. This has led to criticisms of state policies by the private sector. For example, the Ontario Welfare Council (1981, 2–3) has strongly criticized the implementation of the provincial government's policy of deinstitutionalization because

> the province has initiated a process of movement to community based care without providing the comprehensive enabling legislation, policy guidelines, technical assistance and adequate funding that could permit the implementation of a *coherent, caring system.*
>
> We believe that the province has placed too high a priority on the short-term objective of reducing government expenditure on institutional care. This has not only created confusion around the concept

and practice of community based care, but we fear that the short term "solution" will be more expensive in the long run.

In 1972, the Ontario Association for the Mentally Retarded also expressed its concern over the need for improved community-based services to the Provincial Task Force on Mental Retardation: "We believe that mental retardation is not primarily a health problem. . . . We believe that community services must be broadened and expanded in order to have a viable system to carry out the philosophy of returning to the community wherever possible every retarded person who does not require a health facility" (OAMR 1972; cited in Anglin and Braaten 1978, 65).

The private sector has therefore stepped in to fill the gap created by the state's failure to provide those elements necessary to a coherent system. A case in point is the growing demand for emergency shelters in many urban centers in Ontario. Where appropriate residential care facilities are not available, the high costs of rent, the difficulties in finding paid employment, and the inadequacies of Ontario's income-maintenance programs have together resulted in an increasing number of homeless people (City of Toronto 1986). In 1986 the homeless population in Ontario was about ten thousand people (Ontario TFRBL 1986). The voluntary sector is the main source of accommodation for these people, many of whom have psychiatric or some other medical history. Commercial operators have also established homes for people who are without permanent shelter because of shifts in state policy. Deinstitutionalization has meant that people have to find accommodation in the community in which they can find the aftercare service on which they rely. The lodging-home industry now serves a significant proportion of these people (MTFDPP 1984; HWDSS 1986). The locus of care for these special-needs groups is being shifted, by default, from the public to the private sector.

Clearly, deinstitutionalization and privatization were key components of the huge increases in welfare expenditures that were occurring throughout the 1960s and early 1970s. This highlights that these processes were at work prior to the onset of the state's fiscal problems, so arguments that emphasize the role of the fiscal crisis need to be questioned. This trend also suggests that, far from superseding the private sector, the development of the welfare state has in fact encouraged the growth of private activity in the provision of welfare services (Mishra, Laws, and Harding 1989). But, during the recessionary period from the mid-1970s until the early 1980s, privatization became a more explicit means by which the government of Ontario dealt with its fiscal problems. Several government reports released in the mid-1970s pointed to the usefulness of promoting the private sector (see, for example, Ontario SPRC 1975). Such reports were often the end product of review processes that afforded a formal opportunity for community groups to express their concerns regarding social service delivery and thus influence the development of social policy. For example, the Visiting Homemakers' Association of Hamilton-Wentworth presented a brief to the Special Programs Review Committee (SPRC) arguing for increased services under the Visiting Homemakers and Nursing Services Act: "The Home Care Program of the Ministry of Health has recently limited Homemaker Services to a patient to 80 hours. Not only does this appear to contradict the Government's policy to extend care-in-the-home services, but it puts *pressure on Homemaker Services to respond to needs in situations in which the Government has abdicated responsibility*" (VHAHW 1973, 4; emphasis added).

The state did not respond immediately to such calls. Lobbying around this particular issue of home care continued through the 1970s, and in 1986 the province's New Agenda for seniors' services consolidated all of these changes, which had been made in a piecemeal fashion, in one program, the already existing Visiting Homemakers' program. Now both the Ministry of Health and the Ministry of Community and Social Services are involved in this program, but it still operates under purchase-of-service contracts with private agencies (Van Horne 1986).

A critical element of deinstitutionalization is the development of community-based residential facilities. As noted earlier, in Ontario these have mostly been provided by the private sector. By focusing on the privatization of the residential component of community care we are able to begin to understand the impact of this process on local communities.

The Privatization of Residential Care Facilities in Hamilton, Ontario

How have these processes of restructuring affected the development of the welfare state in local urban places and how has the state responded to these new local forms? Here, the example of Hamilton, Ontario, will be used to illustrate the ways in which privatization and deinstitutionalization have resulted in new forms of the local-level welfare state and how they have thus contributed to the uneven spatial development of the welfare state.

Hamilton is the site of a large psychiatric hospital, which has witnessed a significant reduction in its inpatient population over the last two decades. In 1969, the capacity of the hospital was 1,451 beds; by 1980 the bed size had been reduced to 502. Similarly, the year-end inpatient population declined from 1,063 in 1969 to only 325 in 1986. This has created a demand for community-based residential care facilities. At the same time, like most other industrial societies, Hamilton's population is aging, thereby increasing demand for supportive housing for the elderly.

Residential care in Hamilton for persons who may previously have found refuge in an institution is provided both within specific facilities (e.g., nursing homes and lodging homes) and within an individual's home with the assistance of some outside agency. For the purposes of this chapter, residential care facilities are defined as those facilities that provide some level of assistance in the activities of daily living in a noninstitutional or community-based form of care. Emergency shelters are not included in this discussion. Commercial proprietary operators are involved in the provision of care in nursing homes, homes for special care, boarding homes, and lodging homes. The voluntary sector operates a small but important number of group homes and homes for the aged. The domestic sector is responsible for care within the client's home; for the most part, care is delivered by a member of the household, and thus it is difficult to gauge the precise contribution of this sector. Table 8.5 shows a breakdown of the number of beds provided by different types of residential facilities. In all, some 4,154 beds are available within the Hamilton-Wentworth region, 63 percent of which are provided in commercially operated nursing homes, lodging homes, and homes for special care. Group homes, which are usually operated by the voluntary sector, provide less than 10 percent of the community-based accommodations. The remaining 27 percent is provided by charitable or municipal homes for the aged (Laws 1987).

As with the more general provincial trends discussed above, the demand for community-based accommodations in Hamilton grew throughout the 1970s and early 1980s. As the data just reported indicate, the private sector has responded to these needs. Focusing on the growth of the local lodging-home industry will give some further insight into how the process of privatization has been played out in Hamilton and how it has affected the local community. Beamish

Table 8.5. Adult Residential Care Facilities in Hamilton-Wentworth, 1986

Type	Number of beds	% of total
Lodging homes[1]	1,141	27.5
Nursing homes[2]	1,344	32.4
Homes for special care[3]	144	3.5
Total commercial sector	2,629	63.4
Homes for the aged[2]	1,132	27.3
Group homes[4]	384	9.3
Total noncommercial sector	1,516	36.6
TOTAL	4,145	100.0

Sources: [1]Hamilton-Wentworth Department of Social Services 1986, Personal communication; [2]Ontario Ministry of Health, Personal communication; [3]Hamilton-Wentworth Regional Social Services Department 1986, Personal communication; [4]Author's primary data gathered in fieldwork, December 1986.

(1981) has used early licensing records to trace the development of lodging homes in Hamilton. In 1976 there were thirty-three homes. By 1977 this figure had doubled to sixty-eight, and in 1979 there were ninety-one homes. In 1985, one hundred homes were licensed by the city of Hamilton, of which sixty-seven were designated as second level. This designation grew out of local concerns over the care provided for special-needs residents of lodging homes. A second-level lodging home is a commercially operated home with four or more residents. The operators of these homes must be available twenty-four hours a day to provide "guidance in the activities of daily living" (Hamilton bylaw no. 80–259 [rev. 81–93] 1981). Operators of second-level homes are eligible for per diem payments from the regional Department of Social Services. Thus, local legislation encourages commercial community-based homes to enter into a partnership with the local government in providing alternatives to institutional accommodation. This example illustrates clearly the close link between privitization and deinstitutionalization.

To obtain a second-level lodging-home license the operator agrees to comply with stricter regulations. A second-level lodging home is defined as one "(1) which accommodates four or more residents; (2) where, for a fee, the operator offers to residents guidance in the activities of daily living, and advice and information; (3) where, twenty-four hours a day, at least, the operator is on duty in the home and able to furnish such guidance" (Hamilton bylaw no. 80–259 [rev. 81–93] 1981). It is thus a designation that legitimates the commercially operated home as a residential facility that can provide care for those with special needs.

Surveys conducted in the early 1980s by the local Department of Public Health revealed that one-half of the residents in these facilities had previously been in a psychiatric or general hospital. Many more were elderly. While there continues to be an absence of housing alternatives, many of the clients discharged from the local psychiatric hospital are placed in one of the local lodging homes. Between July and November of 1986, for example, approximately 16 percent of patients discharged from Hamilton Psychiatric Hospital were discharged into lodging homes. Lodging homes were the single largest point of discharge after private homes (table 8.6).

Since the passage of the bylaw on second-level lodging homes in 1981, there has been a rapid growth in the number of homes that have received the second-level designation. In fact, their number has more than doubled since 1981, when there were thirty-four homes thus licensed; by July 1986 there were seventy-two. It is in the interest of the operator to obtain this license because homes with the second-level designation are eligible to enter into a contractual arrangement with the regional Department of Social Services. Under provincial legislation, local government can contract with certain residential facilities to provide accommodation for persons in receipt of provincial income-maintenance payments (General Welfare Assistance and Family Benefits). Once discharged from a hospital, many chronically mentally disabled people receive these payments because they have difficulty in finding full-time employment. Some idea of the importance of this contractual relationship can be gained from the following figures. In 1979, $403,333 was spent by the region in subsidizing accommodation in lodging homes (this was before the introduction of the second-level bylaw). By 1983, the regional budget allocated $800,000 for lodging-home contracts, and in 1986 the budget for these contracts was $2,663,000 (Hamilton-Wentworth Department of Social Services, personal communication).

Table 8.6. Patient Disposition on Discharge from Hamilton Psychiatric Hospital,
July-November 1986

	Outpatient		Inpatient		Total	
	N	%	N	%	N	%
Private						
home or apartment	56	55.4	162	62.3	218	60.4
room	1	1.0	5	1.9	6	1.7
boarding house	22	21.8	36	13.8	58	16.1
Domiciliary hostel	6	5.9	5	1.9	11	3.0
Residential homes						
for special care	1	1.0	1	0.4	2	0.5
Co-op home	1	1.0	0	0	1	0.3
Group home	7	6.9	6	2.3	13	3.6
Nursing home:						
extended care	1	1.0	1	0.4	2	0.5
Home for the aged	1	1.0	0	0	1	0.3
Hostel	2	2.0	7	2.7	9	2.5
Correctional						
institution	0	0	2	0.8	2	0.5
COMSOC[a] facility	0	0	3	1.2	3	0.8
Other[b]	3	3.0	32	12.3	35	9.7
TOTAL	101	.100.0	260	100.0	361	100.0

Source: Hamilton Psychiatric Hospital 1986, Personal communication.

[a]Ministry of Community and Social Services.

[b]Includes no fixed address, not elsewhere classified, and unknown.

Local lodging-home operators have mobilized their resources and
organized effectively to lobby the local welfare state apparatus. For
example, in 1986 Hamilton operators could receive a per diem of
twenty-five dollars per subsidized client. This figure was agreed
upon after active lobbying by the Operators' Association and repre-

sents the maximum payment permitted under the relevant provincial legislation (the General Welfare Assistance Act). Given that operating costs are likely to be higher in other cities (e.g., Toronto with its greater land values), it would appear that local operators have been a very successful lobby group. Their 1986 per diem represents an increase of over 10 percent on the previous year's budget at a time when the regional Social Services' budget was held to a 3.8 percent increase. Clearly, some other component of the Social Services' budget was held constant or cut back while public funds were used to support proprietary homes.

Local communities such as Hamilton have clearly been affected by changes in state policies aimed at accommodating service-dependent groups. In particular, social policies have been partly responsible for, and partly the outcome of, the uneven development of the state. This example shows the ways in which privatization is the result of pressures occurring both internal and external to the state. A state policy of deinstitutionalization has encouraged the active participation of the private sector in the provision of residential care for special-needs groups. At the same time, the actions of private operators have ensured their continued and expanding participation in this area. At the local level, the local state is forced to respond by introducing legislation to regulate the activities of private operators. One consequence of the Hamilton legislation has been to make the city more attractive to operators, since the contractual arrangement lends some stability to their incomes. This illustrates the way in which local conditions may influence the spatially uneven development of the welfare state and is related to the horizontal shift in service provision that has occurred during the recent period of restructuring. Certain localities are service rich, while others are service poor (Geiger and Wolch 1986). People in need are likely to be concentrated in areas where services are available. This pattern tends to breed its own perpetuation. For example, Hamilton Psychiatric Hospital has a catchment area that covers several municipalities in the Niagara Peninsula. However, for patients who are discharged from the hospital, the city of Hamilton is service rich in the postdischarge support services they require. Consequently, a large proportion of the people discharged from Hamilton Psychiatric Hospital remain within the city of Hamilton. Thus, there has been a horizontal shift in the focus of care from the home community to the service-rich neighborhoods, which creates further demand for services in these places, draws more services to locate there, and continues to attract more people from other geographic areas.

Conclusions

Recent restructuring of Ontario's welfare state has been dominated by the related processes of deinstitutionalization and privatization. This has resulted in organizations operating under a variety of auspices delivering care to various groups that were previously served primarily by the state. This chapter has highlighted the ambiguous nature of privatization. Various pressures work to promote private-sector services. And, just as there are many calls for privatization, there are many consequences. We might think of the example of the growth of residential care facilities for Ontario's growing elderly population. Changing demographic characteristics combine with political and economic imperatives to create a service-delivery system that is largely dependent upon the private sector.

A crucial question that must be considered is: Does privatization imply an erosion of the welfare state? Millions of dollars of public funds are finding their way into the private sector via purchase-of-service contracts and subsidies. But these contracts are subject to certain regulations, and so privatization may, in fact, result in an extension of the state's control function. We must not be too hasty to generalize about inevitable consequences of privatization. There may not be an erosion of the welfare state; there may simply be a change in its form, as the case of Ontario indicates.

Privatization of residential care also has interesting implications for urban social and built environments. Because operators of commercial facilities will seek to maximize their profits, they will locate in areas where real estate and operating costs permit this: the inner city with its architecture that facilitates conversion for nonfamily living arrangements. This has contributed to the ghettoization of service-dependent groups in the inner city (Dear 1980) and thus has contributed to a special form of residential segregation. Local community opposition to this concentration and to attempts to accommodate special-needs groups in suburban neighborhoods has created difficulties for planners attempting to increase the housing options for these people. The debate as to whether institutional or community-based accommodation is most appropriate has now been superseded

by arguments about the respective merits of public and private models and about the advantages and disadvantages of commercial
versus non-profit service provision. Privatization has created another dimension to the problem of housing service-dependent
groups at a time when their housing situation is becoming increasingly threatened.

PART THREE

ENVIRONMENTAL HEALTH SERVICES

Chapter 9

Privatization, Federalism, and Cancer Prevention in the United States

Abdicating a Noble Goal

MICHAEL R. GREENBERG

We would not want to raise false hopes by simply the signing of [this] act, but we can say this: That for those who have cancer, and who are looking for success in this field, they at least can have the assurance that everything that can be done by government . . . in this great, powerful rich country, now will be done and that will give hope and we hope those hopes will not be disappointed.

President Richard Nixon, 1971

Richard Nixon's declaration of war on cancer in 1971 was a stroke of political genius. Backed by $1.6 billion in research funds for three years and later by billions more, scientists were to learn enough about cell biology, viruses, and immunology to prevent and cure cancer. Eighteen years later, there is no magic bullet. Nor is there a cancer prevention campaign commensurate with 460,000 American cancer-related deaths a year. The shortcomings of the war on cancer and criticisms of the government's failure to build a prevention program have been demonstrated in great detail (Culliton 1987; Epstein 1979; U.S. DHEW 1979; Highland et al. 1979; Agran 1977).

This chapter first shows that the geography of cancer has changed in the last thirty years. In particular, many places that formerly had low cancer rates now have high ones. They need cancer prevention programs. The second part of the chapter shows that the supply of cancer prevention programs does not geographically match the need—that is, there is an undersupply in some places that badly need programs. Existing government and private efforts, built under the politics of privatization and federalism, leave a major gap in cancer prevention among the economically disadvantaged in poor states, particularly in the South. In the third part of the chapter, I suggest an approach for a joint government-private program to fill the gap.

The Changing Geography of Cancer
Mortality and Socioeconomic Status

The geography of cancer in the United States has dramatically changed during the last two decades, and this change has implications for cancer prevention programs. Urban cancer rates in the United States were more than 50 percent higher than rural ones in the 1950s, but the gap has decreased (Greenberg 1983, 1987a). Data for the white male population thirty-five to sixty-four years old illustrate this change. The population thirty-five to sixty-four is chosen because it is young enough to benefit from prevention programs and is a better indicator of recent cancer trends than the elderly and young populations (Greenberg 1987a). Changes in female rates, shown elsewhere (Greenberg 1983, 1987a), are not as striking, but follow the same trend. Data on nonwhites cannot be used because mortality data prior to the 1960s are unreliable.

In 1939–1941, the average white male cancer mortality rate (age-adjusted to the 1960 population of the United States) in the five states with the highest rates was 190.6 per 100,000. It was 95.2—almost exactly half—in the five states with the lowest rates. The high- and low-rate states fit the expected pattern. Urban New York, New Jersey, Massachusetts, Illinois, and Connecticut had the highest rates; and rural Arkansas, North Carolina, Tennessee, West Virginia, and Kentucky had the lowest ones. Urban/rural differences were less two decades later. Rates in the five urban states rose to an average of 208.8, an increase of 9.5 percent. They rose 80 percent to 170.9 in the five rural states. So the urban/rural gap decreased from 100 to 22 percent. The gap was gone by 1979–1981. The average rate in the five urban states decreased from 208.8 in 1959–1961 to 201.2 in 1979–1981, while the rate in the rural ones increased 32 percent to 225.5.

The reality of the 1980s is that Arkansas, Kentucky, Mississippi, Tennessee, and West Virginia are experiencing marked increases in cancer deaths. The places that almost everyone thinks have high cancer rates have stable or declining ones: New Jersey, New York, Massachusetts, and Connecticut.

The diffusion of life-styles, industry, and people, as well as better diagnosis and records, are factors helping to explain the changing geography of cancer mortality in the United States (Greenberg 1983, 1987a). Low socioeconomic status is a key to understanding the new geography of American cancer mortality. Researchers have shown an association between socioeconomic status and cancer rates (Lilienfeld, Levin, and Kessler 1972; Levin 1974). At the state scale, the five states that increased the most in white male cancer rates—Arkansas, Kentucky, Mississippi, Tennessee, and West Virginia—ranked forty-ninth, forty-fourth, fiftieth, fortieth, and forty-seventh in per capita income in 1981 (U.S. Bureau of the Census 1983). Connecticut, Massachusetts, New Jersey, and New York—the four northeastern states with stable or declining white male rates—ranked second, eleventh, fourth, and twelfth. The five southern states ranked forty-ninth, forty-eighth, forty-seventh, forty-fifth, and fiftieth in percentage of college graduates; the four northeastern ones ranked third, fifth, twelfth, and fifteenth. Per capita income averages 40 percent higher in the four northeastern states than in the five southern states, and 19.2 percent of the people completed college in the former compared with only 11.4 percent in the latter.

Analysis of a national survey of behavioral risk factors among Americans eighteen to thirty-four years old shows remarkable differences associated with socioeconomic status as measured by educational achievement (Greenberg 1987c). Fifty percent of Americans ages eighteen to thirty-four who have less than a ninth-grade education smoke, compared with 25 percent among those who had any college education. Educational achievement also differentiates young adults' use of seat belts and the tendency to be obese and hypertensive (Greenberg 1987c). There is a strong association between poverty and low survival rate, which is explained by the fact that the poor know less about cancer warning signs, have less confidence in the medical community, have less physical and financial access to medical care, and therefore go later than affluent people for diagnosis and treatment. Furthermore, they frequently have inadequate nutrition and receive poorer treatment than the more affluent (U.S. DHHS 1985).

Given that cancer rates in southern rural states are now as high as or higher than in urban northern ones, that socioeconomic status is a factor in getting and dying from cancer, and that we have no national cancer prevention program, can federalism and privatization cope with the cancer geography of the 1980s?

State and Local Government

We first look at state programs, then school and community prevention efforts.

State Cancer Prevention Policies

Nearly 90 percent of formal state cancer prevention policies were promulgated during the period 1975–1984. A study by George Washington University (NHPPGWU 1984) for the National Cancer Institute (NCI) permits a geographical analysis of state cancer prevention policies. The George Washington group surveyed state legislated actions affecting cancer prevention policies through early 1984, dividing them into nine types:

1. Providing health education programs for school systems and the general public aimed at reducing smoking, improving nutrition, and other life-style factors
2. Instituting taxes on tobacco products to reduce smoking and to support cancer research
3. Restricting smoking in public places
4. Organizing registries of cancer incidence and mortality
5. Screening for cancer resulting from specific exposures, for examples, DES (diethylstilbestrol) and cervical cancer
6. Developing centers aimed at studying and controlling the causes of cancer and finding cures
7. Controlling occupational and environmental carcinogens through regulations and providing information to workers
8. Mandating insurance coverage for all or some cancers
9. Instituting other actions, including the use of alternative treatments (e.g., laetrile, marijuana), consent for certain surgeries, cancer commissions or advisory councils, regulation and testing of drugs, and cancer treatments.

It is not possible to say whether state cancer legislation has been successful, nor is it possible to read the legislation and say with certainty that one approach will result in greater reductions in cancer than another because one looks better on paper than another. However, it may be assumed that people living in states with policies are better off than those without them.

There is an obvious regional geography of cancer prevention policies (fig. 9.1). Connecticut, Massachusetts, New Jersey, New York, and Ohio form a Northeast cluster with six or more of the nine possible policies. Florida, Minnesota, Texas, and Nevada are the others with six or more policies (the "many" policy group). Idaho, Wyoming, Utah, North Dakota, and South Dakota form a band of northern Mountain and Plains states with two or fewer policies, as do Alabama, Arkansas, Mississippi, Tennessee, and West Virginia in the South. Iowa, Missouri, Indiana, and New Mexico are the remaining "few" policy states. The remaining twenty-five states have three to five policies and are called the "some" policies states.

Greenberg (1987b) showed that states with many policies had high cancer rates, have been strong supporters of public health and environmental protection policies, and are relatively affluent. States with few cancer prevention policies until recently had low cancer rates, have been less progressive in developing environmental protection and public health programs, and are relatively poor.

The few policies in Alabama, Arkansas, Mississippi, Tennessee, West Virginia, and some other states could be rationalized in 1970 by

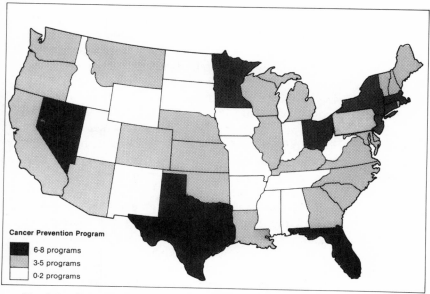

Fig. 9.1. Cancer Prevention Programs in the United States, 1984
Source: Greenberg 1987b. Reproduced courtesy of Pion Ltd.

low cancer rates; that is, these states may have believed that cancer was a problem in the Northeast, not in the South. But as noted earlier, southern states have experienced high increases in cancer mortality rates. Many have to contend with relatively high unemployment and poverty rates. Without federal directives and funds, they can be expected to make cancer prevention a lower priority than jobs, economic development, and dealing with poverty. In short, state governments acting independently of the federal government will bring cancer prevention to the New Jerseys and Connecticuts of the United States, but probably not to the Mississippis and West Virginias.

Local Government

Local governments can help prevent cancer and other chronic diseases by protecting water supplies and by providing health care, nutrition, cancer screening, and land-use controls. Yet health education is their most important opportunity. Historically, the local school district has not embraced the health education role. School health is added on to physical education and biology courses and is usually presented as moral arguments against sex, drugs, and alcohol (Bruess 1978). The unfortunate state of health education in our schools is explained by a lack of effort by health care professionals; lack of support from federal, state, and local governments; and failure to provide curricula and training for teachers (Strategic Planning Group 1984).

The Growing Healthy curriculum offers school systems a health-promotion model (Gotsch and Pearson 1987). Developed in Seattle and California and administered by the National Center for Health Education with help from the American Lung Association, it covers nutrition, smoking, alcohol, and other risk factors for cancer and other diseases for grades K–12. Students learn how today's life-style choices can affect present and future health, how their bodies work, and the relationship between their feelings and health. The center and the American Lung Association will help school districts implement the curriculum. Limited testing suggests that the curriculum reduces behavioral risks. For example, smoking rates increased from 6 to 8 percent among seventh graders exposed to the curriculum; rates among the controls increased from 8 to 13 percent (New York City Department of Health 1986).

About 600 school districts (out of 15,500) in forty-one states are trying Growing Healthy. The number of students using Growing Healthy rose from three hundred thousand to more than five hundred thousand between 1980 and 1983. While Growing Healthy is rapidly being adopted, the geography of its adoption is both predictable and distressing. With the exceptions of Arkansas and New Mexico, suburban and urban residents in populous states are the primary beneficiaries. Alabama, Mississippi, and West Virginia have no, or almost no, participating districts. Strong state cancer and environmental protection programs seem to go along with strong school health education programs. It should be expected that poor and politically conservative communities located in poor and politically conservative states—the very places that are experiencing marked increases in cancer rates—will not adopt the program.

It is hard to be sanguine about community health education programs because there is so little support for them. For example, the Stanford University Heart Disease Program was designed to determine if education through local media and the community would lead to behavioral changes (Farquhar 1984). Communities with programs showed greater reductions in smoking and consumption of saturated fats than control communities. This success led to more pilot programs in California, Minnesota, and Rhode Island. The United States Department of Health and Human Services (DHHS) recognizes excellence in community health-promotion programs by giving awards. Though pilot programs and awards are valuable, there are so few community health programs and there is so little federal and state interest in them that these programs, no matter how well intentioned and successful they may be in their study areas, are tokens that cannot make a dent in the nation's cancer, heart disease, and other chronic disease rates.

Private-Sector Efforts

This section analyzes efforts made by corporations, the health industry, and television to promote cancer prevention.

Corporate Health Promotion

Over one hundred million Americans work. Protecting them against occupational hazards requires an ongoing political effort. Promoting health among workers is a recent idea. Metropolitan Life has offered health-promotion programs for more than a century, but this company is unique. Corporate interest is recent and follows the increase in health insurance costs. Roger Smith, chairman of General Motors summarized the economic rationale behind corporate interest.

> By promoting the concept of preventive health care at the worksite, we won't be solving the problem of soaring health care costs. But we'll be contributing toward a solution—and a fiscally responsible approach to cost containment. More important we'll be promoting good health, longer, more productive careers, and a higher quality of life in general for our employees. . . . The fact is, American industry can't afford not to expand the wellness movement in the workplace. (Smith 1984, 4)

Corporate health-promotion programs aim at smoking cessation, cancer screening, nutrition counseling, stress management, and other behavioral changes that should reduce cancer risk. The U.S. DHHS (1984) expects that 35 percent of all workers will have access to smoking-cessation programs and a slightly larger proportion will have programs aimed at alcohol and drugs, nutrition, and stress control by 1990. DHHS's optimistic forecast is based on the impressive list of Fortune 500 companies with large health promotion programs (e.g., Control Data, IBM, Johnson and Johnson, General Motors).

Corporate promotion of health practices should be applauded. But most Americans work for small companies and may not have access to the programs. For example, the New York City Department of Health (1987) surveyed worksite smoking policies. Twenty percent of companies with at least 500 employees had written smoking policies. This compared with 7 percent of companies with 100–499 employees, 5 percent with 11–99, and only 2 percent with 10 or fewer employees. Preliminary analysis of the geographical distribution of corporate health-promotion programs in the United States shows concentration in large metropolitan regions. Furthermore, they are used primarily by better-educated employees (Cook 1989).

Since corporate programs will not be accessible to every American, we wanted to see how available prevention programs are through sources that should be readily available to the public. We studied smoking-cessation programs that advertise in the Yellow Pages and therefore should be accessible to almost every American (Bellet 1987). Sixty smoking-cessation programs were found in New Jersey during the period 1976–1986. Our preliminary analysis showed that most were located in affluent suburban areas. These were not readily accessible by mass transit. Few were found in low-income areas. In fact, the two best indicators of their location were socioeconomic status and percentage of the population that was white. If our case study is typical, poor minority communities do not have access to private cancer prevention services. In addition, there is a large homeless population that does not even have access to phones, and certainly does not have the money to pay for private smoking-cessation programs.

The Health Care Industry

Physicians, dentists, and other medical care personnel fix problems. But their high credibility means that they can have a major impact on promoting health. The Health Maintenance Act of 1973 requires HMOs to actively provide health education services. Nursing organizations, Blue Cross, the AMA (American Medical Association), the Society for Public Health Education, the Health Insurance Association of America, and the American Cancer Society have adopted health promotion (Gotsch and Pearson 1987).

Hospitals have made the major effort. The typical pre-1980 hospital program concerned nutrition, diabetes, heart disease, mastectomy, and what to do and expect before and after surgery (American Hospital Association 1979). Recent health-promotion programs have expanded to smoking cessation, physical fitness, accident prevention, assertiveness training, and cardiopulmonary resuscitation (Gotsch and Pearson 1987).

As the medical care system moves toward control by for-profit corporations (Starr 1982), prevention will become a way of containing costs. But the Health Policy Agenda for the American People developed over five years by 172 interest groups led by the AMA is illustrative of why some people do not think that prevention can be trusted to the medical care community. Some of the almost two hundred recommendations are about health promotion. But *Nation's Health* (April 1987, 8–9), the voice of the American Public Health Association, characterized the total agenda as one for "medical care," not for "health." The report primarily deals with how to use money for technology, development, biomedical research, professional education, and delivery and regulation of health care services—in other words, ends desired by health care professionals.

The prevention part is the weakest. The document focuses primarily on one-to-one communication rather than on community-based approaches. Health promotion in a one-to-one setting typically

focuses on curing one problem, not on the overall health of the individual. Furthermore, how will this approach reach people who do
not use the medical system? A basic benefit package is recommended, but the package is primarily a way of paying for curative
medical services, not a way of making sure everyone learns how to
promote good health.

Television

Does television convey sufficient information about health and risk
to change people's habits? As part of a study of television coverage of
environmental risk, we analyzed nightly network coverage of cancer-
risk stories.

Using the Vanderbilt index as the data source (Vanderbilt University 1984–1986), we found that during the twenty-six-month period
January 1984 through February 1986, ABC, CBS, and NBC showed
about 100 stories about cancer risk—about one a week. In comparison, there were 482 stories about airplane accidents and 100 about
earthquakes. Cancer stories took three hours and two minutes—
in other words, about three-tenths of one percent of nightly news
coverage. The longest cancer-risk stories were not about cigarette
smoking, asbestos, or other common carcinogens. They were about
NPPD, a suspected carcinogen that was supposedly spread in the
American Embassy in Moscow so the Soviet KGB could follow
American personnel. One NPPD story lasted seven minutes and
twenty seconds, much longer than any story on cigarette smoking.

Obviously, the major source of news for most Americans is not
spending much time teaching them about cancer risk or prevention.
Furthermore, even if it tried, studies show that televised messages
are ignored or misperceived if they conflict with existing attitudes. In
other words, network television may help, but is unlikely to make a
difference in efforts to change behaviors (Sandman et al. 1987; Whitney 1985).

Government-Private Collaboration for
Cancer Prevention

In the context of cancer prevention, privatization and federalism
mean limited federal responsibility for health promotion. Health education, research, screening, worker protection, and pollution control
are left to a few progressive state and local governments, corpora-

tions concerned with minimizing health insurance costs, organizations like the American Cancer Society, and the medical care system. In other words, privatization and federalism mean abandonment of the concept of equal access to prevention and medical care. They emphasize concern with containing costs. Health care becomes an economic good that is subject to supply, demand, and price (Arthur D. Little 1985). Yet I believe there can be a workable cancer prevention program within the constraints of privatization and federalism.

I propose a joint government-private cancer prevention program for the disadvantaged. The federal government would set the agenda, identify areas most in need, and fund the program. It has already accomplished the first two tasks. The agenda is set. In *Cancer Control Objectives for the Nation: 1985–2000* (Greenwald and Sondik 1986), the National Cancer Institute (NCI) claims that cancer mortality would drop as much as 50 percent below 1985 levels if the percentage of smokers and the consumption of fat were reduced; fiber consumption was increased; and breast examinations, Pap smears, and state-of-the-art treatments were adopted. For example, the percentage of adult smokers should decrease from 34 percent in 1983 to 15 percent or less, and the percentage of youths who smoke by age twenty should decrease from 36 to 15 percent or less. NCI's goal is to increase the average consumption of fiber from eight to twelve grams per day to twenty to thirty grams per day and to decrease fat consumption from 37–38 percent to 30 percent or less of total calories. The percentage of women ages twenty to thirty-nine who have a Pap smear every three years would increase from 79 percent to 90 percent, and to 80 percent from 57 percent for women ages forty to seventy. Annual breast examinations for women ages fifty to seventy are targeted to increase from 45 to 80 percent, and mammographies should increase to 15 percent.

For the second task, the NCI and the Environmental Protection Agency have identified counties in need of a program (Riggan et al. 1983). For example, 119 counties were found to have significantly ($p < .05$) more white female breast-cancer deaths than expected during 1970–1979; over 350 had elevated cervical cancer rates; and about 150 had significantly high total white female cancer mortality rates. This research, which has also been done for white males and for nonwhite males and females, can be used to develop an initial list of counties that would automatically be eligible for a cancer prevention program. These would be counties with high rates and many poor and minority people.

The federal government's third role would be to fund cancer prevention. I cannot estimate the cost of this program. In comparison, the federal Superfund program for cleaning up hazardous waste sites costs almost $9 billion. The U.S. Environmental Protection Agency (1987) estimates that there are just over 1,000 cancers a year from exposures to chemicals at hazardous waste sites. This figure compares with 460,000 who annually die from other cancer-related causes. At least 200,000 would not die if NCI's behavioral risk goals were accomplished.

Every public health issue has a constituency and hence a political life of its own, so it would be foolish to call for a new federal cancer program with a cost of tens of billions of dollars. However, it seems reasonable to suggest that the proposed program start in the hundreds of millions of dollars and increase as successful prevention protocols appear.

In the proposed program, states would have the minimal responsibility of distributing federal money to health-promotion providers and evaluators. Many states will want to do more, and this proposal gives them that opportunity. They can request additional funds for counties not in the initial federal list by providing incidence or behavioral risk data that show a problem. For example, they can compare mortality and incidence rates. Counties with high mortality/incidence ratios have a population that is not presenting itself for medical treatment early enough, not getting adequate treatment, or not following treatment regimes. States can survey behavioral risk factors for cancer: smoking, diet, breast self-examinations, Pap smears, and alcohol abuse. Counties with elevated behavioral risks would be eligible for funds.

Private organizations would provide and evaluate the prevention services. Privatization of cancer prevention services allows them the flexibility to work with local religious institutions, public and private schools, social clubs, and other groups, and to design programs to best suit the local population. Such groups are not hampered by a federal government that is unable to take local conditions into account (Portney 1986).

The federal government can save communities from uneconomically reinventing knowledge by making available records of successes and failures. It must also insist that an independent monitoring company certify that behavioral changes have occurred; that is, that smoking has decreased, fiber consumption has increased, and other related behaviors have been improved.

I am working with the New Jersey Department of Health on a

three-phase grant awarded by NCI. The goals are to prevent and end tobacco use, increase breast and cervical cancer detection, increase access to state-of-the-art treatments, and control exposure to carcinogens in the workplace. This type of intervention will move the United States in the direction of my proposed program, but will occur slowly because the government's resources will almost certainly be limited to pilot programs. I recognize that the level of effort proposed in this chapter may be politically infeasible. Accordingly, elsewhere I have argued for a cancer prevention program targeting American blacks, the population with by far the worst cancer problem (Greenberg 1989).

Prevention is not magic (Russell 1986). The wrong messages may be communicated. There is a great deal of controversy about nutrition and cancer (Calkins 1987; Becker 1986), and the medical care system is often criticized by overzealous proponents of health-promotion programs (Roemer 1984). The poor need unambiguous messages about nutrition. They also need to use the medical care system more than they do, especially for detection and treatment of cancers.

Prevention can hurt those whom it should help. Many people are unable to stop smoking, reduce alcohol and drug use, eat more nutritious diets, and follow other recommendations of cancer prevention. Acceptable health behaviors are seen by some as moral behaviors (Becker 1986): if you do not practice them, you are considered immoral; if you are ill, you are at fault—in other words, another form of blaming the victim. Health promoters have to be prepared to be less successful than they would like to be. They must be willing to accept the criticism of conservatives, who will no doubt produce tortured cost-benefit calculations to support dissolving any targeted cancer prevention program. Yet, without such a program there will be a substantial increase in the cancer gap between classes and races.

Prevention was not what President Nixon expected to be the major weapon against cancer. Yet prevention can markedly reduce cancer rates in ten to fifteen years. Privatization and federalism should not be allowed to stop cancer prevention. We must adjust to the swings of the political pendulum in order to start and implement a cancer prevention program that can save dollars and lives.

PART FOUR

DEVELOPING COUNTRIES

Privatization in the Periphery

Chapter 10

Dismantling Public Health Services in Authoritarian Chile

JOSEPH L. SCARPACI

   Authoritarian Chile (1973–present) represents one of the most radical attempts to dismantle an extensive public health care system. This dismantling is unique within Latin America, where, until recently, there has been an uninterrupted trend of growing state participation in economic processes (Glade 1983). State responsibility for the provision, regulation, and accumulation of manifold services and goods has been a heavy one throughout Latin America. But policy shifts in Chile more closely represent the supply-side strategies and deregulation movement of the Reagan administration in the United States, where arguments for restructuring and privatization are quite strong (Vernon 1988). Attempts to cut back state-funded health care are unprecedented in the history of Chile as it was the first country in the Western hemisphere to develop national health insurance for targeted members of the (nonmilitary) labor force.

   State health care financing in Chile culminated with the 1970 presidential victory of socialist Dr. Salvador Allende. A physician by training and a politician, senator, and minister throughout most of his professional life, Allende was the first democratically elected socialist president to hold office in the Americas. His Popular Unity party furthered the state's control of the economy, which had increased in the 1960s. The Christian Democratic administration of Eduardo Frei (1964–1970) had begun what was to be later continued by Allende as Chile's experiment in the "peaceful road to socialism." But this legacy was reversed when the Allende government was overthrown in September 1973 by General Augusto Pinochet. The present authoritarian government, scheduled to relinquish power to a democratically elected civilian government in 1990, has turned away from the more centrally planned economy of previous administrations. Health policies under military rule have been the antithesis of the kind of socialized medical care that prevailed under civilian governments up until 1973 (Roemer 1985, 385). Private medical practices have been encouraged under the sixteen-year Pinochet administration and remain the central feature of the regime's restructuring of health services.

This chapter discusses three aspects of health care privatization enacted by the Chilean military. It first examines the junta's efforts to promote HMO-like private medical plans, an example of a change in health services regulation. Next, it reviews the scaling back of the Environmental Health Services division, a reduction in state provision. Finally, it discusses recent attempts to transfer public primary medical services from national to municipal management, an indication of the changing subsidy of primary care. Collectively, these reduced levels of public regulation, provision, and subsidy form the cornerstone of health services privatization in Chile.

The chapter begins by examining highlights of the national economy in Chile under military rule and by identifying similar economic development strategies in other countries. Seminal health care legislation and movements in Chile prior to the current junta are also reviewed. The three examples of privatization noted above are then examined. The chapter concludes with a review of selected health care privatization experiences in other Latin American countries and a consideration of the significance of the Chilean privatization experience within the Southern Cone region of South America. The characteristics of the bureaucratic-authoritarian regime are then reexamined in light of conventional writings on that type of state apparatus and the way in which the Chilean regime dismantled public health services as compared with other regimes in the region.

Privatizing the National Economy

Attempts by the Pinochet government to decrease the size of the state bureaucracy in Chile have been carried out at ideological, policy, and programmatic levels. At the ideological level, the military regime favors dismantling state enterprises. The regime, comprising ardent capitalists and fervent anticommunists, considers the state's proper role to be that of guard of the national patrimony, as opposed to being an active force in production and service delivery. As noted in chapter 1, adherents of this ideology see the state as inefficient, costly, and generally unfit as a producer of goods and services. This ideology stems in good measure from the ideas of economists Milton Friedman and Friedrich von Hayek, who have been influential in promoting privatization. Throughout the 1970s large numbers of professionals left Chile to train at the University of Chicago and other United States graduate programs where the unabashed free-market ideas of Friedman and Hayek flourished. Upon their return to Chile, those graduates assumed key administrative positions under the Pinochet government (Caviedes 1984). Young economists in Chile, like many of their counterparts in other developing countries, had become disillusioned with their parents' generation—a generation that had resisted decentralized decision making and the power of an efficient market. Raymond Vernon (1988, 6) notes that these youthful economists began "to align themselves with parties of the right, to support measures that built the role of market forces, and to resist forces that built up the powers of government." In Chile they have come to occupy such influential positions as minister of the treasury (hacienda) and economy (economía) as well as head of the Chilean federal reserve board (Banco Central). Antigovernment ideology was also diffused through United States war colleges in Panama and Washington, D.C., where numerous Chilean military officers have trained. The practice of heralding the virtues of the unfettered marketplace is derived from a growing international web of the new laissez-faire philosophy—an ideology common to practitioners and theorists of free-market economics that spans many countries (fig. 10.1; Latin American Bureau 1983, 56–57).

A central thrust of the Pinochet government is the promotion of private-sector participation in industry, commerce, finance and banking, transportation, housing, and health care. Unlike the privatization of other sectors, health care privatization was delayed, partly because of popular opposition rooted in a history of socialized medicine and partly because of the demonstration effect that could be employed if other sectors of the economy were successfully privatized first.

At the programmatic and policy levels, government officials implemented austerity measures during the regime's first two years in power (1973–1975). Many state-owned enterprises were sold. For example, of 460 state enterprises in 1973, only 23 remained in public hands seven years later (Ffrench-Davis 1982). Between 1973 and 1983 the number of public employees was reduced by 25 percent (Martínez and Tironi 1982), and the National Health Service

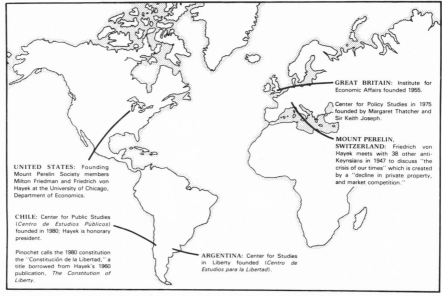

Fig. 10.1.   The International Linkages of the New Laissez-faire
Data Source: Latin American Bureau 1983, 56–57.

physician-to-population ratio was cut by one-fifth (Medina and Kaempffer 1982).

Few restrictions on private business mergers facilitated private-sector accumulation of capital. By 1980 about two-thirds of the country's capital was concentrated among six firms (Gwynne 1986). Tariffs on imported goods (except automobiles) were lowered from around 300 percent to a flat 10 percent (Ffrench-Davis 1982). This laissez-faire model eased the entrance of foreign capital in the form of investment and loans, and between 1977 and 1980 contributed to an average annual growth rate in the gross national product of about 5 percent (Martínez and Tironi 1982). The business community welcomed most of these efforts, including health services privatization, that decreased management's overhead costs and facilitated capital accumulation (Meza 1984; Jiménez de la Jara 1982; Contreras et al. 1986). By 1987 the state was considered to be so successful in the implementation of its free-market development policies that foreign financial analysts were praising Chile's approach to "popular capitalism" (Gwynne 1987).

Table 10.1. Seminal Health Care Legislation and Movements in Chile

Year	Event
1918	Railroad workers and certain industrial workers receive comprehensive medical benefits
1924	First comprehensive national health insurance for selected *obreros* (blue-collar workers) and *empleados* (white-collar workers)
1938	SERMENA (Servicio Médico de Empleados Nacionales) is created, providing comprehensive health services for public employees
1952	National Health Service (Servicio Nacional de Salud) created to coordinate more than fifty private and public health programs
1964-1970	Eduardo Frei presidency (Christian Democrats), increased public medical programs
1970-1973	Dr. Salvador Allende presidency (Popular Unity), proposed Servicio Unico de Salud, which would have eliminated private medical care, but it did not materialize
1973	September 11 coup d'état led by Brigadier General Augusto Pinochet
1974-1976	Austerity measures enlisted under "Operation Shock"
1980s	Restructured health services, privatization, and greater out-of-pocket payments; withholdings (*cotizaciones*) rise from 4 percent in 1984 to 7 percent in 1988 for all nonindigents; Ley de Salud bases primary health care fees on income levels for the first time in Chilean history

Data Sources: Viel 1961; Romero 1977; Scarpaci 1988a.

Seminal Health Care Legislation and Movements in Chile, 1918–1987

The significance of Chilean health services privatization is perhaps best grounded in the history of its health care reforms (table 10.1). Chile became the first nation in the Western Hemisphere to provide comprehensive medical coverage for nonmilitary public workers. State railroad workers began receiving free or low-cost medical care in 1918 (Romero 1977). The stock market crash in 1929 and the ensuing economic depression left Chile (and the rest of Latin America) in a precarious state as its primary-export economy was debilitated by slack demand from the industrial economies. The crisis of the 1930s cast the governments of Brazil, Mexico, Argentina, Uruguay, and Chile into what Cardoso and Faletto (1979) term a "developmentalist" role—that is, they established numerous state-managed development agencies and industries to provide goods and services in sectors of the economy where the private sector could not or chose not to operate.

Although the Second World War boosted demand for Chilean exports, particularly copper and nitrate products, the late 1940s ushered in a bust to that demand cycle. As a result, the issue of nationalized, comprehensive health care, which had been considered by the Chilean parliament at least since the 1930s, returned to the forefront of electoral politics as the need for a strong and healthy labor force during economic booms and busts became apparent. The creation of the National Health Service in Great Britain in 1948 was a sign of encouragement for Chileans, who have long looked toward Europe for political, social, and cultural enlightenment (Viel 1961; Caviedes 1984). Commercial exchange between Chile and Europe, as well as the large numbers of European immigrants in Chile, bolstered public support for a national health service. Reduced to its most fundamental argument, the electorate claimed that a national health service would guarantee minimum health care coverage for blue-collar workers (obreros) and indigents, while the business community recognized that a healthier labor force implied greater worker productivity (Romero 1977).

The political pressures brought on by the 1952 presidential campaign (Jiménez de la Jara 1977), the British example, and the proliferation of public and private medical programs were important catalysts in the formation of Chile's National Health Service (Servicio Nacional de Salud, or SNS) in 1952. The SNS took over the delivery and financing of more than fifty medical programs. It also replaced the functions of many charitable organizations (beneficencias), which had been important (private, non-profit) sources of medical care since the nineteenth century (Roemer 1964, 1985).

Private medical care expenditures in Chile were on the downturn prior to the 1973 coup d'etat. The Christian Democratic government of Eduardo Frei (1964–1970) enlarged public environmental, hospital, and ambulatory care programs. Based on data from the Chilean federal reserve board (Banco Central), Viveros-Long (1982) and Raczynski (1982, 75) determined that 53 percent of health care expenditures in 1969 originated in the private sector. That proportion dropped to 49 percent in 1970 under the Allende government. In contrast, by 1980, after seven years of military rule, private health care expenditures constituted 66 percent of all health care spending.

The level of consumption of medical care in Chile under the Pinochet regime has been, without precedent, strongly correlated with income level and the public or private nature of providers. Three sources of medical care based on income levels can be identified in the 1980s. Income groups constituting the poorest 40 percent of the population (obreros) seek entirely free medical care from the national health services; although a 1987 law mandated charging for care based on income levels, and that will change this traditional entitlement (Scarpaci 1988b). Middle-income white-collar workers (empleados), the next 40 percent of the population, receive care from the National Health Fund (FONASA), which is financed by mandatory wage withholdings, out-of-pocket charges, and employer contributions. The remaining 20 percent of the population (the upper-income group) is treated mainly by private providers (Scarpaci 1985c). Thus, the proportions of out-of-pocket payments and private insurance coverage are strongly and positively correlated with income levels; those with higher income levels used the public system less frequently. It is to this latter category of consumer that Chile's promotion of Health Maintenance Organizations (HMOs) has been targeted. In the section that follows we turn to these HMOs as one of three examples of health services privatization.

Three Examples of Health Services Privatization

Promoting HMOs: Easing Regulation

HMOs are not without precedent in Chile. Organizationally, they are related to medical programs called *cajas de previsión*, which from the 1930s until the early 1980s served as prepaid medical programs only for certain public and private employees. Private firms in banking and finance, construction, and mining provided these medical programs as employee benefits. These cajas offered employees alternatives to crowded and unattractive public facilities used by the general public. Equally important, cajas were less expensive than exclusively private medical care since they were financed by a combination of employee wage withholdings and employer contributions.

The latter were generally greater than levels mandated by law, which greatly increased the quality and quantity of medical benefits versus other programs.

The Pinochet regime changed the regulatory statutes in 1980 and used cajas as HMO prototypes. These new practices, Institutos de Salud Previsional (ISAPREs), are funded by wage withholdings, employer contributions, monthly premiums, and copayments made at the time of service delivery. ISAPREs offer high-amenity medical care and are modeled after HMOs in the United States (Rice and Garside 1986). They are located in the nicest neighborhoods of metropolitan areas. In January 1989, roughly 80 percent of all private-hospital bed use in Santiago was by ISAPRE patients, while in the provinces the figure stood at roughly 20 percent (personal communication, Ramon Martínez, manager, Asociacion Gremial de Clinicas, Hospitales y Otros Establecimientos Privados de Salud, December 21, 1988). Their advertisements emphasize new facilities, private hospital rooms, the latest imaging equipment, and other amenities. Because of their derivation from cajas, ISAPREs were originally formed around certain sectors of workers (e.g., Banmedica for banking and finance employees; Chuquicamata for copper workers), but today they have open enrollments. Prior to the enactment of Law Decree 3626 in November 1981, fewer than 2 percent of all Chileans were enrolled in cajas. By opening enrollments to white-collar workers (empleados) outside these industries, a competitive medical marketplace was expected to emerge. State health planners anticipate that the forces of market competition and the benefits of economies of scale will eventually allow ISAPRE plans to trickle down to middle-income consumers and even to obreros.

Law Decree 3626 permitted wage earners to place their mandatory monthly withholding for medical coverage (cotización) into an ISAPRE of their choice. In 1982, eleven ISAPREs were registered with the government (fig. 10.1), and the three largest ISAPREs captured 74 percent of the ISAPRE market (fig. 10.2). By 1984 the three leading ISAPREs had dropped their market share to 58 percent, suggesting the possible emergence of a more competitive private medical marketplace (Scarpaci 1988c).

Government officials had projected that, by 1984, one million Chileans (about 9 percent of the total population) would be enrolled in one hundred ISAPREs (Jiménez de la Jara 1982; FONASA 1982). However, by 1984, ISAPREs had captured less than half of the original 1980 forecast, and this enrollment figure included at least one

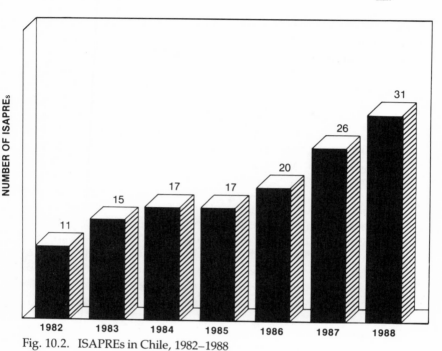

Fig. 10.2. ISAPREs in Chile, 1982–1988

hundred thousand "built-in" affiliates who were transferred from the
cajas of the 1970s. By early 1985, less than 3 percent of all Chileans
belonged to an ISAPRE.

Two important questions must be addressed in analyzing the evolution of ISAPREs in the 1980s. First, what accounted for the slow
growth between 1981 and 1985? Second, what was the state's response to such sluggish growth that in just three years (1986–1988)
had accounted for a twofold increase in the number of ISAPREs and
a trebling of enrollment?

Slow ISAPRE Growth: 1981–1985. Part of the slow growth between 1981 and 1985 can be explained by the spatial concentration of
ISAPRE offices and subscribers in upper-income neighborhoods of
Santiago, Viña del Mar, Valparaíso, and Concepción as well as the
marketing focus on healthy, young, urban professionals with few dependents (Donckaster 1985; Jiménez de la Jara 1982, 170–173). The
Pinochet government had claimed that consumer purchasing power
had been weakened by the national economy's slump, the latter

triggered by low prices for copper, the leading export (personal communication, Office of ISAPRE Coordination, FONASA, Santiago, March 1984). However, such a technical assessment for the slow growth of these private medical programs masks the historical and programmatic reasons for slack HMO growth and casts blame on the invisible forces of the marketplace. At least four other factors must be considered for slow ISAPRE growth between 1981 and 1985.

First, ISAPREs met resistance in marketing efforts because the population had firm opinions about how the traditional cajas operated. Dr. Ruben Acuña, vice-president of the Colegio Médico in 1984, commented that most physicians' objections about ISAPREs "emphasize the inconvenience of introducing . . . a performance measure of market economy in place of solidarity, cooperation and coordination that should exist among all health systems" (El Mercurio, April 24, 1984, sección YA, 12–13). Consultants from midwestern United States HMOs were hired for the delicate matter of advertising for-profit medical programs in a country where such advertising was rare (Colegio Médico 1982; see especially Rice and Garside 1987).

Besides the obstacle of marketing, the business functions of the ISAPREs were not well executed. For example, plans for future building construction and medical equipment purchases that were made during the 1977–1981 boom period proved disastrous for many medical clinics and ISAPREs when the Chilean peso was suddenly devalued in November 1981. ISAPRE debt doubled immediately, and liability was especially high for ISAPREs that had purchased diagnostic equipment in United States dollars as the gap widened between the floating value of the Chilean peso and the dollar. But debt in the private medical sector only mirrored patterns in the rest of the economy. By 1983, two years after ISAPRE creation and the devaluation of the national currency, only oil-rich Venezuela had a higher per capita debt than Chile. Chile is obliged to meet strict repayment schedules outlined by the International Monetary Fund (United States Embassy 1984) and has been one of the most steadfast Latin American nations in debt repayment (CEPAL 1988). ISAPREs, struggling to remain solvent, have had to pass on costs to policyholders. As a result, the unanticipated higher operating costs have also forced ISAPREs to seek even higher income groups than the originally targeted middle- and upper-income groups. Thus, although state-owned enterprises in Latin America are often criticized because they operate only in unprofitable markets (Kelly de Escobar 1988;

Kapstein 1988), it was the state that coaxed ISAPREs into a market that had failed to grow by 1985.

A third weakness in Chile's HMO promotions was that coverage was restrictive, especially for women of reproductive age. Three ISAPREs refuse enrollment to working women in the home (amas de casa) under forty years of age. Still others require women of reproductive age to certify they are not pregnant (as opposed to merely denying maternal coverage to women who become pregnant before enrolling or before satisfying a 270-day waiting period). These exclusionary clauses run against a long tradition in Chile of extremely progressive medical care coverage for women (Meza 1984). One self-employed professional woman (whose earnings fluctuate) who was enrolled in an ISAPRE asked, "Do ISAPREs see us as mere reproductive devices that are dangerous, and without any right to get sick or to reproduce?" In justifying the exclusion of maternity charges and maternity leaves of absence, an ISAPRE administrator stated: "If a women declares a monthly income of 15,000 pesos and suddenly becomes pregnant, and then lists her income at 80,000 pesos [ISAPREs] would have to pay four and a half months [of income] plus [maternity] expenses" (El Mercurio, April 24, 1984 sección YA, 12–13). These complaints by ISAPRE managers notwithstanding, maternity programs in Chile have historically contributed to a high rate of female labor-force participation in the formal sector (Covarrubias and Franco 1978). Gender is not the only restriction. Psychiatric and dental care are not covered in most ISAPREs, nor is treatment for congenital diseases or mental health care provided by nonphysicians. Critics from the Colegio Médico point out that such practices have led to the "institutionalization of discrimination against high-risk persons" (Donckaster 1985, 53).

A fourth factor that accounted for poor ISAPRE performance between 1981 and 1985 stemmed from competition with the semipublic FONASA program, which is mainly used by white-collar and middle-income workers. The FONASA program is divided into three levels of care that are differentiated only in terms of cost; the clinical competence of providers is the same, while only amenities such as waiting rooms and waiting times vary (Scarpaci 1985a). Upper-income FONASA patients have been able to receive care equal in quality to that of ISAPREs, but at lower cost (Scarpaci 1987). The official position of the Colegio Médico is that "ISAPREs should provide at least the same services as FONASA" (Donckaster 1985, 51). Moreover, like ISAPREs and other nonindigent medical programs in

Chile, the FONASA program is financed mainly by monthly wage and salary withholdings (cotizaciones) and matching employer funds. Unofficial estimates from personnel at the World Bank note that ISAPREs consume about 70 percent of all wage and salary withholdings that are extracted from nonindigent workers (personal communication, World Bank, Health Sector, 1988). That less than 10 percent of the national population draws on such a disproportionate amount of funding for such high-amenity medical care attests to the inequity and class bias in medical care financing under the Pinochet regime.

Despite the disproportionate amount of mandatory wage withholdings that the state has allowed ISAPREs to consume, this infusion of capital was still not enough to finance the high-amenity medical programs. Mandatory medical care withholdings rose from 4 percent of gross wages and salaries in 1982 to 5 percent in 1983, to 6 percent in 1984, to 7 percent in 1986, and to 7.5 percent in 1988 (Contreras et al. 1986; Smith 1988)—an 88 percent increase in six years. Significantly, the bulk of these increases in health care withholdings came about between 1979 and the first quarter of 1983 when the medical consumer's purchasing power (defined as the index of salaries and wages divided by the rate of change in the consumer medical price index) fell by one-fifth (Scarpaci and Bradham 1988). This was compounded by a 15 percent fall in real wages during that same time period (Cortázar 1983), which further weakened the medical consumer's purchasing power. In short, the government inadvertently fostered competition between a public and private medical system at a time when real health care costs were rising. By relaxing health service regulation, the regime has diverted large sums of capital to the promotion of a medical program that is strong on nonmedical amenities and weak on allocating health resources efficiently.

The State to the Rescue: ISAPRE Growth, 1986–1988. The 1986 Health Law (Ley de Salud, or Supreme Law 369) was the salvation of ISAPREs. Among its many changes, general tax revenues issued through FONASA replaced ISAPRE funds for the payment of medical and maternity leaves. Since 1986, ISAPRE members have been reimbursed by the ISAPRE from the fourth until the tenth day of illness. The state, through FONASA disbursements, pays for all lost wages due to illness beyond the tenth day of absence from work. In the maternity sector, the state now pays for ninety days of prepartum and postpartum maternity leave. Prior to the Health Law, the maternity leaves were paid exclusively by the ISAPREs and were financed only by the standard wage withholdings, employer contributions, and monthly premiums. Key actors in the Chilean health policy field, ranging from the minister of health, Dr. Juan Giaconi, to the ISAPRE Association president, Dr. René Merino, suggest that, without state intervention to incur the costs of these medical and maternity leaves, ISAPREs would have entered into bankruptcy within a few years (personal communication, December 1988). In short, general tax revenues contributed by all working Chileans have been diverted for the benefit of less than 10 percent of the national population. State intervention in 1986 has been the major reason for the rise in the number of ISAPREs from twenty to thirty-one between 1986 and 1988 and for a threefold increase in ISAPRE affiliates to 1.4 million during that same period (fig. 10.3; see also fig. 10.2).

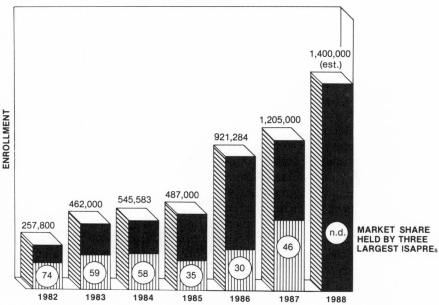

Fig. 10.3. ISAPRE Enrollment and Percentage of Market Share Held by the Three Largest ISAPREs, 1982–1988

Reducing Provision: Cutbacks in Environmental
Health Services Monitoring

De-statizing the economy and reducing public programs and workers have produced noticeable changes in the monitoring of environmental health services. Each of the twenty-seven public health service districts in Chile houses a division of the Environmental Health Service (Servicio de Salud Ambiental). The responsibilities of the Environmental Health Service include monitoring air, water, and land quality, as well as food-service inspection (*New York Times*, July 14, 1987, A-4). But because of the junta's cutbacks in public programs, the monitoring of environmental health has been scaled back.

One of the most deleterious effects of these cutbacks has been the increased rate of hepatitis B and typhoid since 1976 (Colegio Médico 1983). Possible sources of contamination are feces-contaminated streams and unhygienic restaurants (Haignere 1983). These problems have been acute in Santiago, the primate, capital city (estimated 1985 population, 4.6 million), where 42 percent of the nation's population resides. The city's only primary water treatment is a single sewage facility, and there is no secondary or tertiary treatment.

In 1984, personnel cutbacks left only two Environmental Health Service staff available for four hours a week to check fields irrigated by the Mopocho and Maipu rivers in Greater Santiago. Under current regulations, farmers who use contaminated river waters for cultivating leafy vegetables such as lettuce, cabbage, and parsley are asked to cease production within ninety days or be fined. But because there are so few staff to inspect the crops, few sanctions are brought against farmers who harvest small garden crops (*hortalizas*) and sell them in Santiago markets. The Ministry of Health attempts to prevent the spread of hepatitis and typhoid by inserting pamphlets into local newspapers that identify the risks of eating these leafy vegetables. Appropriately, these pamphlets recommend that vegetables be carefully soaked in a commercial disinfectant (about one United States dollar for a six-ounce bottle) or regular household bleach. One pamphlet designed by the Ministry of Health uses the image of "F.T." (*fiebre tifoidea*, or typhoid fever) in a play on words with the movie *E.T.* The cover of the pamphlet (fig. 10.4) announces that "F.T." is a film that "is not recommended." But the health-promotion efforts of the pamphlet are questionable given that it is doubtful whether many Chileans have seen the film, particularly vulnerable and high-risk groups (the poor and young). Despite these efforts,

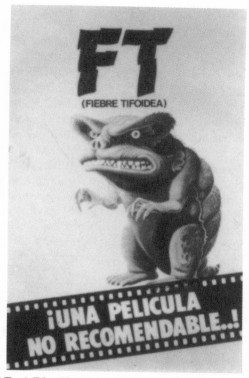

Fig. 10.4. "F.T.: A Film That Is Not Recommended"
Source: Cover of pamphlet put out by the Ministerio de Salud.

Chile, with less than 2 percent of the population, had between 20 and 25 percent of all hepatitis and typhoid cases in the Western Hemisphere in 1983 (Colegio Médico 1983).

Ministry of Health officials recognize the weaknes of their crop surveillance methods. They realize that bringing contaminated crops to market increases the risks of spreading these infections. However, public health officials refuse to destroy the crops in situ or to subsidize farmers who switch to producing another, more salutary crop. Officials refuse to take such measures even though no cost-benefit analyses have examined the opportunity costs associated with crop destruction or subsidies, and none have considered the productivity and profit loss due to employee illness. It has been argued that the public's health could be ensured by immediate crop destruction and a one-time partial subsidy to small farmers who tap the polluted waters to irrigate garden crops (Scarpaci 1985a).

Other sources of infection for hepatitis B are fast-food establishments (*fuentes de soda, kioskos*) and seafood markets and restaurants that sell shellfish (*mariscos*) caught offshore in the nutrient-rich waters of the Humboldt Current. Slightly spoiled clams and oysters and feces-contaminated finger foods such as sandwiches, hot dogs, meat pies (*empanadas*), and pastries are prime sources of infection. Fortunately, seafood consumption in Chile is not high, despite its low cost and availability; the long-standing social preference is for meat. Epidemiologists Medina and Yrarrázaval (1983) reported that random inspections (e.g., for purposes other than license renewal) of food establishments fell from 124 in 1974 to 5 in 1981, a result of decreased levels of funding for Environmental Health Services. In short, reduced provision of environmental health services has been part of a broader strategy to reduce the state's role in health services delivery, the result of which has contributed to an unprecedented rise in certain infectious diseases.

Reducing Subsidies: National-to-Municipal Transfer of Primary Care Clinics

Community participation in the provision of primary care is a cornerstone of effective delivery systems. Health needs are better served when the health care profiles of local areas are incorporated into central planning. To that end, the decentralization of primary care has been a major policy focus throughout the Third World, and was a conference topic at the Tenth Annual Conference of South American Health Administrators held in Montevideo in June 1988 (Gonzalez 1988). However, decentralization has been difficult in Latin America, where centralist and vertical states have long existed (Calderon 1987).

Like the New Federalism of the Reagan administration with its emphasis on states' rights and local-level administration of social programs, the Pinochet regime has transferred many national public health clinics to municipal-government management (*municipalización*). New financing for primary-care visits permits this municipal transfer to be carried out under Law Decree 3060 (Giaconi 1982). By structure and design the transfer reimburses clinics for actual use of goods and services on a slightly higher capitation basis, as opposed to the traditional, lower-cost basis of budget allocations that are based on historical patterns. The ministry claims that this reduces the public bureaucracy and argues that local officials "know the demands and preferences of the people" and can therefore increase clinic efficiency (Ministerio de Salud 1982, 3). During the early years of municipalization, only the best-run clinics were voluntarily transferred to municipal management. One of the first objective analyses of municipalization conducted by an independent, ministry-appointed panel found more mismanagement and inefficiency in maternity and infant care programs in municipalized facilities than in those that were not municipalized (Borgoño et al. 1983). By April 1988, all rural primary care clinics operated by the National Health Service System (SNSS) and 91 percent of all urban clinics had been transferred from national to municipal (i.e., county) management.

The incentive for local governments to assume control lies in the ability to reinvest the reimbursement transfers from the national government. After covering costs, local government can reinvest the surplus (national government transfer fees less operating costs). However, by law the local government can only invest the surplus in nonsalary personnel items or capital improvements. When these transfers began in 1981, there was no limit on the number of primary care treatments a facility might provide. But problems were reported—for example, blood-pressure and cursory dental examinations were reimbursed at the same level as a twenty-minute primary care visit. The Ministry of Health responded to these abuses by placing a ceiling *(techo)* on the number of primary care examinations that a clinic could provide and by issuing guidelines that distinguished primary care from non–primary care treatment.

These abuses aside, it was mainly clinics in the middle- and upper-income municipalities of Nunoa and Las Condes that came under municipal control during the early 1980s (Contreras et al. 1986; Smith 1988). Patients in these neighborhoods tend to be healthier, visit for shorter periods of time, and require fewer tests and prescription drugs. Municipal governments were reluctant to assume management if the illness level of the community would inhibit their ability to provide low-cost care. An independent consulting team contracted by the Ministry of Health, consisting of a nurse, an economist, a sociologist, and two physicians, evaluated municipalized clinics in the municipality of Las Condes in Santiago and concluded that, because the levels of reimbursement from the national government were insufficient, "under the present circumstances there is no possibility that the municipal administration of health [services] is able to finance itself without a deterioration in service delivery" (Infante et al. 1983, 6).

Other skeptics suggest that the national government has transferred these clinics to municipal management in an incremental process that will place health services beyond arm's length from the
state. This arrangement would set the stage for private management
to begin charging for services at primary care facilities (Jiménez de la
Jara 1982). This notion was strongly insinuated in a policy paper issued by the junta shortly after the 1973 coup d'etat (Spoerer 1973),
and the spirit of this policy was finally legislated in 1986 with the is-
suance of the Health Law (Ley de Salud). The law requires that all
SNSS users carry employer-certified income cards. This salary information will allow the application of a progressive scale of charges to
primary care users of public clinics.

But SNSS clinics are not "closer to the needs of the people" as the
normative processes of decentralized primary care suggests. On the
contrary, the Ministry of Health under the Pinochet regime views
community participation in identifying the health needs of the population as political activity. The public primary model remains curative
in focus and physician dominated by design (Jiménez de la Jara and
Gili 1988). Physician directors are routinely dismissed who engage in
community outreach activities that address the real needs of shanty-
town dwellers such as impetigo, body lice, respiratory infections,
and prenatal and postnatal control. Recognition and legitimation of
these real needs would be an indictment of a public health care system that lacks the fiscal resources to do an adequate job. Since clinic
directors of municipalized clinics contract with county governments,
they can be hired and fired by county mayors (who, in turn, are
named by President Pinochet). Ostensibly, then, municipalization
would seem to be an ideal medium for decentralizing primary care,
but it has actually become quite politicized. In fact, municipalization
is now referred to as the "mayorization" of health care (alcadización)
because the real decisions rest in the office of the mayor.

Chilean Privatization in Latin American Context

Industries and Services

The privatization of industries and services in Latin America has
moved at an uneven pace, ranging from rhetorical cries for the dismantling of public enterprises to well-executed policies of regulatory,
provision, and subsidy changes that have tipped the scales toward

the private sector. The rhetorical cries for privatization have been thwarted in some countries because of the high level of professionalization and technical competence of some state industries. Venezuelan petroleum industries, a Chilean copper company, a number of Brazilian public enterprises, and government-owned banks in Mexico have been recognized for "upgrading managerial quality" (Glade 1983, 96). These regional success stories grew out of the *desarrollismo* style of development that was common in the 1950s and 1960s. State capitalism stimulated structural change and economic growth. The public frequently supported public control over such national patrimony as oil in Mexico, copper in Chile, or high-tech industries in Brazil; they become the source of foreign revenues and the pride of national production.

These successes of state-owned industries notwithstanding, well-executed polices of privatization have received a good deal of attention as well, albeit for reasons other than economic efficiency. Brazil responded to attacks on the *estatização* (statization, or growing public sector) of its economy by creating a debureaucratization ministry in 1981. The halting of the Brazilian miracle after the first decade of military rule (1964–1974) became evident when the government announced plans to sell 100 of 564 state-owned enterprises as a means of dismantling the public bureaucracy. But large industrial nations have not been the only ones in Latin America to pursue such a course of action. Jamaica, following the 1980 election of Seaga, began to draw more on foreign capital than on domestic sources for development initiatives. Debt-burdened Uruguay, Costa Rica, and Argentina have seized on privatization as a means of passing on the rising costs of public utilies to the private sector, thus freeing the government to negotiate with the International Monetary Fund on firmer ground. Slack demand for petroleum products has elicited different results in Venezuela and Mexico; the former was able to sell off numerous state firms in the 1980s, while the latter actually loaned money to the large Grupo Alfa consortium so that the consortium could remain solvent.

Health Services

Chile has traditionally had less of a two-tiered society than most Latin American countries. Most Latin Americans have the medical care needs of a destitute population, but organize their services like industrial societies (Horn 1985; Ugalde 1985; Mesa-Lago 1985). Health services privatization in Chile is noteworthy in several regards. Its most distinctive feature is that the decision to cut back state support was determined without consulting the electorate or the congress. Supporters of state cutbacks claim that social public programs have two weaknesses. First, legislation is often passed in election years as a concession to unions, provinces, political parties, or occupational groups. To be sure, most health care and social security legislation in Latin America derives from electoral and political pressures, which in turn are closely bound to class relations (Mesa-Lago 1978). It is not unexpected, therefore, that health care is unevenly distributed geographically and socially. Second, although democratic governments may have inequitable distributions of health services, until 1973 Chile was actually moving toward a convergence of uniform and comprehensive health care among income groups. This egalitarian effort ended abruptly when the Pinochet regime ushered in austerity measures so that private accumulation and military expenditures could be increased (Garretón 1983).

Current efforts to eliminate the ad hoc method of allocating medical care that evolved under populist governments up until 1973 depend on consumers' abilities to select providers (*libre elección*) and to choose a health system according to their purchasing power. As in the industrial societies of the North Atlantic and Australasia, privatization in Chile emphasizes individual responsibility in procuring medical care in a competitive medical marketplace (Virgo 1987). In Great Britain, for example, segments of electrical and railroad workers have opted for more costly private insurance in order to reduce scheduling time in National Health Service clinics (Le Grand and Robinson 1984). As shown in chapter 3, there is a trend in the traditional welfare states of Western Europe to negotiate wages and salaries, on the one hand, and to offer medical care, retirement, and disability benefits on the other (see also Offe 1984). Whereas privatization efforts in Europe have concentrated on separating real wages from social wages, the Chilean experience emphasizes a graduated out-of-pocket scale for financing medical care.

Comparative Aspects of Technical Planning, Decentralization, and Health Policy

Like the "military modernizers" in Chile, the Brazilian military government (1964–1985) treated health as a branch of science that could be addressed in a technical, apolitical manner by imposing

costs on the working classes (Horn 1985). The health status of the
Brazilian population deteriorated markedly in the 1970s, as indicated
by a dramatic upsurge in malaria, an increase in infant mortality related to widespread malnutrition, an unprecedented outbreak of
meningococcal meningitis in the urban slums, and a rise in anemia
among children (Musgrove 1986, 156; Macedo 1984). The Brazilian
Ministry of Health has identified 60 percent of the population as
"destitute." Significant regional variations in these health statuses exist, however. In the poor and agrarian northeastern state of Piauí, 90
percent of the people are classified as destitute; while in the industrial
state of São Paulo the figure, although lower, is still an alarming 26
percent (Horn 1985). The Brazilian military government placed a considerable portion of state resources in the hands of the private sector,
so that by the early 1980s nearly 75 percent of all state-funded hospital and ambulatory-care services were contracted to private providers
(Cordeiro 1982, 103). Like the Chilean experience, these private-
sector operations have been criticized for lacking well-integrated hier-
archical and complementary services and clearly defined regional
boundaries (Landman 1979; Cordeiro 1982).

The shift of national health services to local management is also evident in Mexico. There, as in Chile, the rationale for these transfers
rests on the belief that local management is more sensitive to community health needs than national management, which tends to be
biased toward large metropolitan populations. Mexico has long been
plagued by a top-down approach to health service delivery. Opponents of this method of finance in Mexico argue that it produces geographically and socially unequal reinvestment patterns of public
monies (de la Madrid et al. 1986).

Health care programs in the Southern Cone of South America
(Argentina, Chile, and Uruguay) have been closely linked to development strategies. Since the Second World War the region has em-
barked on a new course of economic and sociopolitical development
that has been marked by two major events. First, the traditional
comparative-advantage model of economic growth (whereby foreign
earnings were largely generated by primary-commodity exports such
as Chilean copper and Argentine and Uruguayan meat and cereal
products) was replaced with import-substitution industrialization
(see Prebisch 1962). High tariffs on foreign manufactured goods were
imposed in order to protect nascent national industries. Economic
growth was anticipated but, for reasons not to be considered here,
fell short of original goals that were expected to lead to sustained economic growth.

Bureaucratic-Authoritarianism and Health Service Privatization

This poor economic performance exacerbated political tensions and produced the second major postwar event in the Southern Cone: the emergence of a unique type of military government known as the bureaucratic-authoritarian (BA) regime (in Argentina, 1966–1972 and 1976–1983; in Uruguay, 1973–1985; in Chile, 1973–present). BA regimes emerge under conditions of hyperinflation, political instability, fiscal deficits, and economic stagnation. After overthrowing democratically elected governments, they demobilize political parties and unions by prohibiting their organizations and banishing their leaders. BA regimes assume a subsidiary role in relation to the private sector. They forge strong alliances with foreign investors once conducive political and economic climates prevail (O'Donnell 1978; Malloy and Borzutsky 1982; Stepan 1973; Klarén and Bossert 1986). The regimes are exclusionary because they seek to overturn the power of the electorate to make demands by enlisting a technical approach to social and economic planning. Managers with experience in complex bureaucracies (i.e., the armed forces, multinational corporations, national government, or domestic firms) assume key ministerial positions. High on their agendas are policies and programs that reverse what Mesa-Lago (1978) calls the "massification of privileges" in health care and social security. Social public programs enacted by earlier populist governments are blamed for carrying the nation to the brink of financial insolvency. BA regimes increasingly place the burden of health care financing on middle- and low-income groups. The relationship between the state apparatus and health services under BA regimes is noted in table 10.2.

The health care policies of the Chilean regime differ from its Southern Cone neighbors of Argentina, Uruguay, and Brazil in several respects. First, because power has been concentrated in the hands of one individual as opposed to the broader institutional rule in neighboring countries, the dismantling process in the Chilean health care sector has been fairly consistent. In this regard, the BA characterization of impersonal institutional rule of the military over the masses is challenged and questions a central thesis of the bureaucratic-authoritarian model.

Second, the Chilean regime has easily dismissed physician opposition from the largest physicians' group in the nation: the Chilean Medical Association (Colegio Médico). This is no small feat in a coun-

Table 10.2. Characteristics of Bureaucratic-Authoritarianism in the National Health Sector in Chile

Characteristics of Bureaucratic-Authoritarian State	Similarities and Differences found in National Health Sector
Higher government positions occupied by persons who came to them after successful careers in complex and highly bureaucratic organizations such as the armed forces, public bureaucracy, or large private firms	Ministry of Health often headed by military officers
Political exclusion of the popular sector through the imposition of vertical (corporatist) controls by the state	Consolidation and centralization of state-controlled health sector as evidenced by the merger of SERMENA and SNS; expansion of private sector through ISAPREs; municipal transfer of primary care so that pro-junta mayors can exclude community participation
Economic exclusion in that the BA reduces or postpones indefinitely the aspiration to economic participation of the popular sector	Antithetical in health sector; summoning of larger out-of-pocket payments from consumers
Depoliticization; reduces social and political issues to "technical" problems	Health status improvements mainly by the reinforcement of capital-intensive and physician-administered care
Transformation in mechanisms of capital accumulation, which "deepens" process of peripheral and dependent captalism	Altering of payment structure places medical and health care more directly in "free-market" competition; impedes lower-income sector from full participation

Source: After G. O'Donnell 1978, 6; and G. O'Donnell, Schmitter, and Whitehead 1986.

try with perhaps the best organized and most influential physician organizations in Latin America. Chilean physicians, moreover, have occupied the presidency and positions in the senate (Chanfreau 1979). By contrast, the level of physician organization in Argentina, for example, is much weaker. It is strongly dichotomized between Buenos Aires and provincial organizations that often differ markedly in political and philosophical organization. Physician organization in Uruguay is also more fragmented than in Chile. On the one hand, there are the Uruguayan physicians who support lower-cost medical care in a prepaid medical program sponsored by a physician-union organization called CASMU (Centro de Asistencia del Sindicato Médico del Uruguay). Affiliates of the CASMU program constitute one-fifth of all Montevideo residents and 30 percent of all prepaid medical program affiliates in that city. CASMU has been highly active politically since its creation in 1935 during the Great Depression. It was a harsh critic of the military regime in Uruguay (1973–1985) and was one of the first professional associations intervened in by military managers shortly after the 1973 coup. On the other hand, some Uruguayan physicians tend to avoid the physician-union medical programs in favor of multiple staff privileges among other prepaid medical programs. This latter group has given rise to the phenomenon of multiple employment (*poliempleo*, or moonlighting). Health economist Ricardo Meerhoff (1987) noted an average of 3.8 jobs per physician in Uruguay (excluding hospital staff privileges), and most of this average reflects the non-CASMU, politically conservative physician. Although the Chilean Colegio Médico was also organized at the provincial level, it remained part of a larger national organization and has never been seriously challenged by smaller organizations (see Jiménez de la Jara 1984; Scarpaci 1987, 558 n. 2).

Third, the process of dismantling health services has taken place in a country with a well-recognized level of medical education, rivaling some of the most comprehensive teaching and research hospitals in southern Brazil and, on average, probably the most rigorous medical curricula in South America. Such technical competence, it would seem, might have garnered much more support from health professionals outside the United States in opposing the regime, but this has not been the case.

Fourth, the large sector of public medical care users in Chile has allowed for a more apparent and widely publicized dismantling of the public sector than elsewhere in the Southern Cone. Among the so-called welfare states of the Southern Cone, Chile had been by far the most progressive in the health care sector until the military intervened. The reduction of health services regulation, subsidy, and provision noted in this chapter must be seen as a remarkable accomplishment for the BA regime. At the same time, it supports conventional theories of the bureaucratic-authoritarian model, which hypothesize an inverse relationship between the high threat levels and the basic conditions of capitalist society that trigger the introduction of orthodox economic policies (O'Donnell 1978). While the conventional literature on the BA model suggests that the Pinochet regime is unique because it has survived since 1983 despite the apparent collapse of its free-market economic model and because in 1986 Pinochet had the lowest rating of any Chilean leader in that country's recent history (Remmer 1988, 4–8), it is noteworthy that the restructured and privatized health care industry was implemented before 1983. Thus, while the dismantling of public health services came after the privatization of banking, finance, mining, and other sectors of the economy, it has escaped much of the criticism that has been hurled at other sectors of the economy.

Related research by Silvia Borzutsky (1985) has shown that the Chilean BA regime acted with greater autonomy in implementing monetarist policies in social security and health care than did the Argentine or Uruguayan regimes. Likewise, a recent World Bank study noted that in the private manufacturing sector, Chilean entrepreneurs were more determined than their Argentine or Uruguayan counterparts to adapt to the new free-market policies enacted by the BA regime. Chilean entrepreneurs sensed little reversibility in these "reforms" and believed that the regime would remain in power long enough for entrepreneurs to benefit from their policies (Corbo and de Melo 1985). Another difference between Chile and its Southern Cone neighbors is in the altered proportion of state-dependent medical consumers. While about four of every five Chileans receive some portion of their medical care from state-paid providers, the private Argentine *(obras sociales)* and Uruguayan *(mutuales)* systems are financed mainly by employer contributions and employee withholdings. Thus, greater state dominance in policymaking has caused the privatization of health services in Chile to be more far-reaching than in neighboring Uruguay and Argentina.

Conclusions

The dismantling of public health services in Chile is part of a broader development strategy imposed by the bureaucratic-authoritarian regime. The guiding ideology behind health services privatization is the new international laissez-faire. Chilean public enterprises are seen as perennial wastrels by the military rulers, and privatization aims to correct such waste. Managerial autonomy in primary care management, individual discretion, and consumer purchasing power are the cornerstones of the privatization movement. We have seen, however, how the relaxation of medical care regulation and financing, the reduction of environmental health services, and the transfer of National Health Service System clinics to municipal management have produced disproportionate investment in high-amenity HMOs, a rise in infectious diseases, and the municipal management of clinics in selected neighborhoods that stand to profit from capital investments. Dismantling public health services under authoritarian rule has concentrated, perhaps even squandered, the scarce capital of a developing country among its high-income patients while simultaneously resurrecting a morbidity profile of an earlier period. The outcome measures of health service privatization are the pitfalls that other Latin American countries must avoid should they contemplate a model of development along the lines of the Chilean experience.

Three aspects of health care privatization in Chile contrast with neighboring Southern Cone countries that were dominated by bureaucratic-authoritarian rule. First, there is considerable variation in regime structure, which determines the outcomes of the privatization experience. Second, the timing of health care privatization is important. The rapidity of privatizing other sectors of the economy before the health care sector gave the regime a successful track record against which the public health sector could be dismantled. Third, the greater proportion of public users of health services before the Chilean military came to power has made the dismantling of public health services much more noticeable than in Argentina or Uruguay. The regime's ability to resist physician opposition and to privatize other sectors of the economy before turning to the health care sector has facilitated this dismantling, but not without inherent structural problems. The limits to health care privatization are evidenced by the state's policy of financing those programs that shifted the burden of paying for lost wages due to illnesses and maternal leaves from the ISAPREs to general tax revenues. The municipal transfer of primary care clinics, although pregnant with implications of a more effective primary care network, has been thwarted by the regime's reluctance to recognize community organization that may lend itself to some form of political expression. In the environmental sphere, hepatitis and typhoid have risen. While the dismantling of public health services intends to roll back the welfare state in Chile, attendant structural problems have brought the state into a more clearly defined role as the limits to dismantling are noted and a new course of capitalist development is charted.

Notes

Partial funding for this research was provided by the National Science Foundation, Grant SES-8722464.

Chapter 11

The Role of Multinational Pharmaceutical Firms in Health Care Privatization in Developing Countries

WILBERT GESLER

It is well known that health care provision in the less developed countries (LDCs) in Africa, Asia, and Latin America is woefully inadequate. Some progress is being made, however, in modifying the purchase, distribution, and (in some cases) production of pharmaceuticals. In fact, the use of drugs has increased faster in LDCs than it has in the more developed countries (MDCs) of Europe, North America, and Oceania. An important factor behind the relatively large drug expenditures in LDCs is the growing use of drugs for self-medication without a doctor's prescription. A study in Calabar, Nigeria, showed, for example, that 34 percent of the people who sought care for the diseases of their young children went to patent-medicine stores as their principal health care source (Gesler 1979). In many countries, growing literacy rates appear to be linked to increases in self-medication. Although self-medication is desirable because it promotes self-reliance in health care, it can be dangerous if not controlled. An overemphasis on drug taking also detracts from more important aspects of the health care delivery system such as better diet and sanitation. Drugs are an excellent example of the medicalization of health care. Woods (1977) calls drugs "transitional medicine" because they bridge the gap between traditional medicine and biomedicine while drawing people toward the latter.

Most of the pharmaceutical trade in LDCs is handled in the private sector. Some governments in LDCs have tried to gain control of the drug industry, but many have been quite willing to let the private sector take the major responsibility for this type of health care. States in developing areas, because of their position of economic dependency, simply cannot afford to spend very much money on such things as drug purchases and research into and development of new drugs. Multinational corporations (MNCs) engaged in pharmaceutical manufacture and sales, which are based for the most part in MDCs, have shown a great eagerness to supply drugs to LDCs. They have been expanding their operations rapidly and have come to dominate drug production and distribution in LDCs in recent decades. Drug firms have a clear interest in promoting the increase in self-medication mentioned above.

The pharmaceutical industry has experienced tremendous growth over the last few decades. The real boom occurred from the end of the 1960s to the mid-1970s; increases in sales were around 20 percent per year. Since then, annual increases have dropped to around 12 to 14 percent. Worldwide sales in 1975 netted approximately $37.5 billion (Pradhan 1983), whereas projections for 1991 are set at approximately $120 billion (McIntyre 1987). The important point to be made here is that drug consumption has increased much faster in LDCs than in MDCs (Tucker 1984). Two decades ago, pharmaceutical firms could almost totally ignore the LDC market; today that market yields more than a quarter of all sales, and that proportion will probably increase.

Compared with LDCs, MDCs spent four times the proportion of their gross domestic product (GDP) on health care (table 11.1). Per capita expenditure on health care in MDCs was almost forty times more than in LDCs. However, the LDCs spent far greater proportions of their health care budget on drugs (40 percent compared with 7.7 percent). This latter fact is essential to understanding the importance of the heavily privatized drug market for health care delivery in the poorer nations of the world.

Unlike the other contributions to this book, this chapter is not a case study of a particular example of privatization within a single country or group of countries. Rather, it is a study of a specific sector of health care, legal drugs, in a global context. The nature of privatization examined in this chapter includes changes in the regulation of pharmaceutical production, distribution and consumption. The evidence reviewed here shows that most LDCs have given preferential treatment to the needs of capital, especially multinational capital. The chapter also discusses several important aspects of the conflict between private business ventures, whose main goal is profit, and national governments (representing the public sector), one of whose goals is the good health of all their people. The private nature of the international drug companies has created many problems for LDCs, including a concentration of market power, control of domestic drug production, sale of inappropriate drugs and drug dumping, uncontrolled marketing and promotion, high prices for pharmaceuticals, control of research and development activity, overemphasis on over-the-counter sales, undue influence on those who dispense drugs, and inequalities in drug distribution. Study of the pharmaceutical industry quite clearly demonstrates controversial issues such as equity versus efficiency and profits versus needs. Discussion of the roles of various actors—the drug companies, government agencies, doctors, pharmacists, and health consumers—further demonstrates these conflicts, problems, and issues.

Problems and Issues in Pharmaceutical Distribution

Competition Among Drug Firms

Lall, an outspoken critic of pharmaceutical firms, alleges that the structure of the drug industry is oligopolistic; that is, very few countries and firms dominate international production, trade, and innovation. There is both a geographic concentration (in innovation more than in production) and a structural concentration (the top one hundred firms account for about 70 percent of all production). Still, concentration is high relative to other MNC industries because patenting and the costs of research and development tend to localize drugs in certain submarkets (Lall 1981).

There is ample evidence for drug industry concentration. In 1980, when world pharmaceutical sales netted around $76 billion, seven countries (United States, Japan, West Germany, United Kingdom, France, Italy, and Switzerland) garnered 76.2 percent of that total. Also, developed market economies, as opposed to developing ones, were responsible for 95.6 percent of all pharmaceutical exports and 67.6 percent of all imports (Pradhan 1983).

The growth of the pharmaceutical oligopoly can be explained by several factors. Drugs are expensive to research and produce. Large companies have the requisite capital, while most LDC governments do not. MNCs can corner the market in such areas as the supply of raw materials used in manufacturing drugs. Although there may be

Table 11.1. Estimated Pharmaceutical and Overall Health Expenditures, 1981

	Population (millions)	Per capita GDP (U.S. $)	GDP used for health (%)	Per capita health expenditure (U.S. $)
North America	238	12.0	10	1160
Europe (West)	366	9.3	8	800
Far East (Japan)	119	9.0	7	630
Europe (East)	366	5.5	7	385
Subtotal	1089	8.5	8	680
South America	327	1.8	4	72
Africa	383	0.7	2	14
Asia (West)	120	2.9	3	87
Asia (Southeast and China)	2160	0.5	2	10
Subtotal	2990	0.8	2	18
TOTAL	4079	2.8	3.6	100

Source: Adapted from M. Patel 1983, table 1. With permission from Pergamon Press PLC.

regulations prohibiting monopolies in some MDCs, there are no such effective regulations at the international level.

Two further criticisms of pharmaceutical firms related to competition or lack of it should be mentioned. One is that, even though competition may exist to some degree, there is reason to believe that price fixing is still practiced in many LDCs (Tucker 1984). Second, what competition exists is based more on products than on price (Heller 1977). Not surprisingly, the pharmaceutical companies deny accusations of oligopoly. Tucker (1984) says that no company has more than 4 percent of the world market or more than 10 percent of the market in any major country. Concentration may occur, however, if a

Pharmaceuticals expenditures		
Per capita (U.S. $)	As a percentage of total health expenditure	Total (U.S. $ billion)
70.5	6.1	16.7
54.9	6.8	20.1
92.4	14.6	11.0
25.4	6.6	9.3
52.5	7.7	57.1
15.2	21.1	4.9
6.5	46.4	2.5
13.4	15.4	1.6
4.7	47.0	10.2
6.4	40.0	19.2
18.7	18.7	76.3

Note: Subtotals represent averages of individual countries except for population totals which are sums.

company discovers and successfully markets one or two very useful drugs.

Market Power

Drug firms exercise a great deal of control over the drug market, what some call market power. As a result, drug supply leads demand on world markets (Tucker 1984). Because most large firms operate internationally, it is very difficult for individual countries to break this control. MNCs are resilient to decisions by a few countries to rationalize drug purchase and distribution. They can retaliate by withdrawing subsidiary plants (Levinson 1970). Ledogar (1975, 162) states that "the basic obstacles to regulation are not technical ones;

they are endemic to the system of multinational enterprises and its ability to play one developing country off against the other." Drug marketers are clearly aware that there are differences among countries on such issues as brand name drugs versus generics and price controls. They take advantage of the positive aspects of a country's policies and try to circumvent the negative aspects.

Drug Firm Investment in LDCs

Many MNCs manufacture drugs in branch plants located in LDCs. This is an important way in which health care services in many LDCs are produced by the private sector. LDCs compete to produce a relationship among domestic capital, foreign capital, and health care workers (especially physicians and pharmacists) that will attract this type of investment. These relationships, which include cheap labor, limited price controls, and little government interference, perpetuate the market power of MNCs (Thrupp 1984). Most of the domestic benefits accrue to local elites; there is little distribution of investments or profits to the rest of the economy.

Indonesia has gone further than most countries in attracting local manufacturing by outside interests—commonly referred to as offshore production (Pradhan 1983). This Southeast Asia country is more economically developed than most of its neighbors because of its clout as an oil producer and its political stability. The government is attempting to be self-sufficient and has strongly hinted that unless drug companies invest in plants they will be excluded from importing and marketing drugs. However, the government is not anxious to nationalize the drug industry, and it encourages private investment in domestic drug production. By 1976, 95 percent of the drugs consumed in the country were manufactured there. In 1983 there were forty-one international drug companies engaged in local manufacture. The industry suffered from two related problems, however: overcapacity and an insufficient market.

Nigeria, Ghana, Sierra Leone, Liberia, and other members of the Economic Community of West African States (ECOWAS) have a policy of eventually gaining control of all aspects of business. These countries have had a very mixed political and economic history since achieving independence in the 1950s and 1960s. Ghana, for example, tried to be independent of England and attempted a socialist economy, while Nigeria was capitalist oriented and maintained closer ties with England. Many of the West African states have experienced severe economic difficulties and political instability. They must of necessity cooperate with foreign drug companies. Still, states such as Nigeria, Ghana, and Sierra Leone require foreign drug firms to invest capital within their countries. They also encourage local participation in drug manufacture and distribution, and they set quotas on the number of foreign employees. The wholesale business in these countries is run mostly by Africans (Pradhan 1983). The examples of Indonesia and West Africa demonstrate that a variety of strategies for foreign drug investment are used by LDCs with quite different political and economic backgrounds.

Inappropriate Drugs and Drug Dumping

Many of the drugs sold to LDCs are simply inappropriate to the needs of people who are at the beginning of the epidemiologic transition (when contagious diseases are the main health problem). For example, in 1980, 17.8 percent of North Yemen's drug imports were vitamins and tonics, whereas only 1.3 percent were for three of the most prevalent diseases: malaria, schistosomiasis, and tuberculosis (Melrose 1983). A study of the drugs imported into Zaire by seven MNCs found that six did not import any antiparasitic medicine (Glucksberg and Singer 1982). Research on tropical diseases lags, while drugs developed for MDC problems such as heart diseases and cancers are promoted in LDCs (Norris 1982). Cutting back on tropical disease research is one of the threats MNCs may use against uncooperative governments (Tucker 1984).

It is well known that industrialized nations have been dumping products banned by their regulatory bodies in LDCs. A double standard on dangerous drugs has been established. In 1972, for example, the United States Food and Drug Administration (USFDA) took Dipyrone off the American market because it could cause a severe blood disorder. The drug was sold, with no warnings on the product, in Latin America to treat minor ailments. In another case, the United States Department of Defense sent ten million capsules of chloramphenicol, also banned in the United States, to clinics in South Vietnam (Heller 1977). The case of depo-provera is not as clear-cut as these examples. This drug is an injectible contraceptive produced by the Upjohn Company. LDCs were receiving supplies through the United States Agency for International Development until the USFDA banned it due to its potentially dangerous side effects. Many people in the international health field and LDCs, however, were angry about the cessation of sales. They felt that problems such as overpopulation and illegal abortions outweighed the potential harmful effects of the drug and charged the United States with cultural imperialism (Norris 1982). Is it possible that the benefits of drugs such as depo-provera outweigh their dangers in some places?

Marketing and Promotion

The following statement by Silverman (1976, xi) summarizes much of the criticism of pharmaceutical marketing practices in LDCs: "In the promotion of drugs to Latin American physicians, the values of these products have been grossly exaggerated and their hazards glossed over or totally ignored." Thus, as with drug dumping, there is a double standard in advertising: full disclosure in countries such as the United States, but not in many LDCs. Drugs that are restricted to a narrow range of indications by the USFDA and other Western regulatory bodies are recommended for a much wider range of health problems in LDCs. These drugs may be ineffective or produce side effects if used improperly (Ledogar 1975). Chloramphenicol, for example, should be restricted to the treatment of typhoid fever and haemophilus influenzae meningitis, but it is advertised to cure many more diseases in LDCs (Heller 1977). Drug advertisements may also be misleading because they use words such as "power" and "strength" that have connotations of virility (Pradhan 1983). Furthermore, warnings about drugs are not sufficiently set out on packages or explained to physicians and pharmacists.

Thrupp (1984, fig. 1) notes that the pharmaceutical industry spent more on advertising and trade promotion (about 19 percent) than on research (about 10 percent, see fig. 11.1). In fact, some would say that the industry's decline in recent years in one source of power, technology, has led to more emphasis on selling (Lall 1981). Some of the marketing money is spent on glossy brochures, free samples, scientific articles, dinners, and conventions for doctors and others (Thrupp 1984). The bulk of the promotion money is probably spent to hire detail men, who are often paid more than physicians in LDCs (Silverman 1976). The ratio of detail men to doctors is often quite high (one to four in Tanzania). In Haiti, most graduates of the pharmaceutical school become detail men (Fefer 1982). Thus, doctors are pressured through highly orchestrated campaigns to purchase vast amounts of inappropriate drugs (Tucker 1984).

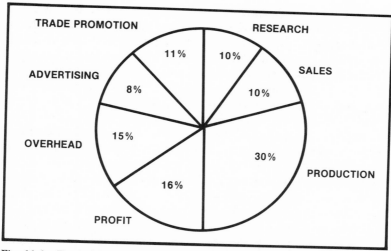

Fig. 11.1. Typical Breakdown of Expenditures for a Pharmaceutical Firm
Source: Thrupp 1984, fig. 1. Reprinted by permission of Baywood
Publishing.

Drug companies respond to criticism about their marketing practices by saying that they advocate the provision of full information
to prescribers, accurate labeling, and warnings about side effects
(Kingham 1982). The marketing code set out by the International
Federation of Pharmaceutical Manufacturers Associations (IFPMA) in
1981 addressed these issues. Critics saw the code as an admission of
guilt (Tucker 1984).

Drug Pricing

Pharmaceutical companies have been the first or second most
profitable manufacturing industries in the world for most years since
1955. They have often been criticized for making excess profits from
drugs whose prices are set too high. A good indication of this is that
prices from country to country vary according to what local markets
will bear (S. J. Patel 1983). Studies in ten Caribbean countries showed
variations in drug prices of 700 percent and higher; these were not
explained by market factors such as size of order (Fefer 1982).

Several reasons may be given for high prices. Intercompany
competition is usually evident in product differentiation and new

products rather than in price. Doctors who prescribe drugs are often not very interested in economizing. Companies spend too much on trivial or imitative research and development (R and D) and on promotion. MNCs discourage competition from small indigenous firms and curtail local R and D by limiting technology transfer (Lall 1981). Pharmaceutical firms also raise prices by using a technique called transfer pricing; that is, by charging inflated prices for raw materials, machinery, and technical assistance sent to their subsidiaries in LDCs (Ledogar 1975). In this way the companies keep profits in their home countries and avoid paying taxes in host countries. A study in Colombia found that the average overpricing of ingredients for intermediate products sent to subsidiaries was 155 percent. Also, drug companies were making an average of 79 percent on products sold but were only declaring 6 percent in profits (Thrupp 1984).

What can LDCs do about high drug prices? One suggestion is to institute a two-tier price system with lower prices for poor nations. Some drug firms have done this (Thrupp 1984). Another type of two-tier system would set lower prices for essential drugs and make up the loss on less important medicines such as vitamins and tonics, which richer people can afford as luxuries (Sallam 1979). Some countries send out tenders for bids on drug sales. Sri Lanka surprised the MNCs by obtaining relatively cheap drugs from new, smaller overseas suppliers. These drugs were tested for quality and were found to be up to standard (Tucker 1984). Table 11.2 shows the potential savings from using five different policies to cut prices (M. S. Patel 1983, 201).

Table 11.2. Potential Savings in Total Drug Expenditures, by Percentage

	Cost Categories				
	Manufacture	Promotion and Distribution	Royalities	General administration	Research and development
Current Policies	28	12	1.5	7	7
Rational choice of drugs	22	10	1.1	5	5
Public distribution system	22	10	1.1	5	5
Imports in bulk	17	8	0.9	4	4
Use of generic names	12	6	0.6	3	3
Domestic production	12	6	0.6	3	3

Source: M. Patel 1983, table 4. Reprinted with permission from Pergamon Press PLC.

Research and Development and Patents

Another way MNCs control the drug market is by dominating R and D activity. If LDCs could engage in their own R and D, many of the problems discussed in this chapter could be alleviated or eliminated. However, development of a totally new drug is very expensive ($30 to $60 million). The pharmaceutical industry spends more than any other industry on R and D, and thus R and D is increasingly only affordable for the largest firms (Heller 1977). Governments in LDCs do not have the necessary capital to pursue their own R and D. Therefore, MNCs argue that only they are capable of carrying out appropriate R and D activities. They complain that LDCs want new drugs, but do not want to pay their share of innovation costs (Parker 1980). Furthermore, MNCs prevent the requisite technology transfer to enable LDCs to carry out R and D. Most drugs manufactured either by indigenous companies or by MNC subsidiaries in LDCs are based on old formulas. Two further criticisms are made of R and D practices by MNCs. One is that most research is on drugs that find their greatest usefulness only in developed countries. The other criticism is that many drugs, marketed as new, are the result of juggling molecules to produce "me-too" variations of old standards (Heller 1977).

Through patent laws, drug companies can protect the prices on their products from being undercut. Patents are necessary, from their point of view, to repay the investment in innovation and to generate further R and D (Wallis 1982). Patents provide innovators with legal monopolies for seventeen to twenty years in most countries. Their role in LDCs is mainly to protect the export markets of MNCs. Some claim that they also provide strong incentives to produce "me-too"

Cost Categories			Savings		
Profit	Retail markup	Total	Domestic currency	Foreign exchange	Total
15	30	100.5	0	0	0 .
11	21	75.1	9	11	20
11	10	64.1	20	11	30
9	9	51.9	20	31	50
7	8	40	20	41	60
7	8	40	9	51	60

drugs (Lall 1981). Several governments in LDCs have tried to do away with or at least minimize patent rights in their countries. Indonesia feels that patents hinder the indigenous drug industry and claims that original research is too far away to require patent protection (Pradhan 1983).

Brand Name and Generic Drugs

In all countries, pharmaceutical companies promote brand name drugs rather than generics. Their position is that, although brands are more expensive, they assure the customer that the drugs are of good quality (Tiefenbacher 1979). Many doctors and pharmacists accept this position and prescribe brands rather than generics (Thrupp 1984). As a result of promotions, many consumers express preference for foreign (MDC) drugs. This was found to be true, for example, among 140 low-income residents of Santiago, Chile (Scarpaci 1985a). To combat this promotional pressure, some LDCs have tried to "rationalize" drug imports by focusing on generics (Lall 1979). Then they are faced with the problem of quality control.

Prescription and Over-the-counter Drugs

In the United States, United Kingdom, and other MDCs, there are strict regulations about which drugs must be prescribed by medical personnel and which can be sold over-the-counter (OTC). This distinction is often blurred in LDCs. Many products requiring a prescription in most Western countries are sold OTC in other parts of the world (Silverman 1976). Pharmacists may sell prescription drugs OTC illegally or out of ignorance (Tucker 1984). OTC sales promote self-medication and are encouraged by MNCs.

All of the practices mentioned in the preceding paragraph mean that LDCs sell a higher proportion of their drugs OTC than is true for MDCs. This is an excellent example of how promotion of laissez-faire economics (i.e., little government regulation of economic affairs) permit individuals to enter pharmacies freely to purchase the drugs they desire. Consumers purchase drugs according to their own perceived needs and income levels. LDC governments often view this situation in a favorable light because it relieves them of some of their responsibility to pay for the health care of their people.

Drug Personnel

Several different kinds of people are involved in dispensing drugs to consumers. The training they receive and the ways in which they respond to pressures from drug salesmen are very important. Inadequate knowledge about pharmaceutical products can be a serious problem. A good example comes from Mexico, where typhoid fever became almost unstoppable because a previously effective drug (chloramphenicol) was so overused that bacteria that were resistant to it developed (Norris 1982).

Physicians prescribe drugs in both public and private settings. Their prescription habits vary widely from area to area, depending on their knowledge, local practices, and consumer preferences (Nyazema 1984). Many doctors in Indonesia work for the government in the morning, at which time they are obliged to prescribe drugs supplied by the government. In the evening they can prescribe freely from private practices (Pradhan 1983). A similar situation was observed by the author in Sierra Leone. Doctors are strongly influenced by the promotional techniques employed by drug concerns (Coleman 1975). Many doctors do not read medical journals, attend scientific meetings, or talk to colleagues in order to find out about the different qualities of various medicines that they recommend to patients. Many of them are thus at the mercy of detail men (Silverman 1976).

Private pharmacists often play a very important role in LDCs because, as health care becomes more costly, they provide an alternative to drug distribution by private physicians and the state. Middle-income consumers often find it convenient to patronize pharmacists. Because doctors are so scarce, especially in small towns and rural areas, pharmacists are often the primary dispensers of medicines. In Latin America, many pharmacists give out drugs illegally while the government looks the other way. Rather than visit a physician, even for free public-sector treatment, many people will go to a pharmacist. Pharmacists and their assistants often are not adequately trained in proper dosage, and they sometimes make inappropriate substitutions (Silverman 1976). A study carried out in West Africa showed that physician prescriptions and the drugs actually dispensed by pharmacists often did not agree (Pradhan 1983). Many pharmacists and other workers in drugstores "diagnose" the diseases of their customers (often on the basis of common symptoms such as fever) and then prescribe erroneously. Still, despite the obvious drawbacks, pharmacists fill a much-needed role in health care (Abosede 1984). What is needed is more education and supervision of drug dispensers. Reform is difficult to achieve, however. Ghana tried to expand the lower ranks of the hierarchy within its pharmacy profession, but the professional pharmacists at the top successfully resisted the attempt (Bennell 1982).

Far more people than physicians and pharmacists prescribe or sell drugs in LDCs. The informal sector is extremely important in promoting drug sales and leads to the further medicalization and privatization of health care. People can buy medicines from market stalls, itinerant peddlers, and people at various levels below doctors and private pharmacists in the medical hierarchy. Many street vendors sell individually wrapped packages of Bayer aspirin, antibiotics, throat lozenges, and other medicines as part of their wares. These drug sources are ubiquitous, and many drugs are thus very accessible.

A fundamental paradox is presented by informal private-sector drug sales. Street vendors fulfill an important health care need because they supply many people who could not afford a bottle of pills from a pharmacy with a few pills to see them through an illness episode. However, the quality of these drugs is often inferior because of exposure to sunlight, humidity, and contaminants. LDC governments are faced with a trade-off in this situation. To what extent should they either encourage or turn a blind eye to a system of drug distribution that relieves them of some health care responsibility and yet can harm their people?

Drug Distribution Infrastructure

A major problem for the delivery of health care in LDCs is the lack of adequate infrastructure. This lack extends to the distribution of medicines. Problems include very limited coverage by facilities such as pharmacies and dispensaries and limited physical access to drug supplies, proper storage, and transport (Lall 1979). Another serious problem is shelf life; many pharmacists continue to sell drugs long after their effectiveness has worn off. Typical examples of poor infrastructure exist in Sierra Leone and Liberia, where 98 percent of the pharmacies are located in the capital cities of Freetown and Monrovia (Pradhan 1983). Isolated pharmacies wait long periods for essential drugs; when they finally arrive, they are sold at prices that make them inaccessible to most.

Illegal Activities Involving Legal Drugs

This study does not involve the illegal trade in such drugs as cocaine and heroin. However, because legally produced drugs are very valuable in both private and public markets in LDCs, they give rise to many illegal activities. Drug theft is very common. It has been reported that about 40 percent of the drugs purchased by the Kenyan government are stolen (Wallis 1982). Many drugs are lost in Nigeria's congested ports. In Indonesia, smuggling is widespread; people are quite willing to buy these cheaper drugs from wholesalers, chemists, and drug stores (Pradhan 1983). Corrupt practices such as bribing government officials to accept tender offers or payoffs to pharmacists are also reported (Ledogar 1975).

Equity Issues

The numerous problems related to drug distribution discussed above lead inevitably to social costs. One way to measure these costs is to examine issues of equity. The core/periphery problems that manifest themselves so often in development issues are clearly apparent here. At the international level there is a wide gap between MDCs and LDCs in drug availability, quality, and appropriateness. Within LDCs there are the familiar problems of inequities both among geographic areas and among subgroups of the population. Drug companies can be quite frank about their interests in this regard. Tiefenbacher (1979) says that pharmaceutical firms cater not just to the elite minority, but also to the emerging middle classes—the most productive people and the future developers in LDCs. International agencies try to serve people on the "social periphery," he says; but this is not productive (Tiefenbacher 1979).

Urban elites, who buy the most drugs, disagree with the rest of the urban dwellers and the rural masses about which drugs are "essential" (Tucker 1984). For example, urban elites might use more Valium, sedatives, sleeping pills, and diet pills than the poor, who buy more simple remedies such as aspirins. In Brazil, drug companies target the wealthy and the urban middle classes, the minority that needs medicines the least. To make matters worse, a study showed that those who earned less than one hundred dollars per month spent proportionately more on drugs than on doctors and dentists (Ledogar 1975). In the Third World, neither the private sector nor the public sector caters drugs to the poor. The growing affluence of a few encourages the private sector, and the public sector lacks the infrastructure to reach the needy. In rural India, investigators found that 40 percent of the patients were sent by medical personnel in clinics to buy drugs that the clinics did not have in stock. Since there were no chemists in their villages, people had to either travel to a city to obtain them or go without. Many people stopped going to the clinics for this reason. The poor often go directly to drug sellers because they cannot afford both medical visits and medicines (Melrose 1983).

The Pharmaceutical Company Position

The stance of the pharmaceutical companies on drug issues has emerged throughout the discussion so far. However, it is useful to summarize some of their principal arguments at this point. Industry spokespersons agree that there is mutual distrust between LDC governments and pharmaceutical concerns, but argue that the drug business is not the guilty party. "To a great extent the blame for this must be ascribed to the politicians, whose emotive and public posturing on industry profits has attracted greater publicity than the industry's rather low-key refutations" (Reekie and Weber 1979, 171). Pharmaceutical companies claim that they meet the standards set by LDCs; any abuses that arise originate within the LDCs themselves (Wallis 1982). The code that IFPMA set up in 1981 on marketing practices provided for full information to prescribers, including drug labeling and warnings on side effects (Kingham 1982).

Drug companies clearly want to deregulate the industry wherever possible. In LDCs, they say, regulation is not for safety, efficacy, or quality so much as it is based on economic and political grounds (Tiefenbacher 1979). The companies point out that regulatory bureaucracies are slow and do not take risks; therefore, market discipline should prevail (e.g., incentives should replace regulations). Technology transfer is another industry concern because it means the loss of competitive advantage (McCulloch 1980).

There is also the issue of self-interest. Many in the drug industry feel that nations with thriving drug companies should treat them as a national asset because they are a source of tax revenue, they earn foreign exchange, and they aid trade balances (Pradhan 1983). While developed countries should show a concern for the health of other people, they must also try to maintain healthy economies (Baroody

1980). Finally, some drug company officials have taken the position that LDCs have become high-risk, low-profit environments for drugs. Therefore, they threaten to withdraw from the markets in these countries (Tiefenbacher 1979).

Attempted Solutions to Drug Distribution Problems

Essential Drugs

There are thousands of different drugs being sold to LDCs. In reaction to this unnecessary proliferation, international organizations and national governments have attempted to make lists of "essential" or "priority" drugs, both branded and generic. As a result, around 30,000 brand name drugs have been cut down to approximately 200 (S. J. Patel 1983). The basic idea is that countries could use fifty to sixty drugs to treat 80 percent of their health problems (Tucker 1984). Mozambique, among other countries, took up the challenge and reduced about 26,000 available drugs to 120, which they then registered for pharmacy sale. They put out bids and found that tenders from a variety of countries varied in price by a factor of twenty (Marzagao and Segall 1983).

The Domestic Drug Industry

Many LDCs feel that one way to lessen the control over drug production and distribution by the MNCs is to produce their own pharmaceuticals. Some countries certainly have the potential for a viable indigenous industry. India is successfully producing drugs for both domestic consumption and export. Egypt has also made some progress along these lines (Heller 1977). These efforts encounter severe problems, however, including lack of requisite capital, training of production workers, and the technology needed to produce quality medicines (Lall 1979). MNCs usually oppose attempts to establish indigenous industry; at best they suggest that self-sufficiency should take place slowly and with their own cooperation (Reekie and Weber 1979). In Brazil, an attempt to develop domestic industry and to distribute drugs to the poor was thwarted by MNC influence within the government (Ledogar 1975).

International Agencies

One way to regulate the international drug trade is through international organizations such as the United Nations (UN), International Labor Organization, International Confederation of Trade Unions, and Health Action International. In the 1950s and 1960s, the World Health Organization (WHO) became involved in a rather passive way with drug regulation. WHO concentrated on quality control of the physical and chemical properties of drugs, provided information, helped to plan the establishment of pharmaceutical industries in LDCs, and drew up its essential drug list. From the early 1970s on, however, WHO began to emphasize the social and economic aspects of drugs. The 1987 director, Halfdan Mahler, took a belligerent attitude toward the MNCs.

Other UN agencies besides WHO have also become involved in pharmaceutical issues. The UN Industrial Development Organization (UNIDO) has tackled technical assistance and domestic drug production; the UN Conference on Trade and Development has examined technology transfer; and UNICEF is engaged in drug procurement for children (Stenzl 1981).

These international efforts have met with several difficulties. UN agencies often depend on MDCs for money and on the drug firms for technology. They are constantly under pressure from companies and developed countries to pull back from regulatory activity. There is divisiveness among the agencies. On the whole the UN has been able to do very little in the way of concrete operations. Its various agencies have formulated policies on such issues as drugs to meet real health care needs and cooperation among LDCs, but have usually not implemented them. As an example, UNIDO worked on a list of essential drugs, but did not publish the list or the report on the working group involved (Stenzl 1981).

Regional and National Strategies

It would appear on the surface that LDCs would benefit if they banded together in regional organizations in order to control the pharmaceutical market. Several countries acting in unison should be able to counteract the market power of MNCs. Such regional organizations do exist. One example is the Pan Arab Pharmaceutical Company (ACDIMA), which has had fair success in such areas as the establishment of priority lists to meet the drug needs of each member country, the development of national agencies that purchase pharmaceuticals; the revision of patent and trademark laws; and the establishment, where possible, of domestic drug industries. By 1977, 44 percent of the drugs used in the Arab World were manufactured there. This example suggests several ways in which regional cooperation can curb the abdication of state responsibility and the increase of the privatization of pharmaceutical items in the LDCs. (Sallam 1979). Regional groups face certain problems, however, as the regional cooperative scheme of the Caribbean Community (CARICOM) discovered. Membership was voluntary, so not every country joined; members could not agree on policy; and countries had different health systems, political ideologies, economic priorities, and social concerns (Thrupp 1984).

National efforts have borne more fruit than regional ones, although success has never been anywhere near complete. As mentioned above, Mozambique is working with an essential drug list. Mexico passed a legislative act that attempted to match the technological level of drugs to its needs. In Pakistan there was an attempt to market only generics (Heller 1977). The socialist government in Cuba has tried to control drugs within the framework of its post-1959 political and social transformation. The Cubans have centralized drug purchase and distribution, have tried to achieve technological self-reliance and quality control, have carried out R and D and educational programs, and have reached agreements with other socialist countries (Thrupp 1984). India, a country with a mixed economy, found that, following independence in 1947, drug imports were becoming a severe drain on foreign exchange. A government committee made an inquiry into the situation. The result was the encouragement of local drug industries, restrictions on imports, and the manufacture of only essential drugs in joint ventures with foreign firms. India now exports drugs, and prices are controlled by the central government (Pradhan 1983).

The recent experiences of two countries, Sri Lanka and Egypt, offer several insights into the struggle between MNCs and LDCs. The government of Sri Lanka made a strong bid between 1972 and 1976 to rationalize its drug market. Six major participants influenced this reform attempt: the Sri Lankan government (basically socialist and for reform, but divided by power struggles); local reformists (elite academics and some doctors); the international drug industry (mostly opposed to reform); local opponents to reform (most of the medical establishment and the educated elite); foreign opponents to reform

(MNCs and their home governments); and foreign supporters of reform (some doctors and government organizations such as the USFDA). Lall and Bibile (1978) traced the activities of these six groups through four issues: centralized drug purchase from a rationalized list, purchase of pharmaceutical chemicals for local manufacture, patents, and brands versus generics. An important conclusion arising from Sri Lanka's experience was that "reform depends on a complex interplay of social, political, and economic factors, as well as upon how they exercise their influence by means of ideology, persuasion, bargaining, or straightforward domination" (Lall and Bibile 1978, 307–308).

The case of Egypt demonstrates how shifts in political economy have affected the privatization of the drug market. During its colonial period, Egypt became increasingly dependent on Western-made drugs and privatization increased. Because of resistance from MNCs, it had great difficulty in starting domestic production. However, an enlightened social awareness that extended to drug issues had developed among the population. After its break with England and France in 1956, the government acted to nationalize drug importation and distribution. The economy was centrally planned and controlled, and drug production and distribution began to shift away from the private sector and toward the public sector. Many problems were created by a change in policy that was too rapid, but public enthusiasm made great gains possible. Since 1975, however, confrontation with MNCs and political nonalignment has been replaced by subdued alignment with the West. Foreign capital and domestic private capital are now encouraged. As a result, the local share of the drug market has declined, and privatization has increased once again (Galal 1983).

Case studies involving countries such as Sri Lanka and Egypt raise the question of the relative success of socialist and nonsocialist governments in dealing with MNCs and the problems they create. In general, socialist governments make more of an attempt to control their drug markets through such measures as essential drug lists (Mozambique), production of pharmaceutical chemicals for use in local drug manufacture (Sri Lanka), and centralized drug purchase and distribution and R and D (Cuba). It is worth noting that Sweden, a developed country and perhaps the epitome of the socialist state, controls its pharmaceutical retail business completely through a national corporation, which does not manufacture drugs but fills all prescriptions. The Swedish compulsory health insurance system provides superb pharmaceutical benefits (Pradhan 1983).

Generalizations about socialist versus nonsocialist drug control are very coarse, however. Ghana, which declared its socialist intentions following independence in 1957, has allowed professional associations, including its pharmaceutical association, to have considerable power and has sought in vain to guide its policies (Bennell 1982). Many LDCs with mixed public and private economies have had some success in dealing with MNCs. Thus, for example, India has a viable domestic drug industry. Furthermore, countries involved in regional economic or pharmaceutical unions such as West Africa (ECOWAS), the Arab World (ACDIMA), and the Caribbean Community (CARICOM) are countries with varying degrees of socialist political economies. In sum, success in controlling drug markets includes other factors besides the socialist/nonsocialist dichotomy, although the dichotomy is important.

Conclusions

The provision of drugs to consumers in LDCs is a rapidly expanding sector of health care delivery in those countries. LDCs spend higher proportions of their total health care budgets on drugs than do MDCs. Self-medication with various medicines is a growing practice. Multinational pharmaceutical companies exert a very strong control over the production and distribution of legal drugs. The result has been to increase the degree of privatization (mainly in the areas of commercialization and deregulation, but also in the promotion of consumer self-care) in health care delivery in many LDCs. What are the implications of the private, international, legal drug business for health care delivery, which is tending toward privatization in many countries around the world?

First, privatization in the form of deregulation and reduced public subsidies for certain drugs creates a complex set of problems that are detrimental to health care delivery. The pharmaceutical oligopoly makes it very difficult for individual or even groups of LDCs to control the production and supply of drugs. LDCs find it very difficult to resist MNC investment in their countries. Privatization has often created an environment in which inappropriate or unsafe drugs are dumped in LDCs. Pharmaceutical firms control R and D activities and use patent laws to protect their products. They encourage brands over generics and OTC sales rather than prescriptions. They often charge inflated prices for drugs; high prices can lead to illegal traffic in drugs. Drug firms spend large sums of money on marketing and promotion and have a strong influence on what the dispensers of drugs (physicians, pharmacists, and others) will sell to consumers. They are in large measure responsible for creating spatial and social inequalities in drug provision. Not all of these problems would disappear if LDC governments took over control of the drug market. Indications are, however, that many of the problems would, in the long run, be alleviated or eliminated.

Second, the responses made to the problems created by privatization will meet with varying success. LDCs have attempted to solve drug control problems in many different ways. Some countries have made lists of essential drugs and purchased only these. Domestic industries have been established in some places. International organizations within the UN have drawn up policies to regulate drug flows, but have done little to implement them. Regional organizations have had some success in drug control, but individual countries, particularly those with socialist political economies, have gone furthest in dealing with MNCs.

Third, private and public interests almost invariably collide over issues of health care delivery; these conflicts cannot be glossed over. The drug industry illustrates very clearly a basic paradox: the right of humans to health care, generally a government or public concern, is controlled by private industry (Levinson 1970). This paradox can also be seen as a conflict between the pursuit of profits by drug firms versus the best interests of people in LDCs, particularly those most in need of health provision (Thrupp 1984). There are several points that can be made in favor of the private drug sector of health care delivery. It is a relatively healthy, growing, and efficient business; it can deliver drugs to people. The public sector, in contrast, is often disorganized, subject to corrupt practices, and wasteful. LDC governments spend very little on health care in general and on medicines in particular. Vast numbers of people turn to private suppliers (physicians, pharmacists, street vendors, and others) as the most convenient (and sometimes the only) drug sources. LDC governments are often very willing to relinquish their health care responsibilities to the private sector. The argument for more public-sector involvement in drugs is that there are issues that transcend efficiency and good business practices. Private-sector drugs are often inappropriate and may be harmful to health; in this sense they too are inefficient and wasteful. Governments have a far better chance of distributing drugs equitably throughout the different regions and social classes within their countries. Privatization fosters all the problems mentioned above in connection with the first implication. If the issue is better health care for the people of a country, it is clear that the public sector wins the argument.

Fourth, in terms of political economy, privatization often leads to or increases a dominance/dependency relationship beween the private and public sectors in health care delivery. The struggle taking place between the multinational firms and national governments over control of drug markets has interlocking political and economic components. Overall, the drug companies maintain the upper hand. MNCs have the political backing of MDCs. It takes tremendous political will on the part of LDC governments to endanger alliances with MDCs by threatening to curb privatization in drug delivery. As noted in chapter 1, LDC governments typically are tempted to relinquish part of their health care delivery obligations to private drug firms, an example of the state deferring to the needs of private capital. Socialist countries have shown the greatest ability to exercise the requisite political will to overcome this temptation. The economic side of the struggle involves access to and control of capital. Here again, drug firms have a distinct advantage. We have seen time and again that MNCs have the ability to spend large sums on such things as chemical raw materials, R and D, and sales promotion. LDCs simply do not have these resources.

Finally, the arguments made for the benefits of privatization are often belied by actual experience. One argument is that privatization will bring about more competition, which will lower health care costs. International drug firms claim that they are competitive, but the evidence points toward oligopoly. Furthermore, competition is over products rather than price, and there is evidence of price fixing. A second argument for privatization is that it will encourage consumer participation in, and some measure of consumer control over, health care delivery. Again, the evidence is that drug firms encourage consumer spending through huge expenditures on advertising campaigns, but are not interested in consumer participation in, much less control over, the drug market. A third argument is that governments and private firms can achieve a mutually beneficial partnership for the delivery of health care. This partnership has taken many forms throughout the world in the area of legal drugs. In many instances, the roles of private and public interests have become blurred. However, we have seen that, for the most part, the private drug industry has dominated the partnership and prevented it from being beneficial to the health of people. In addition, it is very easy for the partnership to become a collusion for mutual profit.

All of the points made in the preceding discussion lead to one overall conclusion: multinational pharmaceutical firms provide a great deal of evidence for the argument that health care privatization in the industrial societies usually has detrimental effects on the health of the masses of people in developing countries. Part of the struggle of individuals, organizations, and nations to achieve adequate health care in the developing world will continue to be against the medical hegemony imposed by this form of health care privatization.

Chapter 12

Conclusions

Lessons on the Methodological and Conceptual Issues of Health Services Privatization

JOSEPH L. SCARPACI

We began this book by arguing that the process of health services privatization takes on many forms, defying neat conceptualization as a monolithic process of economic restructuring. Case studies of privatization provide a vehicle for examining the operations of international health systems. The mounting portion of health care resources merits careful documentation and analysis of how the state shifts its responsibilities to both the private sector and local governments. How welfare state functions are executed in the advanced capitalist nations carries much import in the health care sector of developing nations as the latter struggle to deliver essential human services while maintaining some degree of fiscal soundness.

The various sections of this book exemplify different aspects of this general process of privatization in industrial societies where chronic diseases and biomedical models of health services prevail. The changing role pattern among the state, labor, capital, consumers, and health practitioners indicates the increased tension that has arisen as the modern biomedical model takes firm root in most health care systems. We began with hospital services in part 1 because they consume the largest portion of health services resources. Chapter 2 showed how the pattern of for-profit hospital expansion in the United States is closely related to the availability of investment capital. Bohland and Knox examined the close relationship between capital availability and hospitals' accessibility to paying customers. They showed how these were key determinants for the growth of proprietary hospitals in two periods during the last century. In both the United States and New Zealand, the for-profit hospital market may be reaching a point of saturation. Also, the appearance of national-government deregulation and reduced provision coincides with private-sector expansion, thus underscoring the cyclical nature of health services privatization. While the state in both countries may reduce service provision, there is growing evidence that their regulation of hospital services is increasing. J. Ross Barnett and Pauline Barnett showed that New Zealand's hospital regulations, like deinstitutionalization in Ontario and parts of the United States, represent patterns of reprivatization. John Mohan pointed out in the case of Great Britain that the state could satisfy the demands of the health care market if given the resources to do so. This coincides with work by Taylor-Gooby (1986), who argues that while there is consumer dissatisfaction with the National Health Service in Great Britain, it is inevitably attributable to underfunding. Sara McLafferty's study of hospital closures in New York City indicated that small hospitals in low-income neighborhoods are the most susceptible to losing hospital services. The best that consumers in those districts can hope for is to minimize the deleterious effects of hospital closures through local community action. In the end, however, for-profit hospital services are no match for isolated neighborhood struggles that try to keep hospital services geographically and financially accessible.

Part 2 examined mental health services in the United States and Canada. Significantly, the process of deinstitutionalization that began in the 1950s through the use of psychotropic drugs marked the beginning of state withdrawal from this industry. The shift from public to private providers, which first occurred in the 1950s and recurred in the 1980s, provides points of contrast in the cases presented for Canada and the United States. In Chapter 7, Glenda Laws critically assessed the magnitude of deinstitutionalization in Ontario, where the state is pumping millions of dollars into the private sector. She argued that the welfare state has not been eroded; rather, the public and private sectors must necessarily work in tandem. All that remains truly private in Ontario is facilities management. Private contract awards merely augment the influence of the state in a particular kind of parastatal privatization. This form of privatization exacerbates the ghettoization of dependent groups.

Across the border, Christopher Smith noted in chapter 7 that the substitution of Community Mental Health Centers (CMHCs) as primary mental health providers for corporate psychiatry has placed the stockholder in a position formerly held by the community. Smith argued that the tenets of industrial psychology, a major force in the shift to HMO- and PPO-sponsored mental health services, mean that the homeless and others of the permanent underclass will not benefit from this restructuring. Corporate-sponsored mental health services will allow employers to deal more effectively with problems of substance abuse, absenteeism, and low productivity, while those who are unable to partake in this benefit package will be relegated to underfunded public facilities. The implications of this argument are rich in that they suggest that this shift to a Bismarckian version of mental health care financing will allow private business to deal more effectively with labor unrest and low productivity, while undermining the spirit and purpose of community-based service delivery that characterize CMHCs.

A single chapter constituted part 3, Environmental Health Services. Environmental health has been understudied in the privatization debate. Michael Greenberg documented a more subtle shift in the federal government's role in health services provision. This shift stemmed from the Reagan administration's emphasis on state and local, rather than federal, sponsorship of cancer prevention programs. Although the evidence is still out on the efficacy of federal versus local cancer prevention programs, Greenberg argued that a partnership of private and public agencies could effectively monitor environmental quality and promote health education. This echoes a similar finding in the study of environmental health services in Chile in chapter 10. With the United States government reluctant to entertain any such ventures, a potentially efficient health-promotion strategy forged by the Centers for Disease Control, the National Institutes of Health,and non-profit health care agencies and universities is being missed.

Part 4 presented the extensions of health services privatization in developing countries through health policy adoption and multinational drug companies. Gesler and Scarpaci examined how policies and practices traditionally confined to the advanced capitalist nations have spread to the far corners of the globe. Privatization appeals to developing countries, who often lack the well-defined modern health services of the industrial nations and whose foreign debt tends to place greater pressures on state financing and delivery of service. Chapter 10 examined the anachronistic health plan of the Chilean ministry in a period of fiscal austerity. The chapter discussed the decrease in health services provision, subsidy, and regulation and illustrated how an ardent free-market economy was implanted in a developing country that lacked both consumer purchasing power and electoral input into the dismantling of health services. The Chilean experience may be instructive for other nations situated at an intermediate level of economic development and industrialization.

Chapter 11, by Gesler, showed how dependence on private drug firms greatly undermined the role of traditional health care practices. While multinational firms take advantage of Third World consumers' preferences for name-brand drugs, host governments pay little attention to the appropriateness of those drugs. Until the creation and enforcement of essential drug lists come about, over-the-counter drugs will continue to emphasize costly, drug-related curative care services at the expense of more effective community-based primary care. Gesler's chapter revealed the most insidious outcome of the medicalization of the world's consumers and the key role that private providers play in that distortion.

The overall conclusion is that the tensions and conflict created within capitalist economies reveal general tendencies. The state withdraws from health services provision erratically and in a piecemeal manner, only to notice later that problems were created in the process. Conflict stems from the demands of electoral politics, consumer preferences, and relations between local and national governments. Clearly, no universal metric can gauge the pace in the shift to the private provision of health services. In national politics in New Zealand, for example, the rise in private hospital and geriatric care has evolved gradually since the Second World War, but community opposition to hospital closures in New York City has arisen over a shorter period of time and within a smaller geographic area. Within the United States, the growth of proprietary hospitals has depended on a particular type of investment capital and has needed particular locational criteria for hospital markets. Private hospital care in both countries indicates the state cannot fully withdraw from its present commitments without a collapse in social relations. At the very least, social reproduction would change markedly if the rhetoric of privatization were taken seriously.

Nor can the privatization process be classified as a new phenomenon, as illustrated by the recurrent problems of mental illness in New York and Ontario and by the historical cycle of for-profit hospitals in the United States. Unlike cutbacks in manufacturing or retail trades, the immediate impacts of cutbacks in public health care budgets are not readily noticed. Indeed, as degenerative and chronic illnesses continue to dominate the morbidity profiles of the world's population, the lag time in tracing health services financing, delivery, and outcome makes the task much more difficult. That drawback notwithstanding, these case studies of health services privatization have tried to relate the arguments inherent in theories of why the welfare state should be rolled back to the realities of the limits to rollbacks. We have seen clearly defined limits to this privatization process in economies as diverse as New Zealand, Great Britain, Western Europe, and the Southern Cone region of South America. It seems evident from the debates borne out here that, while the public-private debate is often caustic in political and academic circles, the welfare state will remain a permanent feature of industrial capitalism. We may have turned the corner in the 1980s in terms of squandering precious health care funds for unnecessary, high-amenity services and products, brightly lit reception areas, and brand-name drugs. In fact, at the time of this writing there are rising expectations that a meaningful detente may be achieved by the world superpowers that would facilitate a shift away from military and defense spending and toward funding essential social services. This optimistic forecast (for some) has been painfully evident in public demands for state-mandated research on AIDS. Only as the focus on efficiency in health services privatization becomes more widely associated with concepts of social justice and equity can we begin to assess the value of health services as a universal right, and not as a commodity.

The empirical evidence reviewed here suggests that the state cannot intervene in health services merely in a time of crisis, for the costs are far too great. Although key findings of published WHO research as far back as 1951 noted that health care expenditures could no longer be treated as consumption items (but should be regarded as investments in the productivity of labor), those lessons seem to have been forgotten in the privatization debate in recent years (see Winslow 1951).

Locational conflict has been an inherent feature in health services privatization at various scales of analysis. Local-level conflict surfaces in the struggle between community residents in districts where hospital closures are imminent. It stems from the contradiction of seeking health care as a right and regarding health care as a commodity. As McLafferty's review of urban neighborhoods showed, all that local groups can hope for is to extract a few concessions from either the state or for-profit providers, especially in highly regulated environments like New York City. Consumers of garden vegetables in metropolitan Santiago are exposed to infectious diseases because the state maintains the rights of small farmers over the health of the metropolitan area. And, the skid row areas of inner-city Hamilton are forced to incur the social costs of providing intermediate services for the homeless and mentally ill, thereby defeating the concept of a truly public city.

The use of a geographical perspective in the study of health services privatization uncovers other common processes. From the outset we have argued that health services privatization is neither a uniform nor a monolithic process. The classic welfare states of Western Europe, for instance, are diverse mixed economies with clear limits on how far the state can withdraw from essential service delivery. As John Eyles argued in chapter 3, only the liberal regime of England can seriously contemplate a significant degree of privatization given the structural constraints for private market expansion elsewhere on the continent. Similarly, certain regions of the United States, the South and the West, are ripe for proprietary hospital investment. Thus, we reject the idea of a global privatization conspiracy, yet recognize the common practice of cutting back social programs in times of economic crisis. To end the discussion of the methodological and conceptual issues of health services privatization at this level, however, would be premature because these case studies underscore the importance of examining the relationship between subnational and national levels of health services delivery and finance. Neither Reagan's new federalism, with its attendant emphasis on states' rights, nor multinational corporations' promotion of over-the-counter drugs, nor Thatcher's attacks on Regional Health Areas, nor Pinochet's attempt to pass on primary care clinics to county or private management can fully mask attempts to undercut national public services so that private, subnational health care systems appear prosperous. The conventional notion that decentralization is meritorious, or at least the way in which it has been implemented in health services privatization, has been challenged. The luxury of truly having free choice in the health care field remains confined to a small group of privileged consumers in industrial societies. The historical record to date suggests that the pendulum will gradually shift to more state control as the conceptual and methodological lessons of health services privatization are learned.

Notes

I wish to thank Fred Shelley, Glenda Laws, J. Ross Barnett, and Wil Gesler for their engaging discussion about this topic at the meetings of the Association of American Geographers, Phoenix, May 1988.

Reference List

Abel-Smith, B. 1984. *Cost containment in health care.* London: Bedford Square Press.

———. 1985. Who is the odd one out? *Milbank Memorial Fund Quarterly* 63:1–17.

Abosede, O. 1984. Self-medications: An important aspect of primary health care. *Social Science and Medicine* 19:699–703.

Abramowitz, M. 1986. The privatization of the welfare state: A review. *Social Work* 37:257–263.

Adam Smith Institute. 1981. *Health and the public sector.* London: Adam Smith Institute.

———. 1984. *The omega health papers.* London: Adam Smith Institute.

Agran, L. 1977. *The cancer connection.* Boston: Houghton Mifflin.

AIH (Association of Independent Hospitals). 1987. *Survey of independent hospitals in the acute sector.* London: Association of Independent Hospitals.

Aken, J.; Guilkey, D.; Griffin, C.; and Popkin, B. 1985. *The demand for primary health services in the Third World.* Totowa, N.J.: Rowman and Allanheld.

Alba, R., and Batutis, M. 1983. *The impact of migration on New York state.* Albany, N.Y.: Public Policy Institute.

Alexander, J.; Lewis, B.; and Morrisey, M. 1985. Acquisition strategies of multihospital systems. *Health Affairs* 4:49–66.

Alexander, J.; Morrisey, M.; and Shortell, S. 1986. Physician participants in the administration and governance system of freestanding hospitals: A comparison by type of ownership. In *For-profit enterprise in health care,* ed. B. Gray, 402–421. Washington, D.C.: National Academy Press.

Alford, R. 1975. *Health care politics.* Chicago: University of Chicago Press.

Altenstetter, C. 1987. An end to a consensus on health care in the Federal Republic of Germany? *Journal of Health Politics, Policy, and Law* 12:505–536.

Altman, D. 1983. Health care for the poor. *Annals of the American Academy of Political and Social Science* 468:103–121.

Altman, L., and Frisman, L. 1987. Preferred provider organizations and mental health care. *Hospital and Community Psychiatry* 38:359–363.

American Hospital Association. 1979. *Survey of inpatient education.* Atlanta: U.S. Public Health Service.

Andrews, K. 1984. Private rest homes in the care of the elderly. *British Medical Journal* 288:1518–1520.

Anglin, B., and Braaten, J. 1978. *Twenty-five years of growing together: A history of the Ontario Association for the Mentally Retarded.* Downsview, Ontario: Ontario Association for the Mentally Retarded.

Arthur D. Little, Inc. 1985. *The health care system in the mid-1990s.* Washington, D.C.: Health Insurance Association of America.

Ascher, K. 1987. *The politics of privatisation: Contracting-out public services.* London: Macmillan.

Ashbaugh, J. W., and Bradley, V. J. 1979. Linking deinstitutionalization of patients with hospital phase-down: The difference between success and failure. *Hospital and Community Psychiatry* 30:105–110.

Ashbaugh, J. W.; Leaf, P. J.; Manderscheid, R. W.; and Eaton, W. 1983. Estimates of the size and selected characteristics of the adult chronically mentally ill population living in U.S. households. In *Research in community and mental health,* ed. J. Greenley, vol. 3, 3–26. Greenwich, Conn.: J.A.I. Press.

Atkinson, J., and Meager, N. 1986. *New forms of work organization.* Institute of Manpower Studies, Report 121. Brighton: University of Sussex.

Australia Bureau of Statistics. 1986. *Australia yearbook, 1985.* Canberra: Government Printer.

Baker, J. 1986. Problem of cost control in a "liberal" health care system: The case of France. In *The year book of social policy in Britain, 1985–86,* ed. M. Brenton and C. Ungerson. London: RKP.

Barkin, S. 1977. European union agreements provide framework for public policy. *Monthly Labor Review* 100:62–64.

Barnes, J. A. 1986. The failure of privatization. *National Review* 38:38–40.

Barnett, J. R. 1984. Equity, access, and resource allocation: Planning hospital services in New Zealand. *Social Science and Medicine* 18:981–989.

Barnett, J. R.; Ward, D.; and Tatchell, M. 1980. Hospital resource allocation in New Zealand. *Social Science and Medicine* 14D (June): 251–261.

Baroody, W. 1980. Foreword to *The international supply of medicines,* ed. R. Helms, iv–v. Washington, D.C.: American Enterprise Institute for Public Policy Research.

Barter, J. 1983. California—Transformation of mental health care: 1957–1982. In *Unified mental health systems: Utopia unrealized,* ed. J. Talbott, 7–18. San Francisco: Jossey Bass.

Bassuk, E., and Gerson, S. 1978. Deinstitutionalization and mental health services. *Scientific American* 238:46–53.

Batra, R. 1986. *The great depression of 1990.* Dallas: Venus Books.

Battistella, R. 1987. Politics of government supported health services: Necessity for a new approach. In *Restructuring health policy: An international challenge,* ed. J. Virgo, 55–72. Edwardsville, Ill.: International Health Economics and Management Institute, Southern Illinois University.

Bays, C. 1983. Why most private hospitals are nonprofit. *Journal of Policy Analysis and Management* 2:366–385.

Beamish C. 1981. Space, state and crisis: Towards a theory of the public city. Master's thesis, Department of Geography, McMaster University.

Beanland, K. 1987. Running a profitable operation. *Dominion Sunday Times*, 22 March 35.

Becker, E., and Sloan, F. 1985. Hospital ownership and performance. *Economic Inquiry* 23:21–36.

Becker M. 1986. The tyranny of health promotion. *Public Health Reviews* 14:15–23.

Bellet L. 1987. Location of private smoking cessation programs that advertise. Public Health Program, Rutgers University. Mimeo.

Bellush, J. 1979. Indispensable facilities: In defense of municipal hospitals. *New York Affairs* 5:111–119.

Bennell, P. 1982. Professionalisation: The case of pharmacy in Ghana. *Social Science and Medicine* 16:601–607.

Bergstrand, C. R. 1982. Big profit in private hospitals. *Social Policy* 13:49–54.

Bergthold, L. 1987. Business and the pushcart vendors in an age of supermarkets. *International Journal of Health Services* 17:7–26.

Berkowitz, E. 1980. *Creating the welfare state: The political economy of twentieth-century reform.* New York: Praeger.

Bice, T. 1984. Health planning services and regulation. In *Introduction to health services,* ed. S. J. Williams and P. R. Torrens, 373–402. New York: Wiley.

Biegel, A. 1984. The remedicalization of community mental health. *Hospital and Community Psychiatry* 35:1114–1117.

Birkbeck, C. 1979. Garbage, industry, and the "vultures" of Cali, Colombia. In *Casual work and poverty in Third World cities,* ed. R. Bromely and G. Bromely, 161–183, New York: Wiley.

Bish, R. L. 1971. *The public economy of metropolitan areas.* Chicago: Markham.

Bittker, T. 1985. The industrialization of American psychiatry. *American Journal of Psychiatry* 142:149–154.

Blacksell, S.; Phillips, D.; and Vincent, J. 1987. Spatial concentration of residential homes for the elderly: Planning responses and dilemmas. *Transactions Institute of British Geographers* 12:73–83.

Bluestone, B., and Harrison, B. 1982. *The deindustrialization of America.* New York: Basic.

Bodenheimer, T. 1984. The transnational pharmaceutical industry and the health of the world's people. In *Issues in the political economy of health care,* ed. J. McKinlay, 187–216. New York: Tavistock.

Bogue, D. 1985. *The population of the U.S.: Historical trends and future projections.* New York: Free Press.

Bohland, J.; Knox, P.; and Shumsky, L. 1987. Spatial restructuring of San Francisco's medical services: 1870–1880. Paper presented at conference, The History of Medical Geography, sponsored by the Institute of British Geographers and the Wellcome Institute, September 24, London.

Boland, R., and Young, M. 1983. A qué precio la atención primaria de salud? *Foro Mundial de Salud* 4:151–54.

Borgoño, J.; Domínguez, N. J.; Aldea, A.; and Acuña, C. 1983. Condiciones de eficiencia de los consultorios periféricos de atención materno-infantil. *Cuadernos Médico-Sociales* 24:13–24.

Borus, J. F. 1981. Deinstitutionalization of the chronically mentally ill. *New England Journal of Medicine* 305:339–342.

Borus, J. F.; Olendzki, M. C.; Kessler, L.; Burns, B. J.; Brandt, U. C.; Brover-man, C. A.; and Henderson, P. R. 1985. The "offset effect" of mental health treatment on ambulatory medical care utilization and charges. *Archives of General Psychiatry* 42:573–580.

Borzutsky, S. 1985. Politics and social security reform. In *The crisis of social security and health care in Latin America*, ed. C. Mesa-Lago, 285–304. Pittsburgh: Center for Latin American Studies, University of Pittsburgh.

Bosanquet, N. 1983. *After the new right*. London: Heinemann.

Bowden, M. 1967. The dynamics of city growth: An historical geography of the San Francisco central district, 1850–1931. Ph.D. diss., University of California, Berkeley.

Bow Group. 1983. *Beveridge and the Bow Group generation*. London: Bow Group.

Brady, J.; Sharfstein, S.; and Moszynski I. 1986. Trends in private insurance coverage for mental illness. *American Journal of Psychiatry* 143:1276–1279.

Bremmer, M. 1968. *Dependency and the family: A psychological study in preferences between family and official decision-making*. London: Institute of Economic Affairs.

Brenton, M. 1982. Changing relationships in Dutch social services. *Journal of Social Policy* 11:59–80.

Broadbent, E. 1987. The incentive management programs. In *Restructuring health policy: An international challenge*, ed. J. Virgo, 341–354. Edwardsville, Ill.: International Health Economics and Management Institute, Southern Illinois University.

Brown, E. R. 1982. *Rockefeller medicine men: Capitalism and medicine in America*. Berkeley and Los Angeles: University of California Press.

―――. 1984. Medicare and medicaid: Bandaids for the old and poor. In *Reforming medicine*, ed. V. Sidel and R. Sidel, 50–78. New York: Pantheon.

Brown L. 1987. Introduction to a decade of transition. In *Health policy in transition: A decade of health politics, policy, and law*, ed. L. Brown, 1–16. Durham, N.C.: Duke University Press.

Brown, P. 1985. *The transfer of care*. New York: Routledge and Kegan Paul.

―――. 1988. Recent trends in the political economy of mental health. In *Location and stigma: Contemporary perspectives on mental health and health care*, ed. C. Smith and J. Giggs, 58–80. London: Allen and Unwin.

Brown, P., and Smith, C. J. 1988. Mental patients' rights: An empirical study of variations across the United States. *International Journal of Law and Psychiatry* 11 (2):157–165.

Bruess, C. 1978. National scope of school health education. In *Conference proceedings of school health education: A shared responsibility*. Rutgers University, University of Medicine and Dentistry of New Jersey, Piscataway.

Bulgaro, P., and Webb, A. 1980. Federal-state conflicts in cost control. *Proceedings of the American Academy of Political Science*, no. 33.

Bunker, J. P. 1970. Surgical manpower: A comparison of operations and surgeons in the United States and in England and Wales. *New England Journal of Medicine* 282:135–144.

BUPA (British United Provident Association). 1986. *Provident Association statistics, 1986*. London: BUPA Research Division.

Burrow, J. 1977. *Organized medicine in the Progressive Era*. Baltimore: Johns Hopkins University Press.

Butler, J. 1984. On the relative efficiency of public and private enterprises: Some evidence from hospitals. In *Economics and health 1983*, ed. P. M. Tatchell, 228–256. Canberra: Australian National University.

Calderón, F. 1987. Prologo to *Descentralización del estado: Movimiento social y gestión local*, by J. Borja, T. Valdes, H. Pozo, and E. Morales, 7–10. Santiago: FLACSO.

Caldwell, L. 1970. Authority and responsibility for environmental administration. *Annals of the American Academy of Political and Social Science* 399:107–115.

Califano, J. 1981. *Governing America*. New York: Simon and Schuster.

———. 1986. *America's health care revolution: Who lives? Who dies? Who pays?* New York: Random House.

Calkins, B. 1987. Life-style and chronic disease in western society. In *Public health and the environment*, ed. M. Greenberg, 25–75. New York: Guilford.

Cameron, D. R. 1982. On the limits of the public economy. *Annals of the American Academy of Political and Social Science* 459:46–62.

Campbell, A. J.; Shelton, E. J.; Caradoc-Davis, T.; and Fanning, J. 1984. Dependency levels of elderly people in the institutional care in Dunedin. *New Zealand Medical Journal* 97:12–15.

Canterbury Hospital Board. 1987. *Service development plan for health of the elderly*. Christchurch: Canterbury Hospital Board.

Cardoso, F., and Faletto, E. 1979. *Dependency and development in Latin America*. Berkeley and Los Angeles: University of California Press.

Carpenter, N. 1980. Left orthodoxy and the politics of health. *Capital and Class* 11:74–98.

Carrier, J., and Kendall I. 1977. The development of welfare states. *Journal of Social Policy* 6:271–290.

Castells, M. 1978. *City, class, and power*. London: Macmillan.

———. 1983. *The city and the grassroots*. Berkeley and Los Angeles: University of California Press.

Caviedes, C. 1984. *The southern cone*. Totowa, N.J.: Rowman and Allanheld.

CEPAL (Comisión Económica para América Latina y el Caribe). 1988.

Resultados preliminares de la Economia Latinoamericana. Santiago: CEPAL, United Nations.

Chan, J. B., and Ericson, R. V. 1981. *Decarceration and the economy of penal reform.* University of Toronto: Center of Criminology.

Chanfreau, D. 1979. Professional ideology and the health care system in Chile. *International Journal of Health Services* 9:86–105.

Chávez, V. 1977. *La materia médica en el incanato.* Lima: Editorial Mejía Baca.

Chetwynd, J.; Fougere, G.; Salter, M.; and Hunter, W. 1983. Private medical insurance in New Zealand: Issues of membership and growth. *New Zealand Medical Journal* 96:1052–1055.

City of Toronto. 1986. *Draft report of the sub-committee on the housing needs of the homeless population.* Toronto: Mayor's Office, City of Toronto.

Coddington, D.; Palmquist, L.; and Trollinger, W. 1985. Strategies for survival in the hospital industry. *Harvard Business Review,* May–June, 129–138.

Coelen, C. 1986. Hospital ownership and comparative hospital costs. In *For-profit enterprise in health care,* ed. B. Gray, 322–343. Washington, D.C.: National Academy Press.

COGP (Committee on Government Productivity). 1971. *Report of the Committee on Government Productivity,* vol. 3, Toronto: COGP.

Cohodes, D. 1983. Which will survive? The $150 billion capital question. *Inquiry* 20:5–11.

———. 1986. America: The land of the free and the home of the uninsured. *Inquiry* 23:227–235.

Cohodes, D., and Kinkead, B. 1984. *Hospital capital formation in the 1980s.* Baltimore: Johns Hopkins University Press.

Colegio Médico. 1982. Impacto del modelo económico en la salud. *Vida Médica* 33 (December): 35–39.

———. 1983. *Alguns consideraciones sobre la salud en Chile.* Santiago: Colegio Médico de Chile.

Coleman, V. 1975. *The medicine men.* London: Temple Smith.

Contreras, R.; Duhart, S.; Echeverría, M.; and López H. 1986. *Salud pública privada y solidaria en el Chile actual.* Santiago: Programa de la Economía del Trabajo, no. 44, Academia de Humanismo Cristiano.

Cook, L. 1989. Workplace health promotion programs: Individual behavior, health-care cost containment, and workplace dynamics. M.A. thesis, Department of Geography, Rutgers University.

Cooper, M. 1975. *Rationing health care.* London: Croom Helm.

Corbo, V., and de Melo, J. 1985. *Scrambling for survival: How firms adjusted to the recent reforms in Argentina, Chile, and Uruguay.* Washington, D.C.: World Bank, Staff Working Papers no. 764.

Cordeiro, H. 1982. Politicas de saude no Brasil, 1970–1980. In *Saude e Trabalho no Brasil.* Rio de Janeiro: Editora Vozes Ltda.

Cortázar, R. 1983. Chile: Resultados distributivos, 1973–82. *Notas Técnicas,* no. 57. Santiago: CIEPLAN.

Covarrubias, P., and Franco, R. 1978. *Chile: Mujer y sociedad.* Santiago: Fondo de las Naciones Unidas para la Infancia.

Coyle, A. 1985. Going private: The implications of privatisation for women's work. *Feminist Review* 21:5–23.

Crouch, C. 1985. Can socialism achieve street credibility? *Guardian,* 14 February, 9.

CSSL (Committee to Save Saint Luke's). 1986. Untitled flier, December 18. Mimeo.

Culliton, B. 1987. GAO report angers cancer officials. *Science* 236:380–381.

Culyer, A. 1983. Public or private health services: A skeptic's view. *Journal of Policy Analysis and Management* 2:386–402.

Davis, C., and Fesbach, M. 1980. *Rising infant mortality in the USSR in the 1970s.* U.S. Department of Commerce, Bureau of the Census, ser. P-95, no. 74. Washington, D.C.: GPO.

Davis, K., and Schoen C. 1978. *Health care and the war on poverty.* Washington: Brookings Institution.

Davis, P. 1981. *Health and health care in New Zealand.* Auckland: Longman Paul.

—————. 1984. Policy outcomes in health and health care. In *In the public interest: Health, work, and housing in New Zealand,* ed. C. Wilkes and I. Shirley, 102–115. Auckland: Benton Ross.

Day, P., and Klein, R. 1985. Towards a new health care system? *British Medical Journal* 291:1291–1293.

—————. 1987. The business of welfare. *New Society* 80 (1277): 11–13.

Dear, M. 1980. The public city. In *Residential mobility and public policy,* ed. W. Clark and E. Moore, 219–241. Beverly Hills: Sage.

Dear, M., and Laws, G. 1986. Anatomy of a decision: Recent land use zoning appeals and their effect on group home locations in Ontario. *Canadian Journal of Community Mental Health* 5:5–17.

Dear, M., and Wolch, J. 1987. *Landscapes of despair.* Cambridge: Polity.

Deiker, T. 1986. How to ensure that the money follows the patient: A strategy for funding community services. *Hospital and Community Psychiatry* 37:256–260.

de Janvry, A. 1985. Social disarticulation in Latin American history. In *Debt and development in Latin America,* ed. K. Kim and D. Ruccio, 32–73. Notre Dame, Ind.: University of Notre Dame Press.

de la Madrid, M.; Soberón, A.; Ruiz, J.; Kumate, J.; Martuscelli, J.; and Sandoval, S. 1986. *La descentralización de los services de salud: El caso de México.* Mexico City: Grupo Editorial Miguel Angel Porrua.

Demkovitch, L. 1986. Controlling costs at General Motors. *Health Affairs* 5:58–67.

De Pouvoirville, G. 1986. Hospital reforms in France under a socialist government. *Milbank Memorial Fund Quarterly* 64:392–413.

De Pouvoirville, G., and Renaud, M. 1985. Hospital system management in France and Canada. *Social Science and Medicine* 20:153–166.

Dever, G. E. 1980. *Community health analysis.* Rockville, Md.: Aspen.

Diderichsen, F. 1982. Ideologies in the Swedish health sector today. *International Journal of Health Services* 12:191–200.

Doll, R., and Peto, R. 1981. *The causes of cancer.* New York: Oxford University Press.

Donckaster, R. 1985. Las Isapres y los médicos. *Vida Médica* 36 (2): 50–54.

Doyal, L., and Pennell, I. 1979. *The political economy of health.* Boston: South End Press.

Duerksen, C. 1983. *Environmental regulation of industrial plant siting: How to make it work better.* Washington, D.C.: Conservation Foundation.

Dumont, J. P. 1982. *La securite sociale tourjours en chantier.* Paris: Editions Ouvrieres.

Dunleavy, P. 1986. Explaining the privatization boom: Public choices versus radical approaches. *Public Administration* 64:13–34.

Durkheim, E. 1938. *Rules of sociological method.* Chicago: University of Chicago Press.

Ehrenreich, J., and Ehrenreich, B. 1970. *The American health empire.* New York: Vintage Books.

Eisenberg, L. 1984. The case against for-profit hospitals. *Hospital and Community Psychiatry* 35:1009–1012.

———. 1986. Health care: For patients or for profits? *American Journal of Psychiatry* 143:1015–1019.

Elling, R. 1981. The fiscal crisis of the state and state financing of health care. *Social Science and Medicine* 15C:207–217.

Elliott, S. 1985. *Bless this house: Municipal impediments to the establishment of group homes for ex-offenders in residential neighbourhoods.* UEST Working Paper no. 24, Institute of Urban and Environmental Studies, Brock University.

Emerson, H., and Phillips, A. 1925. *Hospitals and health agencies of San Francisco, 1923: A survey.* Report for the Committee on Hospital and Health Agencies of the Council of Social and Health Agencies. San Francisco.

English, J. T.; Sharfstein, S. S.; Scherl, D. J.; Astrachan, B.; and Muszynski, I. L. 1985. Diagnosis-related groups and general hospital psychiatry: The A.P.A. study. *American Journal of Psychiatry* 143:131–139.

Epstein, S. 1979. *The politics of cancer.* Garden City, N.Y.: Sierra Club Books.

Erickson, R.; Gavin, N.; and Cordes, S. 1986. Service industries in the interregional trade: The economic impacts of the hospital sector. *Growth and Change* 17:17–27.

Ermann, D., and Gabel, J. 1984. Multi-hospital systems: Issues and empirical evidence. *Health Affairs* 3:52–54.

———. 1985. The changing face of American health care. *Medical Care* 23:401–420.

Esping-Andersen, G. 1985. Power and distributional regimes. *Politics and Society* 12:223–256.

Eyer, J. 1984. Capitalism, health, and illness. In *Issues in the political economy of health care,* ed. J. McKinlay, 23–59. New York: Tavistock.

Eyles, J. 1986. Images of care, realities of provision and location: Services for the mentally ill in Northampton. *East Midlands Geographer* 9:53–60.

———. 1987. *The geography of the national health*. London: Croom Helm.

Eyles, J.; Smith, D.; and Woods, K. 1982. Spatial resource allocations and state practice: The case of health service planning in London. *Regional Studies* 16:239–253.

Eyles, J., and Woods, K. J. 1983. *The social geography of medicine and health*. New York: St. Martin.

———. 1987. Who cares and what care?: An inverse interest law? *Social Science and Medicine* 23:1087–1092.

Farquhar, J. 1984. Risk factor reduction from community education: Preliminary results of the Stanford Five City Project. Paper presented at the American Heart Association meetings, Tampa, Florida.

Fefer, E. 1982. Pharmaceutical products and their impact on developing countries. In *Pharmaceuticals and developing countries: A dialogue for constructive action*, 9–13. Washington, D.C.: National Council for International Health.

Feldstein, P. 1986. The emergence of market competition in the U.S. health care system: Its causes, likely structure, and implication. *Health Policy* 6:1–20.

Fergusson, D.; Horwood, L.; and Shannon, F. 1986. Reasons for holding health insurance: A study of a group of Christchurch families. *New Zealand Medical Journal* 99:371–373.

Ffrench-Davis, R. 1982. El experimento monetarista en Chile. *Colección Estudios CIEPLAN* 9:5–40.

Fincher, R., and Ruddick, S. 1983. Transformation possibilities within the capitalist state: Cooperative housing and decentralized health care in Quebec. *International Journal of Urban and Regional Research* 7:44–71.

Flora, P., and Alber, J. 1982. Modernization, democratization, and the development of welfare states in Western Europe. In *The development of welfare states in Europe and America*. ed. P. Flora and A. J. Heidenheimer, 37–81. New Brunswick, N.J.: Transaction.

Flora, P., and Heidenheimer, A. J. 1982. The historical core and changing boundaries of the welfare state. In *The development of welfare states in Europe and America*, ed. P. Flora and A. J. Heidenheimer, 17–34. New Brunswick, N.J.: Transaction.

Foley, H., and Sharfstein, S. 1983. *Madness and government: Who cares for the mentally ill?* Washington, D.C.: American Psychiatric Press.

FONASA (National Health Fund). 1982. Antecedentes financieros Santiago. Santiago, Chile. Mimeo.

Forsyth, M. 1983. *Reservicing health*. London: Adam Smith Institute.

Fougere, G. 1978. Undoing the welfare state: The case of hospital care. In *Politics in New Zealand*, ed. S. Levine, 406–417. Sydney: Allen and Unwin.

———. 1984. From market to welfare state?: State interventions and medical care delivery in New Zealand. In *In the public interest: Health, work, and housing in New Zealand*, ed. C. Wilkes and I. Shirley, 76–89. Auckland: Benton Ross.

Fox, K. 1983. Health care for the elderly: Population, services, and resources in North Canterbury. Planning and Research Series, no. 11. Christchurch, New Zealand: Health Planning and Research Unit.

Fraser, G. 1984. An examination of factors in the development of New Zealand's health system. In *In the public interest: Health, work, and housing in New Zealand*, ed. C. Wilkes and I. Shirley, 53–75. Auckland: Benton Ross.

Freeman, R. 1981. *The wayward welfare state.* Stanford, Calif.: Hoover Institution Press.

Friedman, J. 1973. Structural constraints on community action: The case of infant mortality rates. *Social Problems* 21:230–245.

Friedman, M., and Friedman, R. 1980. *Free to choose: A personal statement.* New York: Harcourt Brace Jovanovich.

Galal, E. 1983. National production of drugs: Egypt. In *Pharmaceuticals and health in the Third World*, ed. S. J. Patel, 237–241. Oxford: Pergamon.

Gallagher, P. 1986. The Presbyterian story: The people pull the strings for a change. *Health PAC Bulletin* 15:5–13.

Gamble, A. 1979. The free economy and the strong state. *Socialist Register* 16:1–25.

Garretón, M. A. 1983. *El proceso politico Chileno.* Santiago: FLACSO.

Gay, G. 1905. Abuse of medical charity. *Boston Medical Surgery Journal* 152: 295–305.

Gaylin, S. 1985. The coming of the corporation and the marketing of psychiatry. *Hospital and Community Psychiatry* 36:154–159.

Geiger, R., and Wolch, J. 1986. A shadow state?: Voluntarism in metropolitan Los Angeles. *Environment and Planning D: Society and Space* 4:351–366.

Gershuny, J., and Miles, I. 1983. *The new service economy: The transformation of employment in industrial societies.* New York: Praegar.

Gershuny, J., and Pahl, R. 1979. Work outside employment. *New Universities Quarterly* 34:120–136.

Gesler, W. 1979. Barriers between people and health practitioners in Calabar, Nigeria. *Southeastern Geographer* 19:27–41.

———. 1984. *Health care delivery in developing countries.* Washington, D.C.: Association of American Geographers.

Giaconi, J. 1982. Funcionamiento del sistema de servicios de salud. In *Desarrollo social y salud en Chile*, ed. H. Lavados, 3:91–100. Santiago: CPU.

Gibson, R., and Waldo, D. 1982. National health expenditures, 1981. *Health Care Financing Review* 4:1–35.

Ginsburg, P. 1972. Resource allocation in the hospital industry: The role of capital financing. *Social Security Bulletin* 35:20–30.

———. 1976. Inflation and capital investment. In *Health: A victim or a cause of inflation?* ed. M. Zubkoff, 164–178. New York: Milbank Memorial Fund Quarterly.

Ginzberg, E. 1983. The delivery of health care: What lies ahead? *Inquiry* 20:201–217.

———. 1984. The monetarization of medical care. *New England Journal of Medicine* 310:1162–1165.

———. 1985. *The U.S. health care system: A look to the 1990's.* Totowa, N.J.: Rowman and Allanheld.

Ginzberg, E., and Ostow, M. 1985. Health care in New York City: A system in flux. *New York Affairs* 9:58–73.

Glade, W. 1983. The privatisation and denationalisation of public enterprises. In *Government and public enterprise*, ed. G. R. Reddy. London: Frank Cass.

Glucksberg, H., and Singer, J. 1982. The multinational drug companies in Zaire: Their adverse effect on cost and availability of essential drugs. *International Journal of Health Services* 12 (3): 381–387.

Godber, C. 1984. Private rest homes: Answers needed. *British Medical Journal* 288:1473–1474.

Goldman, H.; Adams, N.; and Taube, C. 1983. Deinstitutionalization: The data demythologized. *Hospital and Community Psychiatry* 34:129–134.

Goldsmith, J. 1980. The health care market: Can hospitals survive? *Harvard Business Review*, September–October, 100–112.

———. 1985. The changing role of hospitals. In *The U.S. health care system: A look to the 1990's*, ed. E. Ginzberg, 48–69. Totowa, N.J.: Rowman and Allanheld.

González, A. 1988. La regionalización desde el punto de vista geográfico. Paper presented at the meeting, Regionalización de los Servicios de Salud [Health Services Regionalization], Montevideo, June 8, 1988.

Good, C. 1987. *Ethnomedical systems in Africa.* New York: Guilford.

Gotsch, A., and Pearson, C. 1987. Education-for-health: Strategies for change. In *Public health and the environment*, ed. M. Greenberg, 293–330. New York: Guilford.

Gough, I. 1979. *The political economy of the welfare state.* London: Macmillan.

———. 1983. The crisis of the British welfare state. *International Journal of Health Services* 13:459–477.

Gough, I., and Steinberg, A. 1981. The welfare state, capitalism, and crisis. *Political Power and Social Theory* 2:141–171.

Gould, J. 1982. *The Rake's progress?: The New Zealand economy since 1945.* Auckland: Hodder and Stoughton.

Governor's Health Advisory Council (New York). 1984. *Alternative futures for mental health services in New York: 2000 and beyond.* Albany, N.Y.: New York State Health Planning Commission.

Governor's Select Commission (New York). 1984. *Final report of the Governor's Select Commission on the future of the state-local mental health system.* Albany, N.Y.: New York State Office of Mental Health.

Grant, C. 1985. Private health care in the United Kingdom: A review. Economist Intelligence Unit, Special Report no. 207. London.

Gray, A. M. 1984. European health care costs. *Social Policy and Administration* 18:213–228.

Gray, B., ed. 1986. *For-profit enterprise in health care*. Washington, D.C.: National Academy Press.

Greenberg, M. 1983. *Urbanization and cancer mortality*. New York: Oxford University Press.

———. 1987a. The changing geography of major causes of death among middle age white Americans, 1929–1981. *Socioeconomic Planning Sciences* 21:223–228.

———. 1987b. Research policy and review 17. Geographical disparities in state-cancer prevention policies: The need for strong federal intervention. *Environment and Planning A* 19:715–718.

———. 1987c. Urban/rural differences in behavioral risk factors for chronic diseases. *Urban Geography* 8:146–151.

———. 1989. Black male cancer and American urban health policy. *Journal of Urban Affairs* 10:121–138.

Greenwald, P., and Sondik, E. 1986. *Cancer control objectives for the nation: 1985–2000*. NIH pub. 86–2880. Washington, D.C.: National Institutes of Health.

Griffith, B.; Iliffe, S.; and Rayner, G. 1987. *Banking on sickness: Commercial medicine in Britain and the USA*. London: Lawrence and Wishart.

Griffith, B.; Rayner, G.; and Mohan, J. 1985. *Commercial medicine in London*. London: GLC.

Group for the Advancement of Psychiatry. 1978. *The chronic mental patient in the community*. New York: Mental Health Materials Center.

GTIC (Governor's Task Force on Indigent Health Care, Virginia). 1987. *Interim report to the governor and General Assembly*. Report for the Governor's Task Force on Indigent Health Care. Blacksburg, Va.

Gusfield, J. 1984. On the side: Practical action and social constructivism in social problems theory. In *Studies in the sociology of social problems*, ed. J. Schneider and J. Kitsuse, 31–51. Norwood, N.J.: Ablex.

Gwynne, R. 1986. *Industrialization and urbanization in Latin America*. Baltimore: Johns Hopkins University Press.

———. 1987. Practical privatisation in Chile: Pinochet government pushes private purchasing power to the forefront. *Financial Times* (London), 16 June, 25.

Haberlein, L. 1988. The changes in the distribution of for-profit hospitals, 1970–1985. Master's thesis, Department of Urban Affairs and Planning, Virginia Polytechnic Institute and State University.

Habermans, J. 1976. *Legitimation crisis*. London: Heinemann.

Haignere, C. 1983. The application of the free-market economic model in Chile and the effects on the population's health status. *International Journal of Health Services* 13:389–405.

Hall, S., and Jacques, M. 1983. *The politics of Thatcherism*. London: Lawrence and Wishart.

Hanft, R. 1985. Physicians and hospitals: Changing dynamics. In *The health policy agenda: Some critical questions*, ed. M. Lewin, 99–114. Washington, D.C.: American Enterprise Institute.

Harman, H. 1987. No place like home: A report of the first year's work of the Registered Homes Tribunal. House of Commons. London. Mimeo.

Hastings, S., and Levie, H. 1983. *Privatisation?* Nottingham: Spokesman.

Hatch, J., and Eng, E. 1984. Community participation and control. In *Reforming Medicine*, ed. V. Sidel and R. Sidel, 223–244. New York: Pantheon.

Havighurst, C. 1987. The changing focus of decision making in the health care sector. In *Health policy in transition: A decade of health politics, policy, and law*, ed. L. Brown, 129–167. Durham, N.C.: Duke University Press.

Hay, I. 1985. The caring commodity: Transformations in the exchange character of medicine in New Zealand, 1840–1985. Master's thesis, Massey University, Palmerston North.

Haynes, R. 1986. *The geography of health services in Britian*. Beckenham: Croom Helm.

Heald, D. 1985. Will the privatisation of public enterprises solve the problem of control? *Public Administration* 63:7–22.

Health Benefits Review. 1986. *Choices for health care*. Wellington, New Zealand: Government Printer.

Heclo, H. 1972. Policy analysis. *British Journal of Political Science* 2:83–108.

Heller, T. 1977. *Poor health, rich profits: Multinational drug companies and the Third World*. Nottingham: Spokesman.

Hernández, M. 1981. *The capital structure of the hospital industry in the 80's*. New York: Kidder, Peabody.

Hernández, M., and Henkel, A. 1982. Need for capital may squeeze freestanding institutions into multi-institutional arrangements. *Hospitals* 56:75–77.

Hernández, S., and Kaluzny, A. 1983. Hospital closure: A review of current and proposed research. *Health Services Research* 18:419–436.

Heseltine, G. 1983. Towards a blueprint for change: A mental health policy and program perspective. Toronto Ministry of Health Discussion Paper.

Higgins, C. S. 1985. Pathways to longterm care. *New Zealand Medical Journal* 98:646–649.

Higgins, J. 1984. The public control of private health care. *Public Administration* 62:218–224.

Highland, J.; Fine, M.; Harris, R.; Warren, J.; Rauch, R.; Johnson, A.; and Boyle, R. 1979. *Malignant neglect*. New York: Knopf.

Hillman, D. 1985. Strategies in the fifty states. In *Current Strategies for Containing Health Care Expenditures*, ed. J. Christianson, 85–107. New York: Spectrum.

Hindess, B. 1987. *Freedom, equality, and the market*. London: Tavistock.

Hirschman, A. 1970. *Exit, voice, and loyalty: Responses to decline in firms, organizations, and states*. Cambridge: Harvard University Press.

Hirschoff, P. 1986. The privatisation drive. *Africa Report* 31 (July–August): 89–92.

Hollingsworth, J., and Hollingsworth, E. 1987. *Controversy about American hospitals: Funding, ownership, and performance.* Washington, D.C.: American Enterprise Institute.

Horn, J. 1985. Brazil: The health care model of the military modernizers and technocrats. *International Journal of Health Services* 15:47–68.

Horowitz, M. G. 1988. Humana's rising costs divert attention from revenues. *Healthweek* 2 (1): 6.

Horwitz, A. 1982. *The social control of mental illness.* New York: Academic Press.

Hunter, D. 1983. The privatisation of public provision. *Lancet* 1 (June 4): 1264–1268.

Hustead, E.; Sharfstein, S.; Muszynski, S.; Brady, J.; and Cahill, J. 1985. Reductions in coverage for mental and nervous illness in the federal employees health benefits program, 1980–1984. *American Journal of Psychiatry* 142:181–186.

Huws, U., and de Groot, L. 1985. A very ordinary picket. *New Socialist,* January, 8–10.

HWDSS (Hamilton-Wentworth Department of Social Services). 1986. *A brief prepared for the Provincial Social Assistance Review Committee.* Hamilton, Ontario: Department of Social Services, Regional Municipality of Hamilton-Wentworth.

Idenburg, P. A. 1985. The Dutch paradox in social welfare. In *The year book of social policy in Britain, 1984–85,* ed. M. Brenton and C. Jones. London: RKP.

Illich, I. 1975. *Medical nemesis: The expropriation of health.* London: Calder and Boyars.

Incomes Data Services. 1984. *Private health insurance.* IDS Report no. 317. London.

Infante, A.; Jansana, L.; López, H.; Valdivia, M.; and Vergara, C. 1983. Estudio de perfectabilidad para la reformulación de una red de consultorios de salud en la Comuna de Las Condes, informe final. Mimeo.

Issel, W., and Cherny, R. 1986. *San Francisco, 1865–1932: Politics, power, and urban development.* Berkeley and Los Angeles: University of California Press.

Jessop, B.; Bonnett, K.; Bromley, S.; and Ling, T. 1984. Authoritarian populism, two nations, and Thatcherism. *New Left Review* 147:32–60.

Jiménez de la Jara, J., ed. 1977. *Medicina social en Chile.* Santiago: Editorial Aconcagua.

———. 1982. Desarrollo y perspectivas del sector privado en salud. In *Desarrollo social y salud en Chile,* ed. H. Lavados, 3:154–175. Santiago: CPU.

———. 1984. *Salud pública: Bibliografía Chilena, 1974–1983.* Santiago: CPU.

Jiménez de la Jara, J., and Gili, M. 1988. Municipalización de la atención primaria en salud. *Documento de Trabajo*, no. 16/CPU. Santiago: Corporación Promoción Universitaria.

Joseph, A., and Flynn, H. 1988. Regional and welfare perspectives on the public-private hospital dichotomy in New Zealand. *Social Science and Medicine* 26 (1): 101–110.

Joseph, A., and Phillips, D. 1984. *Accessibility and utilization: Geographical perspectives on health care delivery*. New York: Harper and Row.

Judge, K., and Knapp, M. 1985. Efficiency in the production of welfare: The public and private sectors compared. In *The future of welfare*, ed. R. Klein and M. O'Higgins, 131–149. Oxford: Blackwell.

Kapstein, E. 1988. Brazil: Continued state dominance. In *The promise of privatization*, ed. R. Vernon, 122–148. Washington, D.C.: Council on Foreign Relations.

Kaser, M. 1976. *Health care in the Soviet Union and Eastern Europe*. Boulder: Westview.

Kelly de Escobar, J. 1988. Venezuela: Letting in the market. In *The promise of privatization*, ed. R. Vernon, 57–90. Washington, D.C.: Council on Foreign Relations.

Kennedy, L. 1984. The lesson in profits: How proprietaries affect public and voluntary hospitals. *Health PAC Bulletin* 15:5–13.

King, B.; Fletcher, M.; and Main, L. 1985. Institutional provisions for the aged. New Zealand Department of Health Special Report Series, no. 74. Wellington: Government Printer.

Kingham, J. 1982. The involvement of U.S. pharmaceutical manufacturers in developing countries. In *Pharmaceuticals and developing countries: A dialogue for constructive action*, 21–26. Washington, D.C.: National Council for International Health.

Kirby, A. 1983. A comment on "Urban structure and geographical access to public services." *Annals of the Association of American Geographers* 73:289–295.

———. 1984. Health care and the state: Britain and the United States. In *Public Service Provision and Urban Development*, ed. A. Kirby, P. Knox, and S. Pinch, 213–230. New York: St. Martin.

Klarén, P. F., and Bossert, T. J. 1986. *Promise of development: Theories of change in Latin America*. Boulder, Colo.: Westview.

Klarman, H. 1978. Health planning: Progress, prospects, and issues. *Milbank Memorial Fund Quarterly* 56:78–112.

Klee, L. 1983. Culture and disease in nineteenth-century San Francisco. Ph.D. diss. University of California, San Francisco.

Klein, R. 1982. Private practice and public policy: Regulating the frontiers. In *The public-private mix for health*, ed. G. McLachlan and A. Maynard, 95–128. London: Nuffield Provincial Hospitals Trust.

———. 1983. Strategies for comparative social policy research. In *Health and welfare states of Britain*, ed. A. Williamson and G. Room. London: Heinemann.

————. 1984. Privatization and the welfare state. *Lloyds Bank Review* 151: 12–29.

Klerman, G. 1977. Better but not well: Social and ethical issues in the deinstitutionalization of the mentally ill. *Schizophrenia Bulletin* 3:617–631.

Knowles, R. 1985. The welfare state: Social and spatial implications for the working class elderly. Master's thesis, Department of Geography, McMaster University.

Knox, P. 1986. Review of *Accessibility and utilization*, by A. E. Joseph and D. R. Phillips. *Annals of the Association of American Geographers* 76 (3): 438–440.

Knox, P.; Bohland, J.; and Shumsky, N. L. 1983. The urban transition and the evolution of the medical care delivery system in America. *Social Science and Medicine* 17:37–43.

————. 1984. Urban development and the geography of personal services: The example of medical care in the United States. In *Public service provision and urban development*, ed. A. Kirby, P. Knox, and S. Pinch, 152–175. London: Croom Helm.

Kofman, E., and Lethbridge, J. 1987. Family, community, and care: Ideology and practice in Conservative Britain. Paper presented at the Institute of British Geographers (IBG) Annual Conference, Portsmouth, England.

Kohn, R., and White, K. 1976. *Health care: An international survey.* New York: Oxford University Press.

Lall, S. 1979. Problems of distribution, availability, and utilization of agents in developing countries: An Asian perspective. In *Pharmaceuticals for developing countries: Conference proceedings*, 236–249. Division of International Health, Institute of Medicine. Washington, D.C.: National Academy of Sciences.

————. 1981. Economic considerations in the provision and use of medicines. In *Pharmaceuticals and health policy*, ed. R. Blum et al., 186–210. London: Croom Helm.

Lall, S., and Bibile, S. 1978. The political economy of controlling transnationals: The pharmaceutical industry in Sri Lanka, 1972–1976. *International Journal of Health Services* 8 (2): 299–328.

Lamb, H. 1984. *The homeless mentally ill: A task force report of the American Psychiatric Association.* Washington, D.C.: American Psychiatric Association.

Landman, J. 1979. Tendencias de assistencia médica. In *Enontros de Saude no Brasil.* Belo Horizonte, Brazil: Editora Universidade de Brasilia.

Larson, J. 1980. The role of private enterprise in providing health care: The lessons of the American experience. *National Western Bank Quarterly Review* 80:58–65.

Lash, S., and Urry, J. 1987. *The end of organized capitalism.* Cambridge: Polity.

Latin American Bureau. 1983. *Chile: The Pinochet decade. The rise and fall of the Chicago boys.* London: Latin American Bureau.

Law, C., and Warnes, A. 1984. The elderly population of Great Britain:

Locational trends and policy implications. *Transactions Institute of British Geographers* 9:37–59.

Laws, G. 1987. Restructuring, privatization, and the local welfare state. Ph.D. diss., Department of Geography, McMaster University.

Ledogar, R. 1975. *Hungry for profits: U.S. food and drug multinationals in Latin America.* New York: IDOC.

Lee, K., and Mills, A. 1983. *The economics of health in developing countries.* New York: Oxford University Press.

Le Grand, J., and Robinson, J. 1984. *Privatisation and the welfare state.* London: Allen and Unwin.

Lerman, P. 1982. *Deinstitutionalization and the welfare state.* New Brunswick, N.J.: Rutgers University Press.

Levenson, A. 1985. The for-profit system. In *The new economics and psychiatric care,* ed. S. Sharfstein and A. Beigel, 151–163. Washington, D.C.: American Psychiatric Press.

Levin, B., and Glasser, J. 1984. A national survey of prepaid mental health services. *Hospital and Community Psychiatry* 35:350–355.

Levin, D. 1974. *Cancer rates and risk.* Washington, D.C.: GPO.

Levine, M. 1981. *The history and politics of community mental health.* New York: Oxford University Press.

Levine, S. 1987. The changing terrains in medical sociology. *Journal of Health and Social Behavior* 28:1–6.

Levinson, C. 1970. *The multinational pharmaceutical industry.* Geneva: International Federation of Chemical and General Workers' Union.

Levy, E.; Bungener, M.; Dumenil, G.; and Fagnani, F. 1983. *La croissance des depenses de sante.* Paris: Economica.

Light, D. W. 1986. Corporate medicine for profit. *Scientific American* 255:38–45.

Light, D. W.; Phipps, E. J.; Piper, G. E.; Rismiller, D. J.; Mobilio, J. N.; and Ranieri, W. F. 1986. Finding diagnosis-related groups that work: A call for research. *American Journal of Psychiatry* 143:622–624.

Lilienfield, A.; Levin, N.; and Kessler, I. 1972. *Cancer in the United States.* Cambridge, Mass.: Harvard University Press.

Loxley, J. 1984. Saving the world economy. *Monthly Review,* September, 22–34.

McCallum, J. 1986. Salt in the wound. *New Zealand Listener,* 23 August, 28–30.

McCulloch, R. 1980. The multinational pharmaceutical industry: Evidence of product diffusion and technology transfer. In *The international supply of medicines,* ed. R. Helms, 3–4. Washington, D.C.: American Enterprise Institute for Public Policy Research.

Macedo, R. 1984. Brazilian children and the economic crisis: Evidence from the state of São Paulo. *World Development* 12 (3): 203–222.

McGuire, T. 1981. Financing and demand for mental health services. *Journal of Human Resources* 16:501–522.

Mach, E. 1978. The financing of health systems in developing countries: Discussion paper. *Social Science and Medicine* 12 (1C/2C): 7–11.

McIntyre, L. 1987. Drugs. In *U.S. Industrial Outlook*, 17.1–17.7. U.S. Department of Commerce. Washington, D.C.: GPO.

McKeown, T. 1976. *The role of medicine: Dream, mirage, or nemesis*. London: Nuffield Provincial Hospitals Trust.

McKinlay, J. 1980. Evaluating medical technology in the context of a fiscal crisis: The case of New Zealand. *Milbank Memorial Fund Quarterly* 58 (2): 217–267.

———, ed. 1984. *Issues in the political economy of health care*. New York: Tavistock.

McKinlay, J., and McKinlay, S. 1977. The questionable contribution of medical measures to the decline of mortality in the United States in the twentieth century. *Milbank Memorial Fund Quarterly* 55:405–428.

McLachlan, G., and Maynard, A., eds. 1982. *The public-private mix for health: The relevance and effects of change*. London: Nuffield Provincial Hospitals Trust.

McLafferty, S. 1982. Neighborhood characteristics and hospital closures. *Social Science and Medicine* 16:1667–1674.

———. 1986. The geographical restructuring of urban hospitals: Spatial dimensions of corporate strategy. *Social Science and Medicine* 23:1079–1086.

McPherson, K.; Strong, P.; Epstein, A.; and Jones, L. 1981. Regional variations in the use of common surgical procedures: Within and between England and Wales, Canada, and the United States of America. *Social Science and Medicine* 15A:273–288.

Maguire, D., and Mohan, J. 1986. *Devon in maps: A social and economic profile*. Special Publication, South West Papers in Geography. Devon.

Maidenberg, H. 1985. Prospects. *New York Times*, 17 February, sec. 3, 1.

Malloy, J. M., and Borzutsky, S. 1982. Politics, social welfare policy, and the population problem in Latin America. *International Journal of Health Services* 12:77–91.

Mamula, R., and Newman, N. 1973. *Community placement for the mentally retarded: A handbook for community agencies and social work practitioners*. Springfield, Ill.: Charles C. Thomas.

Manhattan Health Working Group. 1987. Position statement, 2 February. Mimeo.

Manning, W. G., Jr.; Wells, K. B.; Duan, N.; Newhouse, J. P.; and Ware, J. E., Jr. 1984. Cost sharing and the use of ambulatory mental health services. *American Psychologist* 39:1077–1089.

Marmor, T. R. 1986. American medical policy and the "crisis" of the welfare state. *Journal of Health Politics, Policy, and Law* 11:617–631.

Marmor, T.R.; Hoffman, W.; and Heagy, T. 1975. National health insurance: Some lessons from the Canadian experience. *Policy Sciences* 6:447–466.

Marmor, T. R., and Morone, F. 1980. Representing consumer interests: Imbalanced markets, health planning, and the HSAs. *Milbank Memorial Fund Quarterly* 58:125–162.

Martínez, J., and Tironi, E. 1982. *Materiales para el estudio de las clases medias en la sociedad Chilena, 1960–1980*. Santiago: SUR.

Marzagao, C., and Segall, M. 1983. Drug selection: Mozambique. In *Pharmaceuticals and health in the Third World*, ed. S. J. Patel, 205–216. Oxford: Pergamon.

Mason, T., and McKay, F. 1974. *U.S. cancer mortality by county: 1950–1969*. DHEW Pub. no. (NIH) 74-615. Washington, D.C.: GPO.

Massey, D., and Meegan, R. 1982. *The anatomy of job loss*. London: Methuen.

Maxwell, R. J. 1974. *Health care, the growing dilemma: Need versus resources in Western Europe, the U.S., and the U.S.S.R.* New York: McKinsey.

———. 1981. *Health and wealth*. Lexington: D. C. Heath.

———. 1987. Private medicine and public policy. In *Health care UK 1987*, ed. A Harrison and J. Gretton. Newbury: Policy Journals.

Mayer, D. 1988a. HCA says poor fourth quarter doesn't reflect restructuring. *Healthweek* 2 (5): 28.

———. 1988b. Shareholders assail AMI for "lackluster" performance. *Healthweek* 2 (2): 13.

Maynard, A. 1983. Privatizing the National Health Service. *Lloyds Bank Review* 148:28–41.

———. 1986. Public and private interactions: An economic perspective. *Social Science and Medicine* 22:1161–1166.

Maynard, A., and Williams, A. 1984. Privatisation and the National Health Service. In *Privatisation and the welfare state*, ed. J. Le Grand and R. Robinson, 95–110. London: Allen and Unwin.

Medina, E., and Kaempffer, A. 1982. La Salud en Chile durante la década del setenta. *Revista Médica de Chile* 110:1004–1115.

Medina, E., and Yrarrázaval, M. 1983. Fiebre tifoidea en Chile: Consideraciones epidemiológicas. *Revista Médica de Chile* 111:609–615.

Meerhoff, R. 1987. Encuesta sobre trabajo médico. Montevideo, Uruguay. Mimeo.

Melrose, D. 1983. Double deprivation: Public and private distribution from the perspective of the Third World poor. In *Pharmaceuticals and health in the Third World*, ed. S. J. Patel, 181–186. Oxford: Pergamon.

Mesa-Lago, C. 1978. *Social security in Latin America*. Pittsburgh: University of Pittsburgh Press.

———, ed. 1985. *The crisis of social security and health care in Latin America*. Pittsburgh: Center for Latin American Studies, University of Pittsburgh.

Meza, M. E. 1984. Isapres: El dilema ante la maternidad. *Paula* 420:60–65.

Miller, R. 1978. The recapitalisation of capitalism. *International Journal of Urban and Regional Research* 2:202–212.

Minford, P. 1984. State expenditure: A study in waste. *Economic Affairs* 4 (3): i–xix.

Ministerio de Salud, República de Chile, Departamento de Planificación. 1982. *Manual para postas y consultorios generales urbanos y rurales traspasados a la administración municipal.* Santiago: Ministerio de Salud.

Mishra, R. 1984. *Welfare state in crisis: Social thought and social change.* Brighton: Wheatsheaf Books.

Mishra, R.; Laws, G.; and Harding, P. 1989. Privatization: The case of Ontario's social services. In *Privatization and provincial social services in Canada: Policy, administration, and delivery,* ed. J. Ismael and Y. Vaillencourt, 119–139. Calgary: University of Alberta.

Mohan, J. 1984a. Geographical aspects of private hospital developments in Britain. *Area* 16 (3): 191–199.

————. 1984b. State policies and the development of hospital services of Northeast England, 1948–82. *Political Geography Quarterly* 4:275–295.

————. 1985. Independent acute medical care in Britain: Its organization, location, and prospects. *International Journal of Urban and Regional Research* 9:467–484.

————. 1986a. The political geography of NHS privatisation. Geography Department, Queen Mary College. Mimeo.

————. 1986b. Private medical care and the British Conservative government: What price independence? *Journal of Social Policy* 15:337–360.

————. 1988. Spatial aspects of health care employment in Britain. 1: Aggregate employment trends. *Environment and Planning A* 20:7–23.

Mohan, J., and Woods, K. 1985. Restructuring health care: The social geography of health care under the British Conservative government. *International Journal of Health Services* 15:197–217.

Moran, A.; Freedman, R.; and Sharfstein, S. 1984. The journey of Sylvia Frumkin: A case study for policymakers. *Hospital and Community Psychiatry* 35:887–893.

Morel, B.; Ravault, M. C.; Weill, C.; Hatton, J.; and Moatti, J. P. 1985. *La sante en France.* Paris: Documentation Française.

Morrissey, J. P. 1982. Assessing interorganizational linkages. In *The chronically mentally ill: Assessing community support programs,* ed. R. C. Tessler and H. H. Goldman, 159–192. Cambridge, Mass.: Ballinger.

Morrissey, J., and Gounis, K. 1988. Homelessness and mental illness in America: Emerging issues in the construction of a social problem. In *Location and stigma: Contemporary perspectives on mental health and health care,* ed. C. Smith and J. Giggs, 483–512. London: Allen and Unwin.

MTFDPP (Mayor's Task Force on Discharged Psychiatric Patients). 1984. *The final report of the Mayor's Task Force on Discharged Psychiatric Patients.* Toronto: Toronto City Council.

Musgrove, P. 1986. The impact of the economic crisis on health and health care in Latin America and the Caribbean. *WHO Chronicle* 40 (4): 152–157.

Nadelson, C. 1986. Presidential address: Health care directions: Who cares for patients? *American Journal of Psychiatry* 143:949–955.

Nasenius, J., and Veit-Wilson, J. 1985. Social policy in a cold climate. In *The year book of social policy in Britain, 1984–85*, ed. M. Brenton and C. Jones. London: RKP.

National Audit Office. 1986. *Making a reality of community care*. London: HMSO.

———. 1987. *Competitive tendering for support services in the NHS*. London: HMSO.

Navarro, V. 1984. The crisis of the international capitalist order and its implications on the welfare state. In *Issues in the political economy of health care*, ed. J. McKinlay, 107–142. London: Tavistock.

New York City Department of Health. 1984. *Vital statistics*. New York: New York City Department of Health.

———. 1986. The effectiveness of school health education. *Morbidity and Mortality Weekly Report* 35:593–595.

———. 1987. Survey of worksite smoking policies—New York City. *Morbidity and Mortality Weekly Report* 36:177–179.

New York Medical and Health Research Association. 1983. *Towards a better mental health system for New York State*. New York: New York Medical and Health Research Association.

New York State Communities Aid Association. 1983. *Promises to keep: A Mental health agenda for New York State*. New York: State Communities Aid Association.

New York State Office of Health Systems Management. 1982. Institutional cost reports. Albany, N.Y.: New York State Office of Health Systems Management, Division of Health Care Financing.

New York State Office of Mental Health. 1986. *Five year comprehensive plan: Mental health services*. 1987 Update and Progress Report. Albany, N.Y.: New York State Office of Mental Health.

New Zealand Department of Health. 1977. *Planning guidelines for beds and services*. Wellington: Department of Health.

———. 1978. *Hospital management data*. Wellington: National Health Statistics Center.

———. 1985a. *Hospital management data*. Wellington: National Health Statistics Center.

———. 1985b. *Service planning guidelines for health services for the elderly*. Wellington: Department of Health.

———. 1986a. *Hospital management data*. Wellington: National Health Statistics Center.

———. 1986b. *New Zealand medical workforce statistics 1984 and 1985*. Wellington: National Health Statistics Center.

———. 1986c. *The public health*. Wellington: Government Printer.

———. 1988. *Unshackling the hospitals*. Report of the Task Force on Hospital and Related Services. Wellington: Government Printer.

New Zealand House of Representatives. 1907. Appendices to the journals of the House of Representatives H22. Wellington: Government Printer.

NHPPGWU (National Health Policy Project of George Washington University). 1984. *State legislated action affecting cancer prevention: A fifty state profile.* Springfield, Va.: National Technical Information Service.

NIMH (National Institute of Mental Health). 1983. *Mental health, United States 1983.* DHSS Pub. no. (ADM) 83-1275. Rockville, Md.: NIMH.

Norris, R. 1982. *Pills, pesticides, and profits.* Croton-on-Hudson, N.Y.: North River Press.

Nyazema, N. 1984. Towards better patient drug compliance and comprehension: A challenge to medical and pharmaceutical services in Zimbabwe. *Social Science and Medicine* 18:551–554.

OAMR (Ontario Association for the Mentally Retarded). 1972. We believe. Submission to the task force on mental retardation (Secretariat for Social Development) by the Ontario Association for the Mentally Retarded. Mimeo.

O'Connor, J. 1973. *The fiscal crisis of the state.* New York: St. Martin.

O'Donnell, G. 1978. Reflections on the patterns of change in the bureaucratic-authoritarian state. *Latin American Research Review* 13:3–38.

O'Donnell, G.; Schmitter, P.; and Whitehead, L. 1987. *Transitions from authoritarian rule: Comparative perspectives.* Baltimore and London: Johns Hopkins University Press.

OECD (Organization for Economic Cooperation and Development). 1977. *Public expenditure on health.* Paris: OECD.

————. 1985a. *Measuring health care 1960–83.* Paris: OECD.

————. 1985b. *Social expenditure 1960–90.* Paris: OECD.

————. 1985c. *The welfare state in crisis.* Paris: OECD.

————. 1986. *Living conditions in OECD countries.* Paris: OECD.

Offe, C. 1984. *Contradictions of the modern welfare state.* London: Hutchinson.

O'Higgins, M. 1983. Rolling back the welfare state. In *The year book of social policy in Britain, 1982,* ed. C. Jones and J. Stevenson. London: RKP.

Ontario. 1985. *Hospital statistics.* Toronto: Government of Ontario.

Ontario. Various years. *Public accounts of Ontario.* Toronto: Government of Ontario.

Ontario Department of Public Health. 1954. *Annual report.* Toronto: Ontario Department of Public Health.

————. 1961. *Annual report.* Toronto: Ontario Department of Public Health.

Ontario Ministry of Health. 1986. Ministry of Health presentations to the Select Committee on Health, August 25–26, Ontario. Unpublished document available from the Ontario Ministry of Health.

Ontario SPRC (Special Programs Review Committee). 1975. *Report of the Special Programs Review Committee.* Toronto: SPRC.

Ontario TFRBL (Task Force on Roomers, Boarders, and Lodgers). 1986. *Housing for roomers, boarders, and lodgers: The "state of knowledge."* Toronto: Ontario TFRBL.

Ontario Welfare Council. 1981. *Community based services: The need for a planned approach.* Toronto: Ontario Welfare Council.

Otto, S., and Orford, J. 1979. *Not quite like home: Small hostels for alcoholics and others*. Chichester: Wiley.

Panzetta, A. 1985. Whatever happened to community mental health: Portents for corporate medicine. *Hospital and Community Psychiatry* 36:1174–1179.

Parker, J. 1980. Pharmaceuticals and Third World concerns: The Lall report and the Otago study. In *The international supply of medicines*, ed. R. Helms, 135–146. Washington, D.C.: American Enterprise Institute for Public Policy Research.

Parry, N., and Parry, J. 1976. *The rise of the medical profession*. London: Croom Helm.

Parson, T., and Fox, R. 1952. Illness, therapy, and the modern urban family. *Journal of Social Issues* 8:31–44.

Pasnau, R. 1987. The remedicalization of psychiatry. *Hospital and Community Psychiatry* 38:145–151.

Patel, M. S. 1983. Drug costs in developing countries and policies to reduce them. In *Pharmaceuticals and health in the Third World*, ed. S. J. Patel, 195–204. Oxford: Pergamon.

Patel, S. J. 1983. Introduction to *Pharmaceuticals and health in the Third World*, ed. S. J. Patel, 165–167. Oxford: Pergamon.

Pattison, R., and Katz, H. 1983. Investor-owned and not-for-profit hospitals: A comparison based on California data. *New England Journal of Medicine* 309:347–353.

Paul, J. 1986. *Where there's muck there's money: A report on cleaning in London*. London: Greater London Council, Industry and Employment Branch.

Pauley, M., and Redisch, M. 1973. The not-for-profit hospital as a physicians' cooperative. *American Economic Review* 63:87–99.

Pauly, M. 1970. Efficiency, incentives, and reimbursement of health care. *Inquiry* 8:114–131.

Peet, R. 1975. Inequality and poverty: A Marxist-geographic theory. *Annals of the Association of American Geographers* 65:564–571.

Pegels, C. 1980. *Health care and the elderly*. Rockville, Mass.: Aspen.

Pepper, B., and Ryglewicz, H. 1983. Unified services: A New York State perspective. In *Unified mental health systems: Utopia unrealized*, ed. J. Talbott, 39–48. San Francisco: Jossey Bass.

Pfaff, M. 1986. Einige Auswirkungen einer Ubertragung marktwirtschaftlicher Steuerungs—und Organisationsformen auf die gesetzliche Krankenversicherung. *Sozialer Fortschritt* 5/6:105–119.

Phillips, D., and Radford, J. 1985. *Closure of major institutions for the mentally handicapped: Geographical evidence from South West England*. South West Papers in Geography, no. 10. University of Exeter, Plymouth Polytechnic, and the College of St. Mark and St. John.

Phillips, D., and Vincent, J. 1986a. Petit bourgeois care: Private residential care for the elderly. *Policy and Politics* 14:189–208.

———. 1986b. Private residential accommodation for the elderly: Geographical aspects of developments in Devon. *Transactions Institute of British Geographers* 11:155–173.

Pinch, S. n.d. The restructuring thesis and the study of public services. *Environment and Planning A*. Forthcoming.

Pirie, M. 1985. *Dismantling the state: The theory and practice of privatization.* Dallas: National Center for Policy Analysis.

Piven, F., and Cloward, R. 1971. *Regulating the poor.* New York: Random House.

Pleines, K. 1980. Hospital closures: The New York City experience. *Proceedings of the Health Policy Forum on Hospital Closures,* 15–39. New York: United Hospital Fund.

Polyani, K. 1957. *The great transformation.* Boston: Houghton Mifflin.

Pommerhene, W., and Frey, B. 1977. Public and private production efficiency in Switzerland: A theoretical and empirical comparison. In *Comparing urban service delivery systems,* ed. V. Ostrom and F. Bish, 221–242. Beverly Hills, Calif.: Sage.

Portney, P. 1986. Environmental evolution. *Resources,* Fall, 1–4.

Pradhan, S. 1983. *International pharmaceutical marketing.* Westport, Conn.: Quorum Books.

Prebisch, R. 1962. El desarrollo económico de la América Latina y algunos de sus principales problemas. *Boletín Económico de América Latina* 12:3–38.

Pred, P. 1981. Production, family, and free-time projects: A time-geographic perspective on the individual and societal change in nineteenth-century U.S. cities. *Journal of Historical Geography* 7:3–36.

President's Commission on Mental Health. 1978. *Report to the President from the President's Commission on Mental Health.* Washington, D.C.: GPO.

Public Service Association. 1985a. The New Zealand health care system: What's gone wrong? PSA Research Discussion Paper, no. 20. Wellington: Public Service Association.

———. 1985b. Private medicine. PSA Research Discussion Paper, no. 21. Wellington: Public Service Association.

Raczynski, D. 1982. Controversias sobre reformas al sector salud: Chile, 1973–1982. *Notas Técnicas,* no. 52. Santiago: CIEPLAN.

Rafferty, F. 1984. The case for investor-owned hospitals. *Hospital and Community Psychiatry* 35:1013–1018.

Ralph, D. 1983. *Work and madness: The rise of community psychiatry.* Montreal: Black Rose Books.

Rathwell, T.; Sics, A.; and Williams, S. 1985. *Towards a new understanding: A study of working relationships between the public and private health sectors.* Leeds: Nuffield Center for Health Services Studies.

Ray, M. 1987. Where one-third are retired. *Town and Country Planning* 46 (3): 76–77.

Rayner, G. 1986. Health care as a business: The emergence of a commercial hospital sector in Britain. *Policy and Politics* 14:439–459.

———. 1987. Lessons from America? Commercialisation and growth of private medicine in Britain. *International Journal of Health Services* 17:197–216.

Reekie, W., and Weber, M. 1979. *Profits, politics, and drugs*. London: Macmillan.

Regier, D.; Goldberg, I.; and Taube, C. 1978. The defacto U.S. mental health service system: A public health perspective. *Archives of General Psychiatry* 35:685–693.

Reinhardt, U. 1986. Financial capital and health care growth trends. In *For-profit enterprise in health care*, ed. B. Gray, 47–73. Washington, D.C.: National Academy Press.

Relman, A. 1980. The new medical-industrial complex. *New England Journal of Medicine* 303:963–970.

————. 1983. Investor-owned hospitals and health care costs. *New England Journal of Medicine* 309:370–372.

Relman, A., and Reinhardt, U. 1986. Debating for-profit health care. *Health Affairs* 5:5–31.

Remmer, K. 1988. The Chilean military under authoritarian rule, 1973–1987. University of New Mexico, Latin American Institute, Occasional Papers Series, no. 1. Albuquerque

Remmer, K., and Merkx, G. 1982. Bureaucratic-authoritarianism revisted. *Latin American Research Review* 17:3–40.

Reverby, S., and Rosner, D. 1979. *Health care in America*. Philadelphia: Temple University Press.

Rice, D., and Estes, C. 1984. Health of the elderly. *Health Affairs* 3:25–49.

Rice, J. A., and Garside, P. M. 1987. Prepaid health plans in developing countries. In *Restructuring health policy: An international challenge*, ed. J. Virgo, 119–136. Edwardsville, Ill.: International Health Economics and Management Institute, Southern Illinois University.

Riggan, W.; Van Bruggen, J.; Acquarella, J.; Beaubier, J.; and Mason, T. 1983. *U.S. cancer mortality rates and trends, 1950–1979*. Vols. 1–3. Report prepared for the National Cancer Institute and the U.S. Environmental Protection Agency. Washington, D.C.: GPO.

Rimlinger, G. V. 1971. *Welfare policy and industrialization in Europe, America, and Russia*. New York: Wiley.

Risse, G.; Numbers, K.; and Leavitte, J. 1977. *Medicine without doctors: Home health care in American history*. Englewood Cliffs, N.J.: Prentice-Hall.

Roach, W. 1982. Hospitals reorganize to survive the 80s. *Hospitals* 56:78–81.

Robbins, A. 1984. Creating a progressive health agenda: 1983 presidential address. *American Journal of Public Health* 74:775–779.

Roberts, C. 1963. *A report on Ontario's mental health services*. Toronto: Ontario Ministry of Health.

Rodwin, V. G. 1981. The marriage of national health insurance and la medecine liberale in France. *Milbank Memorial Fund Quarterly* 59:16–43.

Roemer, M. I. 1964. *Medical care in Latin America*. Washington, D.C.: Pan American Health Union.

———. 1984. The value of medical care for health promotion. *American Journal of Public Health* 74:243–248.

———. 1985. *National strategies for health care organization: A world overview.* Ann Arbor, Mich.: Health Administration Press.

Roemer, M. I., and Roemer, J. E. 1982. The social consequences of free trade in health care: A public health response to orthodox economics. *International Journal of Health Services* 12:111–129.

Rokkan, S. 1974. Dimensions of state formation and nation building. In *The formation of national states in Western Europe*, ed. C. Tilly, 562–600. Princeton: Princeton University Press.

Romero, H. 1977. Hitos fundamentales de la medicina social en Chile. In *Medicina social en Chile*, ed. J. Jiménez de la Jara, 1–37. Santiago: Editorial Aconcagua.

Rosenberg, C. 1982. From almshouse to hospital: The shaping of Philadelphia General Hospital. *Milbank Memorial Fund Quarterly* 60:108–154.

———. 1987. *The care of strangers: The rise of America's hospital system.* New York: Basic.

Rosenthal, M. M. 1986. Beyond equity. *Milbank Memorial Fund Quarterly* 64:592–621.

Rosner, D. 1982. *A once charitable enterprise: Hospitals and health care in Brooklyn and New York, 1885–1915.* New York: Cambridge University Press.

Roth, G. 1987. *The private provision of public services in developing countries.* New York: Oxford University Press.

Rothman, D. J. 1983. Social control: The uses and abuses of the concept in the history of incarceration. In *Social control and the state: Historical and comparative essays*, ed. S. Cohen and A. Scull, 106–117. Oxford: Martin Robertson.

Russell, L. 1986. *Is prevention better than cure?* Washington, D.C.: Brookings Institution.

Ryan, M. 1978. *The organization of Soviet medical care.* Oxford: Blackwell.

Sabshin, M. 1977. On remedicalization and holism in psychiatry. *Psychosomatics* 18:7–8.

Sainsbury, R.; Fox, K.; and Shelton, E. 1986. Dependency levels of elderly people in institutional care in Canterbury. *New Zealand Medical Journal* 99:375–376.

Salkever, D., and Bice, T. 1976. The impact of certificate of need controls on hospital investment. *Milbank Memorial Fund Quarterly* 54:185–214.

Sallam, A. 1979. Perspectives on the distribution and availability of pharmaceuticals in Africa and the Middle East. In *Pharmaceuticals for developing countries Conference proceedings*, 228–235. Division of International Health, Institute of Medicine. Washington, D.C.: National Academy of Sciences.

Salmon, J. 1985. Profit and health care: Trends in corporatization and privatization. *International Journal of Health Services* 15:395–418.

Salmond, E., and O'Connor, E. 1973. General surgical waiting lists and the management of varicose veins. *New Zealand Medical Journal* 78:394–400.

Saltman, R. B. 1988. National planning for locally controlled health system. *Journal of Health Politics, Policy, and Law* 13:27–51.

Sandman, P.; Sachsman, D.; Greenberg, M.; and Gochfeld, M. 1987. *Environmental risk and the press: An exploratory assessment.* New Brunswick, N.J.: Transaction.

Saunders, P. 1985. Public expenditure and economic performance in OECD countries. *Journal of Public Policy* 5:1–20.

Scarpaci, J. 1985a. Accessibility to primary medical care in Chile. Ph.D. diss., Department of Geography, University of Florida.

———. 1985b. Restructuring health care financing in Chile. *Social Science and Medicine* 21:415–431.

———. 1987. HMO promotion and the privatization of health services in Chile. *Journal of Health Politics, Policy, and Law* 12:551–567.

———. 1988a. DRG calculation and utilization patterns: A review of method and policy. *Social Science and Medicine* 26:111–117.

———. 1988b. Help-seeking behavior, use, and satisfaction among frequent primary care users in Santiago de Chile. *Journal of Health and Social Behavior* 29:199–213.

———. 1988c. *Primary medical care in Chile: Accessibility under military rule.* Pittsburgh: University of Pittsburgh Press.

Scarpaci, J., and Bradham, D. 1988. A three-tiered health care system and its inherent cost inflation: The case of medical care inflation in Chile. *Health Policy* 10:65–76.

Scarpaci, J.; Infante, P.; and Gaete, A. 1988. Planning residential segregation: The case of Santiago de Chile. *Urban Geography* 9:19–36.

Schaeffer, R., and Smith, N. 1986. The gentrification of Harlem. *Annals of the Association of American Geographers* 76:347–365.

Schlesinger, H. J.; Mumford, E.; Glass, G. V.; Patrick, C.; and Sharfstein, S. 1983. Mental health treatment and medical care utilization in a fee-for-service system: Outpatient mental health treatment following the onset of a chronic disease. *American Journal of Public Health* 73:422–429.

Schlesinger, M.; Marmor, T.; and Smithey, R. 1987. Nonprofit and for-profit medical care: Shifting roles and implications for health policy. *Journal of Health Politics, Policy, and Law* 12:427–457.

Schoonover, S., and Bassuk, E. 1983. Deinstitutionalization and the private general hospital inpatient unit: Implications for clinical care. *Hospital and Community Psychiatry* 34:135–139.

Scull, A. 1977. *Decarceration: Community treatment and the deviant, a radical view.* Englewood Cliffs, N.J.: Prentice-Hall.

S.E. Thames RHA (Brighton DHA). 1985. *Financing community hospitals: Possibilities for liaison with the private health sector.* Bexhill, Sussex: S.E. Thames RHA.

Sewell, F., and Hawley, T. 1987. Utilization of private hospital beds in Auckland for long-term geriatric care. *New Zealand Medical Journal* 100:16–18.

Sharfstein, S. 1982. Medicaid cutbacks and block grants: Crisis or opportunity for community mental health? *American Journal of Psychiatry* 139:466–470.

Sharfstein, S., and Biegel, A., eds. 1985. *The new economics and psychiatric care.* Washington, D.C.: American Psychiatric Press.

Sharfstein, S.; Frank, R.; and Kessler, L. 1984. State Medicaid limitations for mental health services. *Hospital and Community Psychiatry* 35:213–215.

Sherman, J. 1984. Who will pick up the tab for Tadworth? *Health and Social Services Journal* 93:398–399.

———. 1985. Waiting for the big bite. *Health and Social Services Journal* 94: 806–807.

Shortell, S.; Morrison, E.; Hughes, S.; Friedman, B.; Coverdill, J.; and Berg, L. 1986. Hospital ownership and nontraditional services. *Health Affairs* 5:97–111.

Shumsky, N. L.; Bohland, J.; and Knox, P. 1986. Separating doctors' homes and doctors' offices: San Francisco, 1881–1941. *Social Science and Medicine* 23:1051–1058.

Sigerist, H. 1947. *Medicine and health in the Soviet Union.* New York: Citadel.

Silverman, M. 1976. *The drugging of the Americas.* Berkeley and Los Angeles: University of California Press.

Siminoff, L. 1986. Competition and primary care in the United States: Separating fact from fancy. *International Journal of Health Services* 16:57–69.

Simmons, H. 1982. *From asylum to welfare.* Downsview, Ontario: National Institute on Mental Retardation.

Simpson, A. 1986. Variations in operation rates in New Zealand. *New Zealand Medical Journal* 99:798–801.

Sloan, F., and Steinwald, B. 1980. Effects of regulation on hospital cost and input use. *Journal of Law and Economics* 23:81–109.

SLRHC (Saint Luke's–Roosevelt Hospital Center). 1981. Market analysis and forecast. Mimeo.

———. 1986. Full review certificate of need application, September 30, 1983; amended August 15, 1986.

Smailes, R. 1987. *Review of surgical services.* Canterbury Hospital Board, Health Planning and Research Unit. Christchurch, New Zealand.

Smith, C. 1983. Innovation in mental health policy: Community mental health in the United States of America, 1968–1980. *Environment and Planning D: Society and Space* 1:447–468.

———. 1986. Equity in the distribution of health and welfare services: Can we rely on the state to reverse the "inverse care law"? *Social Science and Medicine* 23:1067–1078.

———. 1987. *Public problems: The management of urban distress.* New York: Guilford.

Smith, C., and Hanham, R. 1981. Deinstitutionalization of the mentally ill: A time path analysis of the American states, 1955–1975. *Social Science and Medicine* 15:361–378.

Smith, M. 1988. Privatized health system turns away Chile's poor. *Latin-america Press*, 17 March, 6.

Smith, N. 1986. On the necessity of uneven development. *International Journal of Urban and Regional Research* 10:89–103.

Smith, R. 1984. Remarks. In *Program summary of a conference on worksite health promotion and human resources: A hard look at the data*. Washington, D.C.: GPO.

Sorensen, J. 1985. Fiscal survival of community mental health in the 80's. *Community Mental Health Journal* 21:223–227.

Southern Cross Medical Care Society. 1986. *Report on a study of public and private surgical care and private medical insurance*. Wellington: Business and Economic Research.

Spann, M. 1977. Public versus private provision of government services. In *Budgets and bureaucrats: The sources of government growth*, ed. T. Borcherding, 71–89. Durham, N.C.: Duke University Press.

Spector, M., and Kitsuse, J. 1977. *Constructing social problems*. Menlo Park, Calif.: Cummings.

Spoerer, A. 1973. Doctrina y política de salud. Santiago: Ministerio de Salud. Mimeo.

Starr, P. 1982. *The social transformation of American medicine*. New York: Basic.

Starr, P., and Marmor, T. 1984. The United States: A social forecast. In *The end of an illusion*, ed. J. de Kervasdoue, J. Kimberly, and V. Rodwin, 234–254. Berkeley and Los Angeles: University of California Press.

Steinwald, B., and Neuhauser, D. 1970. The role of proprietary hospitals. *Journal of Law and Contemporary Problems* 35:817–838.

Stenzl, G. 1981. The role of international organizations in medicines policy. In *Pharmaceuticals and health policy*, ed. R. Blum et al., 211–239. London: Croom Helm.

Stepan, A. 1973. *Authoritarian Brazil*. New Haven: Yale University Press.

Sternlieb, G.; Hughes, J.; and Hughes, C. 1982. *Demographic trends and economic reality: Planning and markets in the 80s*. New Brunswick, N.J.: Center for Urban Policy Research.

Stockman, D., and Gramm, P. 1980. The administration's case for hospital cost containment. In *New directions in public health care*, ed. C. M. Lindsay. San Francisco: Institute for Contemporary Studies.

Storper, M., and Scott, A. 1986. *Production work and territory*. New York: Allen and Unwin.

Strategic Planning Group, National School Health Education Coalition. 1984. *Obstacles and strategies*. New York: National School Health Education Coalition.

Talbott, J., ed. 1983. *Unified mental health systems: Utopia unrealized*. San Francisco: Jossey Bass.

Tatchell, M. 1982. A comparative examination of the Australian and New Zealand health system. *Community Health Studies* 6:274–291.

Taylor, P., and Hadfield, H. 1982. Housing and the state: A case study and structuralist interpretation. In *Conflict, Politics, and the Urban Scene*, ed. K. Cox and R. Johnston, 241–263. London: Longman.

Taylor-Gooby, P. 1986. Privatization, power, and the welfare state. *Sociology* 20:228–246.

Therborn, G., and Roebroek, J. 1986. The irreversible welfare state. *International Journal of Health Services* 16:319–338.

Thiemeyer, T. T. 1986. Gesundheitsleitungen-Steuerung durch Markt, Staat oder Verbande? *Sozialer Fortschritt* 5–6:98–104.

Thorpe, K. 1987. Does all-payer rate setting work? The case of New York's prospective hospital reimbursement methodology. *Journal of Health Politics, Policy, and Law* 12:391–408.

Thrift, N. 1986. The geography of international economic disorder. In *A world in crisis*, ed. R. Johnston and P. Taylor. Oxford: Blackwell.

Thrupp, L. 1984. Technology and planning in the Third World pharmaceutical sector: The Cuban and Caribbean community approaches. *International Journal of Health Services* 14 (2): 189–216.

Tiefenbacher, M. 1979. Problems of distribution, availability, and utilization of agents in developing countries. In *Pharmaceuticals for developing countries Conference proceedings*, 211–227. Division of International Health, Institute of Medicine. Washington, D.C.: National Academy of Sciences.

Titmuss, R. 1970. *The gift of relationship: From human blood to social policy*. London: Allen and Unwin.

————. 1976. *Essays on the welfare state*. London: Allen and Unwin.

TMI (Tayloe Murphy Institute). 1986. *Projections of median family and household income for Virginia cities and counties, 1986–1990*. Charlottesville: Tayloe Murphy Institute, University of Virginia.

Torrens, P. R. 1982. Some potential hazards of unplanned expansion of private health insurance in Britain. *Lancet* 2 (January 2): 29–31.

Tucker, D. 1984. *The world health market: Future of the pharmaceutical industry*. Guilford, England: Euromonitor Publications.

Tullock, G. 1970. *Private wants, public needs: An economic analysis of the desirable scope of government*. New York: Basic.

Turshen, M. 1984. *The political ecology of disease in Tanzania*. New Brunswick, N.J.: Rutgers University Press.

Ugalde, A. 1985. The integration of health care programs into a national health service. In *The crisis of social security and health care in Latin America*, ed. C. Mesa-Lago, 109–142. Pittsburgh: Center for Latin American Studies, University of Pittsburgh.

U.K. DHSS (Department of Health and Social Services). 1976. *Sharing resources for health in England*. London: DHSS.

————. 1980. *Inequalities in health: Report of a working group*. London: DHSS.

————. 1981. *Care in the community: A consultative document on moving resources for care in England*. London: DHSS.

———. 1983a. *Competitive tendering in the provision of domestic catering and laundry services*. Circular HC (83) 18. London: DHSS.

———. 1983b. *NHS management inquiry report*. London: DHSS.

———. 1986. *Independent sector hospitals, nursing homes, and clinics in England*. London: DHSS.

U.K. Hansard. 1987. *House of Commons Parliamentary Debates: Official Report*, 22 April, 5th ser. Written Answers, cols. 611–618. London: HMSO.

U.K. H.M. Treasury. 1988. *The government's expenditure plans, 1988–89 to 1990–91*. London: HMSO.

U.K. House of Commons. 1985a. *Report from the Social Services Committee: Community care with special reference to adult mentally ill and mentally handicapped people*. London: House of Commons.

———. 1985b. *Sixth report from the Social Services Committee: Public expenditure on the social services*. HC-339. London: House of Commons.

U.K. OPCS (Office of Population Censuses and Surveys). 1985. *General Household Survey, 1983*. London: OPCS.

United States Embassy, Santiago, Chile. 1984. Economic trends report. Mimeo.

Urry, J. 1987. Some social and spatial aspects of services. *Society and Space* 5:5–26.

U.S. Bureau of the Census. 1905. *Benevolent institutions, 1904*. Washington, D.C.: GPO.

———. 1925. *Hospitals and dispensaries, 1923*. Washington, D.C.: GPO.

———. 1983. *County and city data book, 1983*. Washington, D.C.: GPO.

———. 1985. *Statistical abstract of the United States, 1985*. Washington, D.C.: GPO.

———. 1987. *Statistical abstract of the United States*. Washington, D.C.: GPO.

U.S. DHEW (Department of Health, Education, and Welfare). 1979. *Healthy people*. Washington, D.C.: GPO.

U.S. DHHS (Department of Health and Human Services). 1980. *Towards a national plan for the chronically mentally ill*. Report to the Secretary by the Steering Committee on the Chronically Mentally Ill. Washington, D.C.: GPO.

———. 1984. Workplace health promotion objectives: 1990. In National Center for Health Education. *Center* 2:25.

———. 1985. *Report of the Secretary's task force on black and minority health*. Washington, D.C.: GPO.

U.S. EPA. 1987. *Unfinished business: A comparative assessment of environmental problems*. Washington, D.C.: U.S. Environmental Protection Agency.

U.S. Health Care Finance Administration. 1987. National health expenditures, 1986–2000. *Health Care Financing Review* 8:1–36.

Vanderbilt University. 1984–1986. *Television news index and abstracts*. Nashville, Tenn.: Vanderbilt University.

Van Horne, R. 1986. *A new agenda: Health and social service strategies for*

Ontario's seniors. Toronto: Minister for Senior Citizens' Affairs, Queens Park.

VDPB (Virginia Department of Planning and Budget). 1986. *Population projections for cities and counties: 1990–2000.* Richmond: Virginia Department of Planning and Budget.

Veatch, R. 1983. Ethical dilemmas of for-profit enterprise in health care. In *The new health care for profit,* ed. B. Gray, 145–146. Washington, D.C.: National Academy Press.

Vernon, R. 1988. *The promise of privatization: A challenge for American foreign policy.* Washington, D.C.: Council on Foreign Relations.

VHA (Virginia Hospital Association). 1985. *Uncompensated care: Analysis and recommendations.* Report by the Virginia Hospital Association. Richmond, Va.

VHAHW (Visiting Homemakers' Association of Hamilton-Wentworth). 1973. Brief to the Hanson Task Force, Ministry of Community and Social Services, regarding homemaking services and the Homemaker and Nurses Services Act of Ontario. Mimeo.

Viel, B. 1961. *La medicina socializada y su aplicación en Gran Bretaña, Unión Soviética y Chile.* Santiago: Ediciones de la Universidad de Chile.

Virgo, J., ed. 1987. *Restructuring health policy: An international challenge.* Edwardsville, Ill.: International Health Economics and Management Institute, Southern Illinois University.

Viveros-Long, A. M. 1982. Changes in health financing: The Chilean experience. Paper presented at the International Health Conference, June 13–16, Washington, D.C.

Vladeck, B. 1981. Health. In *Setting Municipal Priorities,* ed. C. Brecher and R. Horton, 322–349. New York: Russell Sage Foundation.

———. 1985. The dilemma between competition and community service. *Inquiry* 22:115–212.

Vogel, M. 1980. *Invention of the modern hospital: Boston, 1870–1930.* Chicago: University of Chicago Press.

Vollmer, R. J., and Hoffman, G. 1985. Ermittlung der budget—under pflegesatzfahigen Selbstkoster der Krankenhause. *Ersatzkasse* 65:448–461.

———. 1986. Inhalt und Grenzen des staatlichen Genehmigungvorbehalts. *Ersatzkasse* 66:191–204.

Walker, A., ed. 1982. *Community care: The family, the state, and social policy.* Oxford: Blackwell.

———. 1984. The political economy of privatization. In *Privatisation and the welfare state,* ed. J. Le Grand and R. Robinson, 19–44. London: Allen and Unwin.

Wallace, A. 1988. A strong rebound for hospital stocks. *New York Times,* 3 April, 8F.

Wallis, C. 1982. A double standard on drugs? *Time,* 28 June, 76.

Walton, J. 1987. Urban protest and the global political economy: The I.M.F.

riots. In *The capitalist city*, ed. M. P. Smith and J. R. Feagin, 364–386. Oxford and New York: Basil Blackwell.

Ward, B. 1985. Pollution politics: The importance of being New Jersey. *Environmental Forum* 4:17–20.

Warner, S. 1972. *The urban wilderness: A history of the American city*. New York: Harper and Row.

Watt, J.; Renn, S.; Hahn, J.; Derzon, R.; and Schramm, C. 1986. The effects of ownership and multihospital system membership on hospital functional strategies and economic performance. In *For-profit enterprise in health care*, ed. B. Gray, 260–289. Washington, D.C.: National Academy Press.

Weinstein, A., and Cohen, M. 1984. Young chronic patients and changes in the state hospital population. *Hospial and Community Psychiatry* 35:595–600.

Welfare Research Inc. 1979. *Survey of the needs and problems of adult home residents in New York State*. Albany, N.Y.: Welfare Research.

Weller, G., and Manga, P. 1983. The push for reprivatization of health services in Canada, Britain, and the United States. *Journal of Health Politics, Policy, and Law* 8:495–518.

Wessler, J. 1986. The Mount Sinai story: Down from the mountain and into the streets. *Health PAC Bulletin* 16:12–13.

West, P. 1984. Private health insurance. In *Privatisation and the welfare state*, ed. J. LeGrand and R. Robinson, 111–115. London: Allen and Unwin.

West Midlands County Council. 1986. *The realities of home life*. Birmingham: NUPE/West Midlands CC.

Whiteis, D., and Salmon, J. 1987. The proprietarization of health care and the underdevelopment of the public sector. *International Journal of Health Services* 17:47–64.

Whitney, D. 1985. *The media and the people: Americans' experience with the news media, a fifty-year review*. New York: Gannett Center for Media Studies, Columbia University.

Widem, P.; Pincus, H.; Goldman, H.; and Jencks, S. 1984. Prospective payment for psychiatric hospitalization: Context and background. *Hospital and Community Psychiatry* 35:447–451.

Wiener, C. 1981. *The politics of alcholism: Building an arena around a social problem*. New Brunswick, N.J.: Transaction.

Wilensky, H., and Lebeaux, D. 1965. *Industrial society and social welfare*. New York: Free Press.

Wilensky, H.; Luebbert, G.; Hahn, S.; and Jameison, A. 1985. *Comparative Social Policy*. Berkeley: Institute of International Studies, University of California.

Will, G. 1983. *Statecraft as soulcraft: What government does*. New York: Simon and Schuster.

Williams, B.; Nicholl, J.; Thomas, K.; and Knowelden, J. 1984a. Analysis of the work of independent acute hospitals in England and Wales, 1981. *British Medical Journal* 289:446–448.

_____. 1984b. Contribution of the private sector to elective surgery in England. *Lancet*, 14 July, 88–92.

_____. 1985. Differences in durations of stay for surgery in the NHS and the private sector in England and Wales. *British Medical Journal* 290:978–980.

Williams, C. 1984. *Decades of service: A history of the Ontario Ministry of Community and Social Services, 1930–1980*. Toronto: Ontario Ministry of Community and Social Services.

Winslow, C. 1951. *The cost of sickness and price of health*. World Health Organization Monograph Series, no. 7. Geneva: WHO.

Wolfensburger, W. 1972. *The principle of normalization in human services*. Toronto: National Institute on Mental Retardation.

Wood, T., and Thomas, S. 1986. Private practice in Australian public hospitals. *Hospital and Health Services Review* 82:159–161.

Woods, C. 1977. Alternative curing strategies in a changing medical situation. *Medical Anthropology* 1 (3): 25–54.

World Bank. 1987. *World Development Report*. New York: Oxford University Press.

Yolles, S. 1967. Mental health at work. In *To work is human: Mental health and the business community*, ed. A. McClean, 57–84. New York: Macmillan.

Zelman, W. N.; McLaughlin, C. P.; Gelb, N.; and Miller, E. 1985. Survival strategies for community mental health organizations: A conceptual framework. *Community Mental Health Journal* 21:228–236.

Zuckerman, H. 1983. Industrial rationalization of a cottage industry: Multi-institutional hospital systems. *Annals of the American Academy of Political and Social Science* 468:216–230.

Index

absenteeism, 181, 271
Accident Compensation Corporation (ACC), 94
accidents, 21, 94
accumulation: facilitated by state health care, 18; limited, 64; opportunities for, 7; renewal of, 19
Adam Smith Institute, 14
Addenbrooke's Hospital, Cambridge, 126
administrators, 15
adolescents, unemployed, 181
advanced capitalist countries, 2, 3, 271; and welfare state, 20
advertising, 114, 133, 140
Africa, 22, 245
aged, homes for, 47, 194
AIDS (acquired immune deficiency syndrome), 139, 142, 273
alcohol, 210, 214
alcoholism, 176
alienation, 187
Allende, Salvador, 219
altruism, 22
ambulatory care: categories of, 13–14, 166; in Chile, 224; as retail activity, 8
ambulatory centers, 7. *See also* primary care
American Cancer Society, 211, 213
American Medical Association (AMA), 41, 175, 211
American Medical International (AMI), 28, 115, 127

American Public Health Association, 211
ancillary services, 52; in Ontario, 187–188; subcontracting, in England, 120–124, 127
architecture, 199
Argentina, 224, 237
Asia, 22, 245
asylums, 47
Australia, 14
Austria, 14, 69, 70, 73
authoritarian regimes, 15. *See also* bureaucratic-authoritarianism
average length of stay (ALOS): in England and Wales, 103; for mentally ill, in New York, 161; in New Zealand, 102–103; in psychiatric facilities in Ontario, 184

Barking Hospital, 123
Belgium, 14, 70; health care expenditures, 71
benefits, 124, 132, 134, 136, 212
Beverly Enterprises, 175
biomedical model, 4, 245, 269. *See also* health care
Birmingham, England, 117
Bismarck, Otto von, 8, 271
blacks, 59, 215
blood donation, 22
Blue Cross, 139, 147, 172, 211
Blue Shield, 135, 147, 173
boarding homes, 194